Orthopedic Diseases and Traumatology: Surgical Treatment and Rehabilitation

Orthopedic Diseases and Traumatology: Surgical Treatment and Rehabilitation

Editor

Christian Ehrnthaller

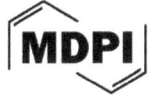

Basel • Beijing • Wuhan • Barcelona • Belgrade • Novi Sad • Cluj • Manchester

Editor
Christian Ehrnthaller
LMU Munich
Munich
Germany

Editorial Office
MDPI
St. Alban-Anlage 66
4052 Basel, Switzerland

This is a reprint of articles from the Special Issue published online in the open access journal *Journal of Clinical Medicine* (ISSN 2077-0383) (available at: https://www.mdpi.com/journal/jcm/special_issues/Orthopedic_Diseases_Traumatology).

For citation purposes, cite each article independently as indicated on the article page online and as indicated below:

Lastname, A.A.; Lastname, B.B. Article Title. *Journal Name* **Year**, *Volume Number*, Page Range.

ISBN 978-3-7258-0941-7 (Hbk)
ISBN 978-3-7258-0942-4 (PDF)
doi.org/10.3390/books978-3-7258-0942-4

© 2024 by the authors. Articles in this book are Open Access and distributed under the Creative Commons Attribution (CC BY) license. The book as a whole is distributed by MDPI under the terms and conditions of the Creative Commons Attribution-NonCommercial-NoDerivs (CC BY-NC-ND) license.

Contents

Christian Ehrnthaller, Klevin Hoxhaj, Kirsi Manz, Yunjie Zhang, Julian Fürmetz, Wolfgang Böcker and Christoph Linhart
Preventing Atrophic Long-Bone Nonunion: Retrospective Analysis at a Level I Trauma Center
Reprinted from: *J. Clin. Med.* **2024**, *13*, 2071, doi:10.3390/jcm13072071 1

Raffael Cintean, Alexander Eickhoff, Carlos Pankratz, Beatrice Strauss, Florian Gebhard and Konrad Schütze
Radial vs. Dorsal Approach for Elastic Stable Internal Nailing in Pediatric Radius Fractures—A 10 Year Review
Reprinted from: *J. Clin. Med.* **2022**, *11*, 4478, doi:10.3390/jcm11154478 13

Carlos Pankratz, Raffael Cintean, Dominik Boitin, Matti Hofmann, Christoph Dehner, Florian Gebhard and Konrad Schuetze
Early Surgical Care of Anticoagulated Hip Fracture Patients Is Feasible—A Retrospective Chart Review of Hip Fracture Patients Treated with Hip Arthroplasty within 24 Hours
Reprinted from: *J. Clin. Med.* **2022**, *11*, 6570, doi:10.3390/jcm11216570 23

Konrad Schuetze, Alexander Boehringer, Raffael Cintean, Florian Gebhard, Carlos Pankratz, Peter Hinnerk Richter, et al.
Feasibility and Radiological Outcome of Minimally Invasive Locked Plating of Proximal Humeral Fractures in Geriatric Patients
Reprinted from: *J. Clin. Med.* **2022**, *11*, 6751, doi:10.3390/jcm11226751 34

Alexander Fisher, Wichat Srikusalanukul, Leon Fisher and Paul N. Smith
Comparison of Prognostic Value of 10 Biochemical Indices at Admission for Prediction Postoperative Myocardial Injury and Hospital Mortality in Patients with Osteoporotic Hip Fracture
Reprinted from: *J. Clin. Med.* **2022**, *11*, 6784, doi:10.3390/jcm11226784 43

Joanna Kapusta and Marcin Domżalski
Long Term Effectiveness of ESWT in Plantar Fasciitis in Amateur Runners
Reprinted from: *J. Clin. Med.* **2022**, *11*, 6926, doi:10.3390/jcm11236926 70

Felix Christian Kohler, Philipp Schenk, Theresa Nies, Jakob Hallbauer, Gunther Olaf Hofmann, Uta Biedermann, et al.
Fibula Nail versus Locking Plate Fixation—A Biomechanical Study
Reprinted from: *J. Clin. Med.* **2023**, *12*, 698, doi:10.3390/jcm12020698 81

Alexander Böhringer, Raffael Cintean, Alexander Eickhoff, Florian Gebhard and Konrad Schütze
Blade Augmentation in Nailing Proximal Femur Fractures—An Advantage despite Higher Costs?
Reprinted from: *J. Clin. Med.* **2023**, *12*, 1661, doi:10.3390/jcm12041661 92

Roslind K. Hackenberg, Fabio Schmitt-Sánchez, Christoph Endler, Verena Tischler, Jayagopi Surendar, Kristian Welle, et al.
Value of Diagnostic Tools in the Diagnosis of Osteomyelitis: Pilot Study to Establish an Osteomyelitis Score
Reprinted from: *J. Clin. Med.* **2023**, *12*, 3057, doi:10.3390/jcm12093057 100

Martin Paulsson, Carl Ekholm, Roy Tranberg, Ola Rolfson and Mats Geijer
Using a Traction Table for Fracture Reduction during Minimally Invasive Plate Osteosynthesis (MIPO) of Distal Femoral Fractures Provides Anatomical Alignment
Reprinted from: *J. Clin. Med.* 2023, 12, 4044, doi:10.3390/jcm12124044 113

Markus Bormann, David Bitschi, Claas Neidlein, Daniel P. Berthold, Maximilian Jörgens, Robert Pätzold, et al.
Mismatch between Clinical–Functional and Radiological Outcome in Tibial Plateau Fractures: A Retrospective Study
Reprinted from: *J. Clin. Med.* 2023, 12, 5583, doi:10.3390/jcm12175583 130

Nevsun Pihtili Tas and Oğuz Kaya
Treatment of Plantar Fasciitis in Patients with Calcaneal Spurs: Radiofrequency Thermal Ablation or Extracorporeal Shock Wave Therapy?
Reprinted from: *J. Clin. Med.* 2023, 12, 6503, doi:10.3390/jcm12206503 142

Christoph Linhart, Dirk Mehrens, Luca Maximilian Gellert, Christian Ehrnthaller, Johannes Gleich, Christopher Lampert, et al.
Gluteal Muscle Fatty Atrophy: An Independent Risk Factor for Surgical Treatment in Elderly Patients Diagnosed with Type-III Fragility Fractures of the Pelvis
Reprinted from: *J. Clin. Med.* 2023, 12, 6966, doi:10.3390/jcm12226966 149

Christoph Linhart, Manuel Kistler, Maximilian Saller, Axel Greiner, Christopher Lampert, Matthias Kassube, et al.
Micro-Structural and Biomechanical Evaluation of Bioresorbable and Conventional Bone Cements for Augmentation of the Proximal Femoral Nail
Reprinted from: *J. Clin. Med.* 2023, 12, 7202, doi:10.3390/jcm12237202 159

Chang-Yu Huang, Chia-Che Lee, Chih-Wei Chen, Ming-Hsiao Hu, Kuan-Wen Wu, Ting-Ming Wang, et al.
The Outcome of under 10 mm Single-Incision Surgery Using a Non-Specialized Volar Plate in Distal Radius Fractures: A Retrospective Comparative Study
Reprinted from: *J. Clin. Med.* 2023, 12, 7670, doi:10.3390/jcm12247670 172

Patricia Hurtado-Olmo, Ángela González-Santos, Javier Pérez de Rojas, Nicolás Francisco Fernández-Martínez, Laura del Olmo and Pedro Hernández-Cortés
Surgical Treatment in Post-Stroke Spastic Hands: A Systematic Review
Reprinted from: *J. Clin. Med.* 2024, 13, 945, doi:10.3390/jcm13040945 185

Alexandre Lädermann, Alec Cikes, Jeanni Zbinden, Tiago Martinho, Anthony Pernoud and Hugo Bothorel
Hydrotherapy after Rotator Cuff Repair Improves Short-Term Functional Results Compared with Land-Based Rehabilitation When the Immobilization Period Is Longer
Reprinted from: *J. Clin. Med.* 2024, 13, 954, doi:10.3390/jcm13040954 207

Grzegorz Starobrat, Anna Danielewicz, Tomasz Szponder, Magdalena Wójciak, Ireneusz Sowa, Monika Różańska-Boczula and Michał Latalski
The Influence of Temporary Epiphysiodesis of the Proximal End of the Tibia on the Shape of the Knee Joint in Children Treated for Leg Length Discrepancy
Reprinted from: *J. Clin. Med.* 2024, 13, 1458, doi:10.3390/jcm13051458 218

Alexander Böhringer, Raffael Cintean, Konrad Schütze and Florian Gebhard
Primary Radial Nerve Lesions in Humerus Shaft Fractures—Revision or Wait and See
Reprinted from: *J. Clin. Med.* 2024, 13, 1893, doi:10.3390/jcm13071893 230

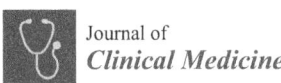

Article

Preventing Atrophic Long-Bone Nonunion: Retrospective Analysis at a Level I Trauma Center

Christian Ehrnthaller [1,*], Klevin Hoxhaj [1], Kirsi Manz [2], Yunjie Zhang [1], Julian Fürmetz [1,3], Wolfgang Böcker [1] and Christoph Linhart [1]

1. Department of Orthopaedics and Trauma Surgery, Musculoskeletal University Center Munich (MUM), University Hospital, LMU Munich, 81377 Munich, Germany; klevin.hoxhaj@campus.lmu.de (K.H.); yunjie.zhang@med.uni-muenchen.de (Y.Z.); julian.fuermetz@med.uni-muenchen.de (J.F.); wolfgang.boecker@med.uni-muenchen.de (W.B.); christoph.linhart@med.uni-muenchen.de (C.L.)
2. Institut für Medizinische Informationsverarbeitung, Biometrie und Epidemiologie (IBE), Medizinische Fakultät, LMU München, Marchioninistr. 15, 81377 München, Germany; manz@ibe.med.uni-muenchen.de
3. Department of Trauma Surgery, Trauma Center Murnau, Professor-Küntscher-Straße 8, 82418 Murnau am Staffelsee, Germany
* Correspondence: christian.ehrnthaller@med.uni-muenchen.de; Tel.: +49-89-4400-73500

Abstract: **Background**: Among the risk factors for nonunion are unchangeable patient factors such as the type of injury and comorbidities, and factors that can be influenced by the surgeon such as fracture treatment and the postoperative course. While there are numerous studies analyzing unchangeable factors, there is poor evidence for factors that can be affected by the physician. This raises the need to fill the existing knowledge gaps and lay the foundations for future prevention and in-depth treatment strategies. Therefore, the goal of this study was to illuminate knowledge about nonunion in general and uncover the possible reasons for their development; **Methods**: This was a retrospective analysis of 327 patients from 2015 to 2020 from a level I trauma center in Germany. Information about patient characteristics, comorbidities, alcohol and nicotine abuse, fracture classification, type of osteosynthesis, etc., was collected. Matched pair analysis was performed, and statistical testing performed specifically for atrophic long-bone nonunion; **Results**: The type of osteosynthesis significantly affected the development of nonunion, with plate osteosynthesis being a predictor for nonunion. The use of wire cerclage did not affect the development of nonunion, nor did the use of NSAIDs, smoking, alcohol, osteoporosis and BMI; **Conclusion**: Knowledge about predictors for nonunion and strategies to avoid them can benefit the medical care of patients, possibly preventing the development of nonunion.

Keywords: nonunion; long bone; fracture healing; femur; pseudarthrosis; delayed fracture healing; atrophic

1. Introduction

Bone healing is a long and complex healing process in the body that depends on many different factors [1]. These include individual characteristics, as well as fracture properties. With a good understanding of these factors, fracture healing can be promoted not only qualitatively, but also in terms of time. In rare cases, however, defective or delayed fracture healing occurs. Delayed fracture healing with the subsequent development of nonunion is one of the most difficult conditions to treat and with a great socio-economic impact in trauma surgery patients [2,3].

To date, there is no clear or exact definition of nonunion. There are differences in terms of the period of fracture healing, with the majority of the literature assuming the state of nonunion after 9 months [4]. Ultimately, not only is the exact healing latency important, but also the correlation between the radiological findings and the clinical situation of the patient [5–7]. Nonunion is generally divided into three different types

- Hypertrophic nonunion;
- Atrophic nonunion;
- Infectious nonunion.

Depending on the underlying pathology, the treatment of nonunion must be approached individually and tailored according to each patient and fracture characteristics. The treatment concept consists of the four pillars: radical surgery; soft tissue and bone management; biomechanical stability; and syst./local antibiotic therapy, also known as the "Diamond Concept", according to Giannoudis et al. [8–10]. Since its introduction over a decade ago, this concept has gained wide acceptance in the assessment and planning of nonunion fracture management. This model takes into account the heterogeneity of the underlying physiological and clinical appearance and supports the individual choice of treatment in order to create the best possible biological and mechanical conditions.

Although there are generally accepted principles for fracture treatment which should help minimize the risk for nonunion development [11], the exact cause for the development of nonunion, especially atrophic nonunion, remains unknown.

A high number of studies have attempted to identify the risk factors for the development of nonunion so far [2,7,12–15]. Most studies have focused on comorbidities and their effect on the development of bone healing delay. Among the generally accepted risk factors are smoking, diabetes, obesity and soft tissue damage, as well as severe fracture classification [13,15]. While the pathophysiological role for these comorbidities and trauma characteristics is relatively clear, these parameters are usually given and not prone to influence by orthopedic surgeons. This study is the first to focus on the traumatological parameters that may contribute to the development of a bone healing delay or nonunion. In daily clinical routine, there is a multitude of theories and opinions regarding which form of treatment is the best and which may contribute to the development of pseudarthrosis. Unfortunately, scientific evidence here is rather limited. Therefore, with this study, we attempted to gain a deeper insight into the true background of the development of nonunion and possibly identify the risk factors which, if considered, could prevent a delay in bone healing.

2. Materials and Methods

2.1. Study Design

As the study design, a retrospective analysis of patients treated conservatively or surgically for nonunion in the period from 2015 to 2020 at the Department of General, Trauma and Reconstructive Surgery—Campus Großhadern and City Campus was chosen. The patient group was identified using the hospital's radiological and clinical databases. Firstly, all patients potentially eligible for the study were selected using the corresponding keywords and ICD-10 codes. Then, duplicate entries and all patients with missing records or inadequate imaging were eliminated. In the end, 327 patients in total were included in the study.

2.2. Inclusion Criteria

- Atrophic, hypertrophic and infectious nonunion
- Age > 18 years
- Conservative or surgical therapy

2.3. Data Collection

After a review of patient records (radiological imaging, surgical protocol, anesthesiologic protocol, patient charts), the following parameters were recorded:

- Age, weight, height, gender;
- Alcohol and nicotine abuse;
- Comorbidities;
- Fracture classification;
- Fracture location;

- Previous surgical/conservative treatments;
- Nonunion type;
- Use of bone supplements, autograft or comminution;
- Postoperative fracture characteristics (anatomic reduction, stability);
- Mechanical complications;
- Wound healing disorders;
- American Society of Anaesthesiologists (ASA) score.

In patients with multiple nonunions, all patient-specific parameters were considered and noted again for each case, even if it was the same patient with another nonunion. Thus, each nonunion including all parameters was evaluated individually, and 167 atrophic (Figure 1), 91 hypertrophic and 69 infectious nonunions were continuously reported in the patient collective.

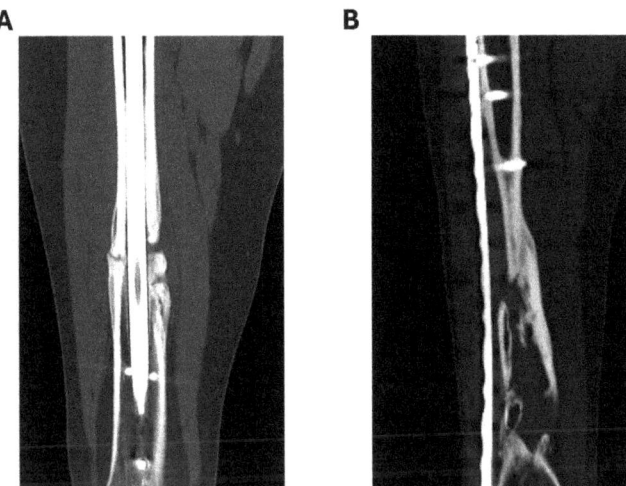

Figure 1. Examples of atrophic femoral nonunions. (**A**) Diaphyseal nonunion after intramedullary nailing; (**B**) diaphyseal nonunion after minimally invasive plate osteosynthesis.

Postoperative fracture characteristics such as anatomic reduction and the definition of postoperative "stability" were assessed by two independent senior consultants of the trauma department according to postoperative radiographs. "Stability" was defined as the presence of osteosynthesis, which would be stable enough to perform at least partial weight-bearing. This was estimated based on the AO principles (Arbeitsgemeinschaft für Osteosynthesefragen) with respect to reduction, implant size and positioning, number of screws and the overall aspect of the osteosynthesis in regard to the fracture situation.

2.4. Statistics

The historical patient data were retrieved from the inpatient database of our hospital (Meona Ltd., Freiburg, Germany) and irreversibly anonymized in a confidential database (Microsoft Excel 2018, Microsoft Corporation, Redmond, WA, USA) before analysis. Our data were processed and analyzed using the statistical program "SPSS" (SPSS Statistics 29, IBM, New York, NY, USA) and "R" (Version 4.2.3, R Project, Vienna, Austria), in compliance with data protection regulations.

We retrospectively recorded the relative frequency of the parameters mentioned for all patients and compared them descriptively to gain a comprehensive insight into the central tendency measures and the dispersion of the variables under consideration. Both the mean and median were calculated for continuous data, and standard deviation was used to quantify the dispersion of the data points around the mean. In addition, we examined the static correlation between different parameters by analyzing linear and logarithmic regressions.

Specifically, logistic regression with a calculation of the odds ratio (OR) with a 95% confidence interval (CI) was used to analyze the incidence of nonunion compared to controls, as well as binary outcome variables. The tests for statistical significance were always performed as "two-tailed", allowing for a comprehensive assessment of the possible differences or correlations in both directions.

The non-parametric Mann–Whitney U test was used to compare the nonunion group with the control group after testing for normality.

Regarding specific questions, we developed a matched-pair (age and gender) patient collective that served as the control group for nonunion of long tubular bones (humerus, radius, ulna, femur, tibia, fibula). Both pure descriptive analysis and direct statistical comparison were performed. Fisher's exact test was used to analyze categorical variables between the groups, particularly in the four field tables.

3. Results

3.1. Descriptive Analysis of the Nonunion Collective

A descriptive analysis of our study collective is shown in Table 1. Three hundred and twenty-seven patients were analyzed, with a wide variety of ages (20–99 years), and predominantly male (60%) patients. Smoking was recorded for almost 30% of the cases, and the most frequent nonunion site was the femur, accounting for 25% of all cases. Atrophic (51%) and 28% hypertrophic nonunions were recorded. Polytrauma and osteoporosis were almost equally represented in 12–13% of the patients. Most often, plate osteosynthesis was performed in 44% followed by intramedullary nailing in 25%. An anatomic reduction was achieved in 61%, and stability was estimated in 75% of cases.

Table 1. Descriptive analysis of the whole nonunion collective.

Factor	Total Numbers	Percentage
Age (years)	20–99 (Mean 57.8)	
Sex (male)	195	59.6
BMI	17–66 (Mean 26.5)	
Alcohol abuse	29	8.9
Smoking	93	28.4
Polytrauma	39	11.9
ASA score		
1	50	15
2	144	44
3	112	34
4	4	1
Osteoporosis	43	13.1
Anti-osteoporotic treatment	34	10.4
Nonunion site		
Femur	83	25
Tibia	71	22
Humerus	33	10
Clavicula	27	8
Foot	21	6
Hand	20	6
Radius	17	5
Ankle	14	4
Fibula	12	4
Ulna	10	3
Dens axis	8	2
Os pubis	5	2
Patella	4	1
Scapula	2	1

Table 1. *Cont.*

Factor	Total Numbers	Percentage
Type of nonunion		
Atrophy	167	51.1
Hypertrophy	91	27.8
infectious	69	21.1
Bone substitute/autograft		
At first surgery	12	3.7
At nonunion surgery	146	44.6
Cerclage wiring (total number)		
1	31	9.5
2	11	3.4
3	1	0.3
4	1	0.3
5	0	0
6	1	0.3
7	1	0.3
Anatomic Reduction	199	60.9
Stability	245	74.9
Implant removal	47	14.3
Soft tissue damage		
Closed	214	65.4
Grade I closed	30	9.2
Grade II closed	21	6.4
Grade III closed	1	0.3
Not specified	162	49.5
Open	36	11
Grade I open	4	1.2
Grade II open	15	4.5
Grade III open	17	5.1
No data	77	23.5
Type of osteosynthesis		
K-wires	5	1.5
External fixator	10	3.1
No data	14	4.3
Conservative	27	8.3
Intramedullary nail	90	27.5
Plate	146	44.6
Cerclage wiring	4	1.2
Screw	24	7.3
Joint replacement	7	2.1

3.2. Descriptive Analysis of Atrophic Nonunions

Further, atrophic nonunions of long bones (humerus, radius, ulna, femur, tibia, fibula) were descriptively analyzed (Table 2). No significant differences could be found when compared to the whole nonunion collective described above. In contrast, sex was almost equally distributed. The nonunion site was also more distributed among long bones, with a smaller amount of femur nonunions (34.7%). There were less patients who achieved an anatomic reduction (59%) and stability of the osteosynthesis (70%) postoperatively. Contrary to the complete nonunion collective, we analyzed the use of aspirin (ASS) and non-steroidal anti-inflammatory drugs (NSAIDs). While 9% of the patients were treated with ASS, only 3% used NSAIDs according to medical records.

Table 2. Descriptive analysis of the atrophic nonunion collective.

Factor	Total Numbers	Percentage
Age	22–100 (Mean 63)	
Sex (male)	47	48
BMI	17.3–66.1 (Mean 24.5)	
Alcohol abuse	7	7.1
Smoking	18	18.4
Polytrauma	14	14.3
ASA score	1–4 (Mean 2)	
Osteoporosis	15	15.1
Anti-osteoporotic treatment	11	11.1
ASS	9	9.1
NSAIDs	3	3.1
Vitamin D (ng/mL)	9.9–57.1 (Mean 24.45)	
Nonunion site		
Femur	34	34.7
Tibia	22	22.4
Humerus	17	17.3
Radius	12	12.2
Ulna	6	6.1
Fibula	3	3.1
Tibia, fibula	2	2.1
Radius, ulna	2	2.1
Bone substitute/autograft		
At primary surgery	4	4.1
At nonunion surgery	47	47.9
Cerclage wiring (total number)		
1	12	12.2
2	5	5.1
3	1	1.1
Anatomic reduction	58	59.1
Stability	69	70
Implant removal	12	12.1
Soft tissue damage		
Closed	68	69.4
Grade I closed	11	11.2
Grade II closed	8	8.1
Not specified	49	50
Open	16	16.3
Grade I open	2	2
Grade II open	3	3.1
Grade III open	4	4
No data	21	21.4
Type of osteosynthesis		
K-wires	2	2.1
External fixator	1	1.1
No data	1	1.1
Conservative	3	3.1
Intramedullary nail	27	27.5
Plate	54	55.1
Plate + Intramedullary nail	1	1.1
Screw	6	6.1
Joint replacement	3	3.1

3.3. Atrophic Nonunion vs. Matched-Pair Control Group

To elucidate and highlight the possible pathomechanisms of atrophic long-bone nonunions, a direct statistical comparison of atrophic nonunions and the matched-pair control group was performed (Table 3).

Table 3. Results from the analysis of atrophic nonunion vs. matched-pair control group.

Parameter	Nonunion No. (%)	Control No. (%)	p-Value
Sex (male)	47 (48.0%)	46 (46.9%)	0.99
Age (years)	64 (46–79)	64 (28–78)	0.88
BMI (kg/m^2)	24.5 (22.5–26.9)	25.7 (22.4–28.6)	0.16
Alcohol abuse	7 (7.1%)	12 (12.2%)	0.33
Smoking	18 (18.4%)	29 (29.6%)	0.09
Polytrauma	14 (14.3%)	18 (18.4%)	0.56
Used implant			
Intramedullary nail	27 (27.6%)	46 (46.9%)	
Plate	54 (55.1%)	39 (39.8%)	0.021
Other	17 (17.3%)	13 (13.3%)	
Use of cerclage wires	18 (18.4%)	26 (26.5%)	0.23
Total number of cerclage wires			
0	80 (81.6%)	72 (73.5%)	
1	12 (12.2%)	9 (9.2%)	0.08
2	5 (5.1%)	11 (11.2%)	
3	1 (1.0%)	6 (6.1%)	
Anatomic reduction			
Yes	58 (59.2%)	88 (89.8%)	
No data	7 (7.1%)	0 (0.0%)	<0.0001
Conservative treatment	3 (3.1%)	0 (0.0%)	
No	30 (30.6%)	10 (10.2%)	
Stability			
Yes	69 (70.4%)	97 (99.0%)	
No data	7 (7.1%)	0 (0.0%)	<0.0001
Conservative treatment	3 (3.1%)	0 (0.0%)	
No	18 (18.4%)	1 (1.0%)	
Vitamin D (ng/mL)	26.8 (15.6–36.7)	18.5 (11.2–26.4)	0.09
Osteoporosis	15 (15.3%)	17 (17.3%)	0.85
Anti-osteoporotic treatment	11 (11.2%)	14 (14.3%)	0.67
Implant removal	12 (12.2%)	27 (27.6%)	0.007
ASA score (mean)	2 (2–3)	2 (2–3)	0.82
NSAIDs	3 (3.1%)	8 (8.2%)	0.21
ASS	9 (9.2%)	16 (16.3%)	0.19

The control group was matched to the nonunion group for age and gender. Like the nonunion group, the control group consisted of 98 patients. The distribution among long bones is shown in Table 3. The femur and tibia were the two most common nonunion sites in the control group, accounting for 34.7% and 23.5%, respectively.

The distributions of the fracture locations are not statistically significantly different between men and women (p = 0.72 (Fisher's exact test)).

3.4. Type of Implant

Intramedullary nailing and plate osteosynthesis were the two most common surgical methods employed (Table 3). If we consider only the two methods, the odds ratio for the development of a nonunion is significantly increased in patients with plate osteosynthesis compared to patients undergoing intramedullary nailing (Figure 2) (OR = 2.36; 95% CI = 1.26, 4.42; p = 0.008).

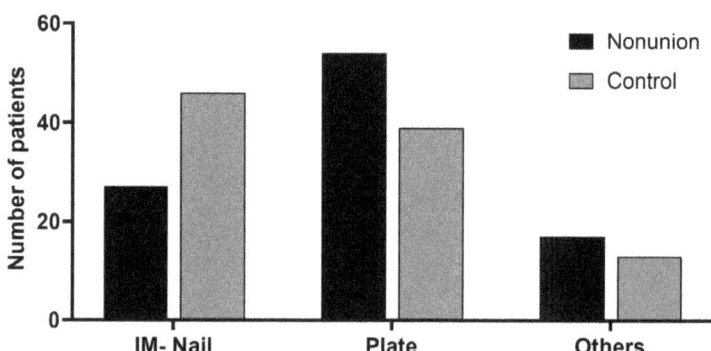

Figure 2. Surgical procedure employed in the nonunion group vs. control group in total numbers.

3.5. Cerclage Wiring

The use of cerclage wiring was of special interest and was analyzed separately. Hereby, we were able to demonstrate that the use of cerclage wiring corresponds to a lower odds ratio for nonunions, although not significantly (OR = 0.62; 95% CI = 0.32, 1.23; p = 0.173).

Further analysis of the number of cerclage wires used showed a different result. Here, the more cerclage wires that were used, the lower the risk for the development of a nonunion was (Figure 3) (OR = 0.66; 95% CI = 0.45, 0.97; p = 0.033).

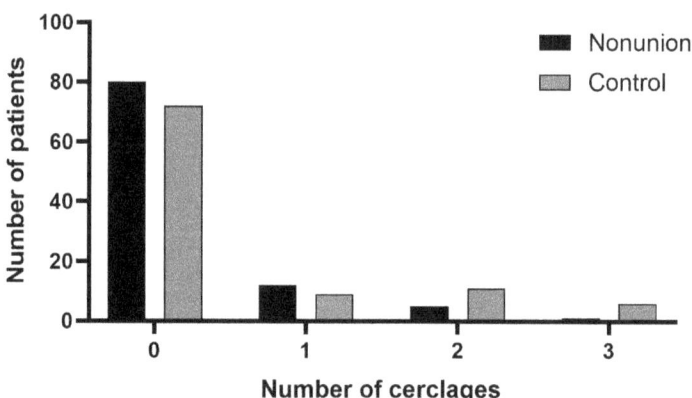

Figure 3. Use of wire cerclages in the nonunion group vs. control group in total numbers.

3.6. Use of Anti-Inflammatory Drugs

Analysis for the use of acetylsalicylic acid (ASS) (OR = 0.52; 95% CI = 0.22, 1.24; p = 0.139) and non-steroidal anti-inflammatory drugs (NSAIDs; ASS excluded) (OR = 0.36; 95% CI = 0.09, 1.38; p = 0.14) showed no significant effect on the development of long-bone atrophic nonunion.

3.7. Anatomic Reduction/Stability

There is a statistically significantly elevated risk for the development of a nonunion in patients where an anatomic reduction (p < 0.0001) or stability after osteosynthesis could not be obtained (p < 0.0001).

3.8. Polytrauma/Osteoporosis/Vitamin D/Smoking/Alcohol Abuse

When comparing atrophic long-bone nonunion with the control cases, one could not find any significant changes when looking at factors such as polytrauma, osteoporosis, vitamin D value (Figure 4), smoking and alcohol abuse (for details, see Table 3).

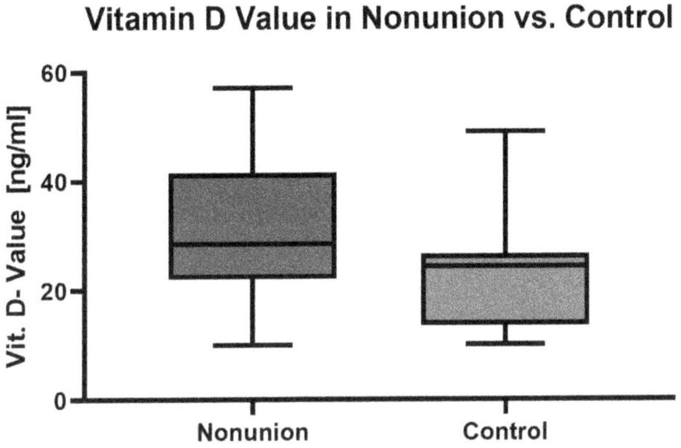

Figure 4. Vitamin D value in ng/mL in the nonunion vs. control group.

4. Discussion

This study was the first to show the factors which could have an influence on the development of delayed fracture healing or nonunion during surgical fracture osteosynthesis. Unfortunately, previous studies have often been limited to comorbidities and patient factors that are not within the surgeon's sphere of influence [2,6,7,13–15]. Due to the lack of evidence in this area, a variety of opinions and theories on the development of nonunions have developed at clinics and institutions, which, on closer examination, do not stand up to evidence-based scrutiny.

Besides obvious reasons such as bad primary surgical treatment with large gaps or failure to achieve sufficient stability, patients even developed nonunion one would have never thought possible at times.

In line with the available literature, this study confirmed that factors such as anatomical reduction and stability have a significant influence on the development of nonunion [13]. Other factors, which are generally assumed to be risk factors, could not be confirmed in this study. For example, there was no significant increase in the risk for smoking, polytrauma, osteoporosis and BMI. This is quite surprising given that, as already mentioned, many studies describe these factors as risk factors for the development of nonunion [2,3,7,12–15].

Smoking is cited as a risk factor in almost all studies; however, there are also several studies that have seen no correlation, as in the present study [16]. Another controversial example is BMI and age. The data situation here is very heterogeneous. In some cases, both advanced age [17] and BMI [13] are seen as risk factors, but in others, there is a clear trend to the contrary, with the frequency of nonunion even decreasing in older age [14].

One reason for the strong fluctuations in the literature could be the different study designs. Almost all available studies do not differentiate between the pathogenesis of nonunion, meaning that the study collectives contain a mixture of infectious pseudarthroses with atrophic and hypertrophic pseudarthroses. Since the underlying problem is completely different depending on the type of nonunion, it is obvious that the risk factor predictors also differ, and it is difficult to analyze them. This is the reason why this study mainly deals with atrophic nonunions of long tubular bones. In our view, the bias of an inhomogeneous study collective can be reduced as much as possible. While we also looked at population-based predictors in this study, the focus was set on factors that can be influenced by the treating physician and that could have an impact on the development of pseudarthrosis as part of its clinical treatment.

The most urgent question in the case of acute shaft fractures of long tubular bones is in regard to the method of fixation to be selected.

While some fractures clearly indicate the use of either an intramedullary (mainly diaphyseal fractures) or an extramedullary (mainly metaphyseal proximal or thistle) implant, the data situation for proximal or distal shaft fractures at the meta-diaphyseal junction is less clear [18,19]. In this case, the choice of implant is primarily dependent on the personal preferences of the surgeon or on the usability and availability of implant types. The present study showed that the use of plate osteosynthesis is a risk factor for the development of a nonunion across all atrophic nonunions of long tubular bones. Some studies also showed evidence for a shorter bone union time [19], whereas others were not able to detect any significant differences [18]. The reason for a possible higher nonunion time after plate osteosynthesis could lie in the implantation technique. Although often implanted, MIPO (minimally invasive plate osteosynthesis) results in a bigger anatomical reduction compared to intramedullary implants usually achieved through direct open visualization. This leads to increased soft tissue trauma and disruption of the environment around the fracture. In line with AO guidelines and biological osteosynthesis principles [20], the fracture area is left untouched with intramedullary implants, and although an anatomical reduction is often not achievable, this appears to be a more advantageous approach in terms of delaying healing. In order to objectify the impact of surgical trauma in patients, a paper dealing with sterile inflammation after surgical therapy was published only recently. Here, the elevated inflammatory impact of additional surgical trauma from open reduction was highly significant [21]. Besides short-term side effects such as prolonged hospital stay and blood loss, it is tempting to speculate that this additional sterile inflammation might also play a role in nonunion development.

An important and very heterogeneously discussed point in everyday clinical practice is the use of cerclage and its role or disadvantage in bone healing. Many surgeons are of the opinion that by tightening and compressing the periosteum, cerclage wires could lead to reduced blood flow, thus preventing fracture healing. The data on this are very controversial. While some studies assume a delay in healing [22,23], others have even found an acceleration in healing times [24] or no significant difference [25]. A major advantage of using cerclage is improvement in the anatomical position of the fracture fragments in relation to each other and the resulting greater stability [23,25], which can have an effect not only on blood flow but also on the success of fracture healing. However, no predictors for the development of nonunion using cerclage wires were found in this study. On the contrary, the risk actually decreased significantly the more cerclage was used. As already mentioned, one possible reason for this could be the more precise reduction and thus the more favorable biomechanical conditions achieved.

Another point that is treated inconsistently in clinical routine is the use of NSAIDs during the postoperative phase. Based on animal studies showing an important role for COX-2 in fracture healing [26], the postoperative pain management protocol has been changed in many hospitals, and NSAIDs have been avoided whenever possible [27]. Meta-analyses and epidemiologic studies show a heterogeneous picture. While some meta-analyses have shown no negative effect on fracture healing [28,29], more recent observational studies have shown that selective COX-2 inhibitors were associated with a delay in fracture healing [30], whereas nonselective COX-2 inhibitors showed no negative effect. In our study, no increase in the nonunion rate was found with the use of NSAIDs; however, we did not analyze selective COX-2 and non-selective COX-2 inhibitors separately because selective COX-2 inhibitors were generally not used at our hospital.

Limitations

Although the investigated collective represents a realistic study group of patients suffering nonunion, some limitations have to be taken into account. Even though a large collective was analyzed, and significant differences were observed between the groups, the number of patients in the subgroups is limited. Matched-pair analysis was carried out with one patient each, and a higher number could have ruled out some selection bias. Due to the retrospective study design, there was no evaluation of the definitive outcome of the chosen treatment regime and no evaluation of PROMs (patient-reported outcome measures). Some parameters, such as "stability" or "anatomic reduction", are dependent on the examiner and therefore prone to bias. To minimize this risk, these subjective factors were evaluated independently by two senior orthopedic surgeons. Lastly, missing information about the patients in the clinical chart might have altered the results.

5. Conclusions

Nonunion, especially atrophic nonunion, is one of the greatest challenges in orthopedic surgery. For the patient, the development of nonunion represents a major impairment and leads to prolonged medical treatment with consequent physical disability and high socioeconomic burden due to medical leave and treatment costs. In addition to the given factors such as type of injury, comorbidities, soft tissue damage and concomitant injuries, the factors prone to influence especially give surgeons the opportunity to avert complications. This study therefore sought to evaluate such factors to possibly minimize the risk for nonunion development.

Besides obvious surgical goals such as anatomic reduction and stable fixation, it is of note that plate osteosynthesis increases the risk for nonunion development, whereas the use of cerclage wires does not seem to affect the development of nonunion in a negative way. Besides other important factors, the often-highlighted negative role of NSAIDs in nonunion development could also not be confirmed. This study is a very good example that in everyday clinical practice, there are many opinions and hospital treatment standards that are intended to help prevent complications such as nonunion, but their scientific background is often not given, or the evidence is scarce. In this regard, consideration of the results presented here could help prevent the development of atrophic nonunion in some patients.

Author Contributions: Conceptualization, C.E. and C.L.; methodology, K.H.; software, K.M.; validation, K.H., C.E. and C.L.; formal analysis, K.H.; investigation, K.H. and J.F.; resources, C.E.; data curation, Y.Z.; writing—original draft preparation, C.E., J.F. and C.L.; writing—review and editing, C.E., J.F. and C.L.; visualization, K.H.; supervision, W.B.; project administration, C.L. All authors have read and agreed to the published version of the manuscript.

Funding: This research received no external funding.

Institutional Review Board Statement: The study was conducted in accordance with the Declaration of Helsinki. Ethical review and approval were not required for this study due to its observational nature.

Informed Consent Statement: Not applicable.

Data Availability Statement: The data presented in this study are available on request from the corresponding author. The data are not publicly available due to privacy reasons.

Conflicts of Interest: The authors declare no conflicts of interest.

References

1. Biberthaler, P.; van Griensven, M. *Knochendefekte und Pseudarthrosen*; Springer: Berlin/Heidelberg, Germany, 2017.
2. Vanderkarr, M.F.; Ruppenkamp, J.W.; Vanderkarr, M.; Holy, C.E.; Blauth, M. Risk factors and healthcare costs associated with long bone fracture non-union: A retrospective US claims database analysis. *J. Orthop. Surg. Res.* **2023**, *18*, 745. [CrossRef] [PubMed]
3. Ekegren, C.L.; Edwards, E.R.; de Steiger, R.; Gabbe, B.J. Incidence, Costs and Predictors of Non-Union, Delayed Union and Mal-Union Following Long Bone Fracture. *Int. J. Environ. Res. Public Health* **2018**, *15*, 2845. [CrossRef] [PubMed]
4. Wittauer, M.; Burch, M.A.; McNally, M.; Vandendriessche, T.; Clauss, M.; Della Rocca, G.J.; Giannoudis, P.V.; Metsemakers, W.J.; Morgenstern, M. Definition of long-bone nonunion: A scoping review of prospective clinical trials to evaluate current practice. *Injury* **2021**, *52*, 3200–3205. [CrossRef] [PubMed]
5. Weinlein, J. *Delayed Unions and Nonunions Fractures*, 14th ed.; Orthopaedics, C.S.O., Ed.; Elsevier: Philadelphia, PA, USA, 2021; pp. 3192–3227.
6. Zura, R.; Xiong, Z.; Einhorn, T.; Watson, J.T.; Ostrum, R.F.; Prayson, M.J.; Della Rocca, G.J.; Mehta, S.; McKinley, T.; Wang, Z.; et al. Epidemiology of Fracture Nonunion in 18 Human Bones. *JAMA Surg.* **2016**, *151*, e162775. [CrossRef] [PubMed]

7. Nicholson, J.A.; Makaram, N.; Simpson, A.; Keating, J.F. Fracture nonunion in long bones: A literature review of risk factors and surgical management. *Injury* **2021**, *52* (Suppl. S2), S3–S11. [CrossRef] [PubMed]
8. Giannoudis, P.V.; Einhorn, T.A.; Marsh, D. Fracture healing: The diamond concept. *Injury* **2007**, *38* (Suppl. S4), S3–S6. [CrossRef] [PubMed]
9. Giannoudis, P.V.; Einhorn, T.A.; Schmidmaier, G.; Marsh, D. The diamond concept--open questions. *Injury* **2008**, *39* (Suppl. S2), S5–S8. [CrossRef] [PubMed]
10. Andrzejowski, P.; Giannoudis, P.V. The 'diamond concept' for long bone non-union management. *J. Orthop. Traumatol.* **2019**, *20*, 21. [CrossRef] [PubMed]
11. Bhandari, M.; Tornetta, P., 3rd; Sprague, S.; Najibi, S.; Petrisor, B.; Griffith, L.; Guyatt, G.H. Predictors of reoperation following operative management of fractures of the tibial shaft. *J. Orthop. Trauma.* **2003**, *17*, 353–361. [CrossRef]
12. Everding, J.; Rosslenbroich, S.; Raschke, M.J. Pseudarthroses of the long bones. *Chirurg* **2018**, *89*, 73–88. [CrossRef]
13. Jensen, S.S.; Jensen, N.M.; Gundtoft, P.H.; Kold, S.; Zura, R.; Viberg, B. Risk factors for nonunion following surgically managed, traumatic, diaphyseal fractures: A systematic review and meta-analysis. *EFORT Open Rev.* **2022**, *7*, 516–525. [CrossRef] [PubMed]
14. Mills, L.A.; Aitken, S.A.; Simpson, A. The risk of non-union per fracture: Current myths and revised figures from a population of over 4 million adults. *Acta Orthop.* **2017**, *88*, 434–439. [CrossRef]
15. Wiss, D.A.; Garlich, J.; Hashmi, S.; Neustein, A. Risk Factors for Development of a Recalcitrant Femoral Nonunion: A Single Surgeon Experience in 122 Patients. *J. Orthop. Trauma.* **2021**, *35*, 619–625. [CrossRef] [PubMed]
16. Hernigou, J.; Schuind, F. Tobacco and bone fractures: A review of the facts and issues that every orthopaedic surgeon should know. *Bone Jt. Res.* **2019**, *8*, 255–265. [CrossRef] [PubMed]
17. Chitnis, A.S.; Vanderkarr, M.; Sparks, C.; McGlohorn, J.; Holy, C.E. Complications and its impact in patients with closed and open tibial shaft fractures requiring open reduction and internal fixation. *J. Comp. Eff. Res.* **2019**, *8*, 1405–1416. [CrossRef] [PubMed]
18. Sensoz, E.; Cecen, G. Comparison of Intramedullary and Extramedullary Fixation Results in Subtrochanteric Femur Fractures. *Cureus* **2023**, *15*, e49258. [CrossRef] [PubMed]
19. Kim, H.S.; Yoon, Y.C.; Lee, S.J.; Sim, J.A. Which fixation produces the best outcome for distal femoral fractures? Meta-analysis and systematic review of retrograde nailing versus distal femoral plating in 2432 patients and 33 studies. *Eur. J. Trauma Emerg. Surg.* **2023**. [CrossRef] [PubMed]
20. Weller, S. Biological osteosynthesis. *Langenbecks Arch. Chir. Suppl. Kongressbd* **1998**, *115*, 61–65.
21. Moldovan, F. Sterile Inflammatory Response and Surgery-Related Trauma in Elderly Patients with Subtrochanteric Fractures. *Biomedicines* **2024**, *12*, 354. [CrossRef]
22. Apivatthakakul, T.; Phaliphot, J.; Leuvitoonvechkit, S. Percutaneous cerclage wiring, does it disrupt femoral blood supply? A cadaveric injection study. *Injury* **2013**, *44*, 168–174. [CrossRef]
23. Karayiannis, P.; James, A. The impact of cerclage cabling on unstable intertrochanteric and subtrochanteric femoral fractures: A retrospective review of 465 patients. *Eur. J. Trauma. Emerg. Surg.* **2020**, *46*, 969–975. [CrossRef] [PubMed]
24. Hantouly, A.T.; Salameh, M.; Toubasi, A.A.; Salman, L.A.; Alzobi, O.; Ahmed, A.F.; Ahmed, G. The role of cerclage wiring in the management of subtrochanteric and reverse oblique intertrochanteric fractures: A meta-analysis of comparative studies. *Eur. J. Orthop. Surg. Traumatol.* **2023**, *33*, 739–749. [CrossRef] [PubMed]
25. Hoskins, W.; McDonald, L.; Spelman, T.; Bingham, R. Subtrochanteric Femur Fractures Treated With Femoral Nail: The Effect of Cerclage Wire Augmentation on Complications, Fracture Union, and Reduction: A Systematic Review and Meta-Analysis of Comparative Studies. *J. Orthop. Trauma* **2022**, *36*, e142–e151. [CrossRef] [PubMed]
26. Simon, A.M.; Manigrasso, M.B.; O'Connor, J.P. Cyclo-oxygenase 2 function is essential for bone fracture healing. *J. Bone Miner. Res.* **2002**, *17*, 963–976. [CrossRef] [PubMed]
27. Geusens, P.; Emans, P.J.; de Jong, J.J.; van den Bergh, J. NSAIDs and fracture healing. *Curr. Opin. Rheumatol.* **2013**, *25*, 524–531. [CrossRef] [PubMed]
28. Dodwell, E.R.; Latorre, J.G.; Parisini, E.; Zwettler, E.; Chandra, D.; Mulpuri, K.; Snyder, B. NSAID exposure and risk of nonunion: A meta-analysis of case-control and cohort studies. *Calcif. Tissue Int.* **2010**, *87*, 193–202. [CrossRef] [PubMed]
29. Kim, H.; Kim, D.H.; Kim, D.M.; Kholinne, E.; Lee, E.S.; Alzahrani, W.M.; Kim, J.W.; Jeon, I.H.; Koh, K.H. Do Nonsteroidal Anti-Inflammatory or COX-2 Inhibitor Drugs Increase the Nonunion or Delayed Union Rates After Fracture Surgery?: A Propensity-Score-Matched Study. *J. Bone Jt. Surg. Am.* **2021**, *103*, 1402–1410. [CrossRef]
30. George, M.D.; Baker, J.F.; Leonard, C.E.; Mehta, S.; Miano, T.A.; Hennessy, S. Risk of Nonunion with Nonselective NSAIDs, COX-2 Inhibitors, and Opioids. *J. Bone Jt. Surg. Am.* **2020**, *102*, 1230–1238. [CrossRef]

Disclaimer/Publisher's Note: The statements, opinions and data contained in all publications are solely those of the individual author(s) and contributor(s) and not of MDPI and/or the editor(s). MDPI and/or the editor(s) disclaim responsibility for any injury to people or property resulting from any ideas, methods, instructions or products referred to in the content.

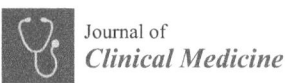

Journal of Clinical Medicine

Article

Radial vs. Dorsal Approach for Elastic Stable Internal Nailing in Pediatric Radius Fractures—A 10 Year Review

Raffael Cintean *, Alexander Eickhoff, Carlos Pankratz, Beatrice Strauss, Florian Gebhard and Konrad Schütze

Department of Trauma-, Hand-, and Reconstructive Surgery, Ulm University, Albert-Einstein-Allee 23, 89081 Ulm, Germany; alexander.eickhoff@uniklinik-ulm.de (A.E.); carlos.pankratz@uniklinik-ulm.de (C.P.); beatrice.strauss@uniklinik-ulm.de (B.S.); florian.gebhard@uniklinik-ulm.de (F.G.); konrad.schuetze@uniklinik-ulm.de (K.S.)
* Correspondence: raffael.cintean@uniklinik-ulm.de

Citation: Cintean, R.; Eickhoff, A.; Pankratz, C.; Strauss, B.; Gebhard, F.; Schütze, K. Radial vs. Dorsal Approach for Elastic Stable Internal Nailing in Pediatric Radius Fractures—A 10 Year Review. *J. Clin. Med.* **2022**, *11*, 4478. https://doi.org/10.3390/jcm11154478

Academic Editors: Christian Ehrnthaller and Christian Carulli

Received: 7 July 2022
Accepted: 29 July 2022
Published: 31 July 2022

Publisher's Note: MDPI stays neutral with regard to jurisdictional claims in published maps and institutional affiliations.

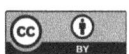

Copyright: © 2022 by the authors. Licensee MDPI, Basel, Switzerland. This article is an open access article distributed under the terms and conditions of the Creative Commons Attribution (CC BY) license (https://creativecommons.org/licenses/by/4.0/).

Abstract: Background: Forearm fractures are one of the most common fractures in children. Over the last years, a tendency towards surgical treatment was seen, especially closed reduction and internal fixation with elastic stable internal nailing (ESIN). Despite an overall low complication rate being described, a risk of intraoperative complications remains. Material and Methods: A total of 237 patients (mean age 8.3 ± 3.4 (1–16) years) with forearm or radius fractures treated with ESIN between 2010 and 2020 were included in the study. The retrospective review of 245 focused on fracture pattern, pre- and postoperative fracture angulation, intra- and postoperative complications, and surgical approach for nail implant. The fracture pattern and pre- and postoperative angulation were measured radiographically. Complications such as ruptures of the extensor pollicis longus (EPL) tendon and sensibility disorders of the superficial radial nerve were further analyzed. Results: In 201 cases (82%), we performed a dorsal approach; 44 fractures (17.9%) were treated with a radial approach. In total, we found 25 (10%) surgery-related complications, of which 21 (8.6%) needed further surgical treatment. In total, we had 14 EPL ruptures (5.7%), 4 sensibility disorders of the superficial radial nerve (1.6%), 2 refractures after implant removal (0.8%), 2 superficial wound infections (0.8%), and 1 child with limited range of motion after surgery (0.4%). No statistical significance between pre- and postoperative angulation correlated to fracture patterns or diameter of the elastic nail was seen. As expected, there was a significant improvement of postoperative angulation. Using radial approach in distal radial fractures showed a lower rate of surgical related complications, 2.3% of which need further surgical treatment as well as better postoperative angulations compared to the dorsal approach (8.5%). Conclusion: Especially due to the low risk of damaging the EPL tendon, the radial approach showed a lower complication rate which needed further surgical treatment. The risk of lesions of the superficial radial nerve remains.

Keywords: ESIN; forearm fractures; EPL; SBRN; nerve damage; tendon lesion; approach; radial fracture; pediatric

1. Introduction

With an incidence of approximately 1 in 100 children per year, forearm fractures are one of the most common fractures in children. Among these injuries, diaphyseal forearm fractures are the third most common long-bone fractures in children [1,2]. Most pediatric fractures have a greater remodeling potential. Due to this fact, nonoperative treatment can be performed in most pediatric nondisplaced or minimally displaced radial and ulnar shaft fractures [3]. Despite this, the operative treatment with closed reduction and intramedullary nailing due to the minimally invasive approach gained popularity in the last 20 years. Cheng et al. reviewed the treatment of pediatric forearm fractures at their institution in the time frame of 10 years between 1985 and 1995 and found a trend towards intramedullary stabilization from 1.8% to 22% as an alternative to closed reduction and cast immobilization in pediatric forearm fractures [4]. Even though literature shows that intramedullary nailing has a generally low complication rate, a risk of intra- and postoperative complications remains. Different studies have shown a complication rate up to 67%. Kruppa et al. reported a complication rate of 8.9% in 202 patients [5], Smith et al. reported a complication rate of 42% [6], whereas other researchers did not report any complications after surgery [7]. Concerning complications in treatment of pediatric forearm fractures, rupture of EPL tendon and lesion of the superficial radial nerve are mentioned. Therefore, controversy exists regarding the preferred entry point for intramedullary nailing at the distal radius [8]. A dorsal approach through the Lister tubercle avoids the possible risk of damaging the superficial radial nerve but sets the EPL tendon at risk for injury [9]. Although studies describe the different approaches and the consecutive risks, a clinical comparative study could not be found in the literature search.

This study was performed to investigate and compare the advantages and disadvantages of both approaches to the distal radius using ESIN.

2. Methods

The study was a retrospective exploratory review at a Level One Trauma Center. Between January 2010 and December 2019, patients with forearm fractures were identified using the ICD-Code (International Statistical Classification of Diseases and Related Health Problems) as well as the OPS Code, which is the German equivalent to the International Classification of Procedures in Medicine (ICPM). We included every patient under 16 years of age treated with open or closed reduction and internal fixation with at least one radial intramedullary nail. Patients with previous fractures of one forearm were included provided there was adequate trauma, no osteosynthesis material was implanted, and the previous fracture was thought to have no influence on the new fracture. Patients with nonoperative treatment, other osteosynthesis techniques, and patients with multiple injuries, pathological fractures, or pre-existing bony conditions (i.e., osteogenesis imperfecta) were excluded. Patients with implanted osteosynthesis material in the fractured arm were excluded. A total of 245 fractures in 237 patients, surgically treated using at least one radial ESIN, were included. All found complications were chart reviewed and categorized.

The study was approved by the institutional ethical committee (89/20-FSt/TR).

2.1. Angulation

All patient charts as well as the pre- and postoperative radiographic data were reviewed by two experienced attending surgeons. The fracture patterns were analyzed on available anterior–posterior as well as lateral performed X-rays. The pre- and postoperative angulations of the radius in both plane anterior–posterior and lateral imaging were measured in the institutional PACS system and categorized in 3 groups with 0 degree pre- and postoperative angulation, between 1 and 5 as well as above 5 degrees in anterior-posterior and lateral plane. The radial diaphysis was subdivided in proximal, medial, and distal thirds for statistical reasons.

2.2. Operative Technique

In all patients, we used the Synthes Titanium Elastic Nail System (West Chester, PA, USA) with diameters of 1.5 mm up to 3.0 mm, generally to be up to 2/3 of the diameter of the intramedullary canal. The ESIN is usually prebend to secure an intramedullary 3-point-fixation. The ulnar ESIN was implanted through a 3 to 5 mm incision at the olecranon distal of the growth plate. The radius was either stabilized through a 3 to 5 mm distal dorsal incision near the Lister tubercle or a distal radial approach proximal of the growth plate was chosen also through a 3 to 5 mm radial incision. The approach as well as the used osteosynthesis was chosen by the attending surgeon's choice by case. During all surgeries, free range of motion (ROM) of the elbow and wrist was tested after stabilization. All surgeries were performed by or under supervision of an experienced attending surgeon.

Postoperatively, the patients were immobilized in a long arm cast for forearm fractures and in a short arm cast only for radial fractures for the first 2–4 days after surgery. Longer cast immobilization was performed individually depending on the intraoperative fracture stability and the surgeon's decision. As it is institutional practice, an anterior–posterior as well as lateral X-ray was performed on the day after the surgery. Most patients were discharged the next day, the mean hospitalization time was 1.69 days (range 1–3 days). Clinical and radiographic follow-up was performed 6 and 12 weeks after surgery if no complication occurred.

2.3. Complications

Complications such as lesions of the superficial branch of the radial nerve (SBRN), ruptures of the extensor pollicis longus tendon, wound infections, postoperative hematoma, refracture after implant removal, restricted mobility after surgery, and lesions of the ulnar and median nerve were recorded. Complications, especially ruptures of the EPL tendon and lesions of the superficial radial nerve, were further analyzed regarding fracture type, surgical treatment, treatment of complication, and final outcome.

2.4. Statistics

Data analysis was performed with IBM SPSS Statistics (V12.0, IBM, Armonk, NY, USA) and Microsoft Excel (V15.2, Microsoft, Redmond, WC, USA). Demographic characteristics were described as mean and standard deviation. Logistic regression was performed for primary outcome measures considering all variables related to the pre- and postoperative angulation and postoperative complications.

3. Results

The average age of our patients was 8.3 ± 3.4 years (range 1–16 years). We found 202 radial and ulnar fractures and 43 radial fractures. In the radiographic analysis of the cohort, we found 182 middle diaphyseal fractures, 23 proximal diaphyseal fractures, and 40 distal diaphyseal fractures treated with ESIN. Three patients presented with a Gustilo–Anderson type I open fracture which needed extended wound debridement [10].

In all 202 cases with radial and ulnar fractures, we performed intramedullary nailing of both radius and ulna; in 46 cases only, the radius was reduced and stabilized. The mean time of surgery was 27.6 ± 12.5 min with a range from 8 to 82 min. In 201 cases, the dorsal approach through the Lister tubercle was performed. After showing a rising incidence of EPL lesions, a change of practice in the institution was done. After that, 44 fractures were operated with a radial approach.

Demographic factors such as age, sex, and side of fracture showed no statistical significance correlated to postoperative angulation or complications. Intraoperative surgical factors such as thickness of the used elastic nail or operative time did not show statistical significance to postoperative angulation or complications.

The follow-up averaged 4.7 ± 4.2 months (range 1.7–28.1 months). Implant removal was performed on average after 3.3 ± 2.8 months (range 1.1–11 months) after clinical and radiographic healing was ensured. A total of 23 patients (9.2%) were lost during follow-up.

3.1. Angulation

In the anterior–posterior plane, the fracture angulation of the radius distributed between 70 radial angulations with a maximum of 35 degrees and 149 ulnar angulations with a maximum of 55 degrees. There was no significant angulation in the anterior–posterior plane of 30 fractures. In the lateral plane, we found 196 dorsal angulations with a maximum of 76 degrees and 46 volar angulations with a maximum of 47 degrees. Three fractures showed no significant angulation in the lateral view. As shown in Figure 1, most fractures were dorsal and ulnar angulated (Figure 1).

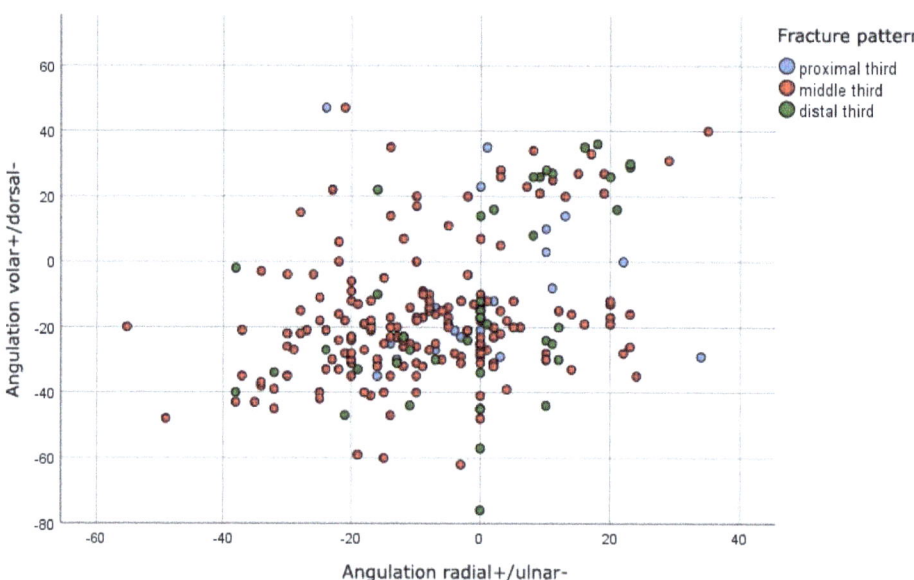

Figure 1. Preoperative distribution of angulations in degrees of fractures in anterior-posterior (x axis) and lateral (y axis) plane.

The postoperative radiographic measurements showed an expected improvement of the angulations, even though angulations up to 18 degrees in all planes could be found (Figure 2). In relation to the surgical approach, no significant difference ($p = 0.129$) was seen. However, we found a significant correlation ($p < 0.001$) between the fracture pattern and the postoperative angulations. Fractures in the distal diaphysis showed a significantly higher postoperative angulation compared to fractures in the proximal and middle diaphysis (Table 1, Figure 3).

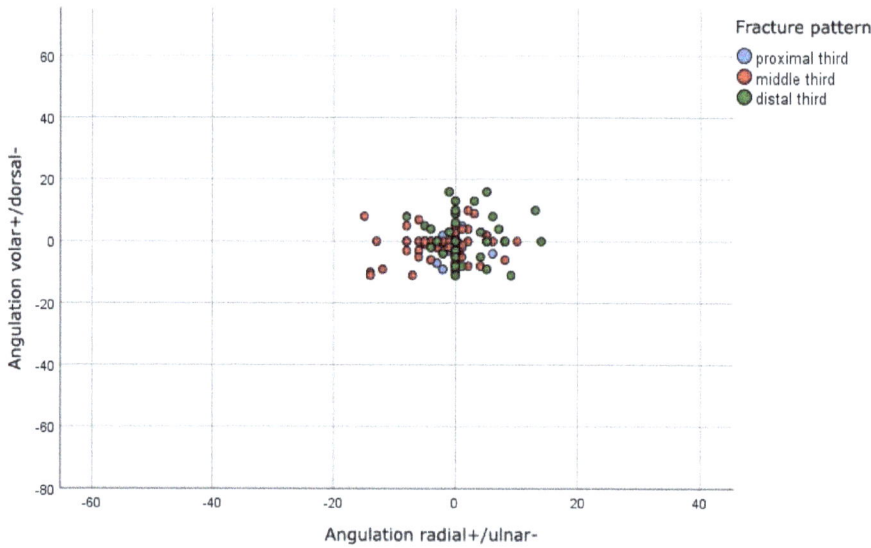

Figure 2. Postoperative distribution of angulations in degrees of fractures in anterior–posterior (x axis) and lateral (y axis) plane.

Table 1. Fracture pattern compared to postoperative angulations.

Postoperative Angulation		Fracture Pattern			Total
		Proximal Third	Middle Third	Distal Third	
0°	N	12	117	8	137
	Percentage	52.2%	64.3%	20.0%	55.9%
>0° to ≤5°	N	6	38	12	56
	Percentage	26.1%	20.9%	30.0%	22.9%
>5°	N	5	27	20	52
	Percentage	21.7%	14.8%	50.0%	21.2%
Total	N	23	182	40	245
	Percentage	100.0%	100.0%	100.0%	100.0%

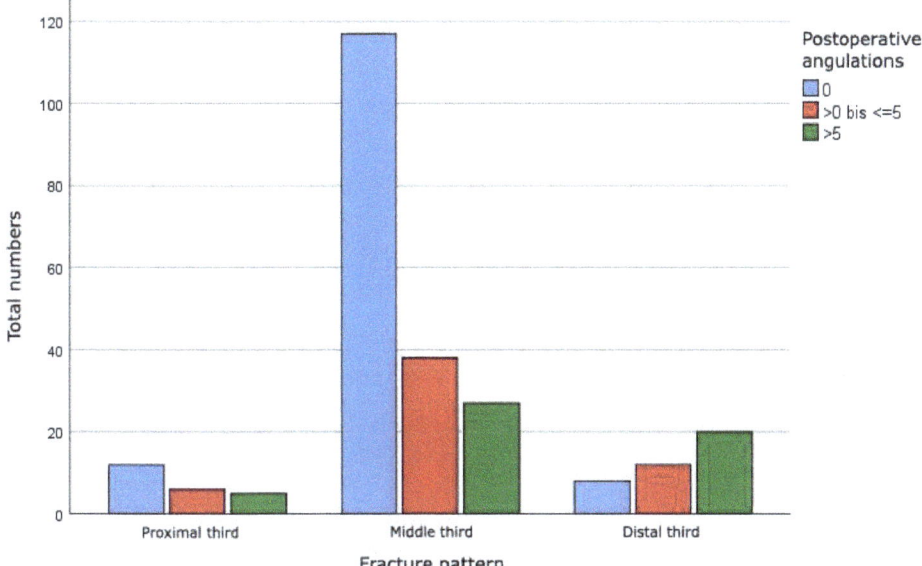

Figure 3. Comparison of fracture pattern and maximal postoperative angulations of diaphyseal radial fractures in degrees in both planes.

In 29 out of 40 fractures of the distal third of the diaphysis, the ESIN was performed through a dorsal approach, 11 fractures were operated on using a radial approach. No significant correlation ($p = 0.414$) between the approach and postoperative angulation of distal forearm and radial fractures was shown. A tendency towards the radial approach in terms of better maximal postoperative angulation in both planes and radiographic outcome was found (Figure 4).

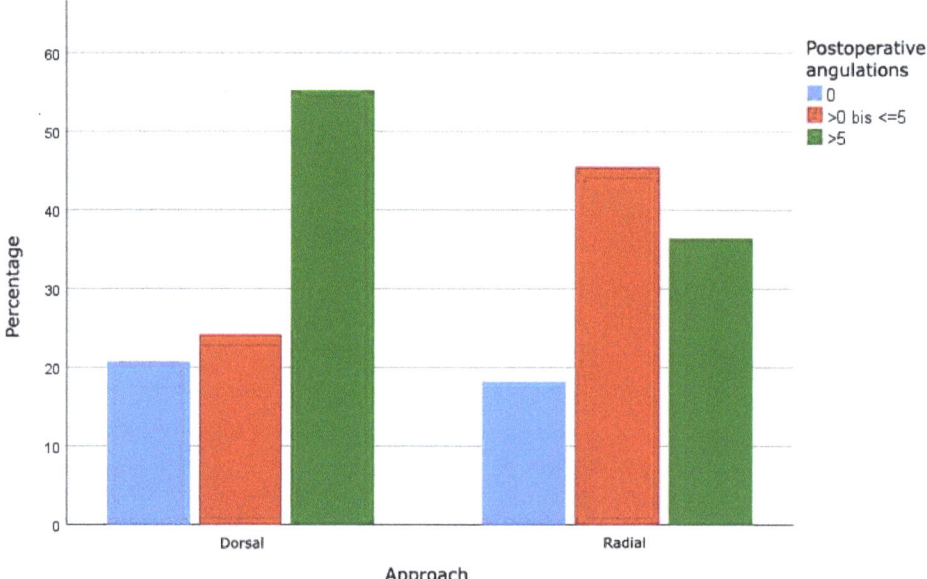

Figure 4. Maximal postoperative angulations in degrees in both planes of distal radial diaphysis fractures operated with dorsal or radial approach.

3.2. Complications

In total, 25 (10.0%) surgery-related complications occurred in the study population. A total of 21 (8.6%) children required further surgical treatment (Table 2).

Table 2. Surgery related complications (EPL = extensor pollicis longus, SBRN = superficial branch of radial nerve, ESIN = elastic stable intramedullary nailing, ROM = range of motion.

Surgery-Related Complications	Total (%)	Dorsal Approach	Radial Approach
EPL rupture	16 (6.5%)	16 (7.9%)	0
Lesion of SBRN	4 (1.6%)	0	4 (9.1%)
Refracture after ESIN removal	2 (0.8%)	1 (0.5%)	1 (2.2%)
Wound infection	2 (0.8%)	2 (1%)	0
Limited ROM	1 (0.4%)	1 (0.5%)	0
Total	25 (10%)	20 (9.9%)	5 (11.4%)

A total of 16 (7.9% of dorsal approaches) ruptures of the extensor pollicis longus tendon were observed and required operative treatment, one child showed an entrapment of the EPL tendon and did not need further treatment after surgical release. In one case, an EPL rupture due to adhesion to the callus formation was observed. One child with EPL rupture was lost during follow-up. The mean time from initial surgery to EPL repair was 3.3 ± 2.4 months (range 21 days–6.3 months). All EPL repairs were treated with a transfer of the extensor indicis proprius (EIP) tendon. A significance ($p < 0.001$) between the chosen approach for ESIN and EPL rupture was found. All of them were operated on using a dorsal approach. No significant correlation between diameter (range 1.5–3.0 mm) of the ESIN and EPL rupture could be found. All children showed good outcome after EPL repair in the clinical follow-ups.

In 4 (9.1% of radial approaches) cases, we observed hypesthesia of the thumb due to lesion of the superficial branch of the radial nerve (SRNB) after ESIN. In all cases, a radial approach with a skin incision of around 5 to 8 mm was performed. Further surgical treatment was required in none of the cases, as sensibility improved over time. After early implant removal and cast immobilization after 1.1 months, one child complained about a persistent mild sensibility disorder which was addressed with physiotherapy. The palsy was consistent after a follow-up of 6 months after ESIN removal. No further surgical treatment was required.

Two (0.8%) refractures occurred due to new adequate trauma at 1.1 and 1.6 months after implant removal. In one case, we decided to perform open reduction and plate osteosynthesis. In one case, a secondary loss of reduction 21 days after ESIN implantation was observed which required early implant removal, open reduction, and plate fixation. No mal- or nonunion occurred.

Two superficial wound infections were observed and required surgical treatment. No compartment syndrome occurred due to trauma or surgery.

One child with a diaphyseal forearm fracture showed limited range of motion (ROM) in supination of >20° after radial and ulnar ESIN implantation. After hardware removal, the ROM improved to almost normal.

Implant removal was performed on average after 3.3 ± 2.8 months (range 1.1–11 months) after clinical and radiographic healing was ensured. Except the 23 patients lost during follow-up, all children got implant removal at our department.

4. Discussion

In this study, both approaches were shown to have unique complications described in the literature. However, it was found that the radial approach to the distal radius was associated with significantly fewer complications that required further surgical revision. Especially for the critical distal diaphyseal fractures, we could additionally demonstrate a better reduction in the radiographic controls.

Fixation with ESIN is already a standard operative technique for both or single bone forearm fractures in children providing a primary definitive treatment [6,11–13]. However, in the literature there is no clear opinion on approaches to the radius for ESIN. Many authors perform the dorsal approach through the Lister's tubercle [7,14,15]. As initially described by Lascombes et al., a radial approach to the distal radius can be performed [15,16].

Although low complication rates were generally reported, a large diversity of complication rates from 8.9% up to 67% are reported in the literature [5,7,11,14,17].

In our study, we included 237 patients with 245 fractures of the forearm treated with at least one radial ESIN with an overall surgery related complication rate of 10%. Focusing on the dorsal approach, we found 16 (7.9% of dorsal approaches, 6.5% in total) ruptures of the EPL tendon, which all occurred using a dorsal approach. Flynn et al. reported EPL injuries from ESIN after dorsal approach in 2 of 103 patients (1.9%) [14]. In a small cohort of 17 patients, Lee et al. reported 3 EPL ruptures after surgical treatment with ESIN and a dorsal approach of pediatric forearm fractures (17.6%) [15]. A recent systematic review by Murphy et al. listed a total of 30 patients with EPL ruptures after ESIN of forearm fractures in 338 children, all using the dorsal approach (8.9%). In their study, the EPL lesion is described as unique complication of the dorsal entry approach [18]. We had similar findings in the present study with all EPL lesions being associated with dorsal approaches. It is recommended when performing the dorsal approach to use a mini-open incision to avoid lesions of the EPL tendon via effective retraction. Varga et al. even recommended intraoperative visualization of the EPL using sonography to avoid lesion of the tendon, though mentioning basic skills in sonography are necessary [19]. Even though in the literature most surgeons use the mini-open technique to avoid damaging the tendon, a high risk of EPL tendon ruptures remains [14,18,20].

Although seeming safer, the radial approach has been associated with complications [16]. Fernandez et al. reported lesions of the superficial branch of the radial nerve in 15 out of 553 patients after implantation or removal of ESIN (2.7%). In 2 patients, it was regressive but persistent. No further surgical treatment was necessary [17]. Lyman et al.

reported 3 superficial radial nerve palsies in 456 patients after ESIN using the radial approach (0.9%). No further surgical treatment was required [15]. Schmittenbecher et al. found 9 lesions of the SBRN in 300 patients (3%) [21]. After showing a rising incidence of EPL ruptures, a change of practice in our institution to radial approach was indicated. We performed the radial approach to the distal radius in 44 cases. We found 4 lesions of the SBRN after radial approach (9%). In one case, the sensibility disorder was regressive but consistent after a follow-up of 6 months. No cases required further surgical treatment. Different studies recommend the radial approach using a mini-open incision to ensure the visualization and effective retraction of the superficial branch of the radial nerve [1,9,17,21]. We considered the lesion of the SBRN a less severe complication not requiring further surgical treatment.

Unrelated to approach, refracture after implant removal showed the third highest complication rate in the present study with 0.8%. All patients with refractures showed an adequate trauma. Similar or higher numbers can be found in the literature. Fernandez et al. reported 13 refractures in 537 patients after implant removal within 2 years (2.4%) [17]. Kruppa et al. reported 7 refractures after ESIN removal in 202 cases (3.5%) [5]. As a main reason for refractures early implant removal is mentioned [9,15,17,21]. We removed ESIN after an average of 3.3 months after clinical and radiographic 4-cortices healing. Literature recommends longer times for implant removal of 6 to 12 months [7,9,15–17]. Due to low incidence in the present study, no statistical correlation between implant removal and refracture could be found. Other authors describe a higher refracture risk after early implant removal [21–23].

The pre- and postoperative angulation showed the expected improvement in all planes. Focusing on the distal diaphyseal fractures, a better postoperative outcome of the maximal angulation in both planes after radial approaches was found. The literature recommends K wire fixation for pediatric metaphyseal or epiphyseal fractures but highlights the difficulties in distal diaphyseal fractures with K wire fixation [22,24,25]. No clear guidelines exist for distal diaphyseal or metaphyseal fractures. Du et al. used anterograde ESIN as it is mentioned that there is not enough space to secure a stable fixation in the distal fragment [24]. We used the same technique in the past. In this study, we found 40 distal diaphyseal fractures treated with retrograde ESIN and found good results in clinical and radiographic outcome. Despite being reported not to be ideal for fractures in distal diaphyseal or metaphyseal fractures, the radial approach showed better results in maximal postoperative angulation in both planes (Figure 4). Together with this and our findings of less complications which need further surgical treatment, we recommend the radial approach for ESIN in most diaphyseal pediatric fractures.

The study shows several limitations. The retrospective aspect of the study comes with its inherent problems. Due to the late change of surgical technique, we only had 44 cases of radial approaches to the distal radius. More cases would provide better data for statistical significance. Due to the wide age range of the included patients, differences between bone healing and maximal angulation may occur. Moreover, some patients may have been missed because of errors in coding.

5. Conclusions

We recommend taking the radial approach into consideration for most radial diaphyseal fractures due to lower complication rate which require further surgical treatment. Care should be taken during nail insertion and removal to avoid damage to the SBRN. Removal can be performed after 3 months and clinical and radiographic healing.

Author Contributions: Conceptualization, C.P. and K.S.; data curation, R.C., A.E., C.P., B.S. and K.S.; formal analysis, K.S.; investigation, R.C.; supervision, F.G.; validation, A.E.; visualization, K.S.; writing—original draft, R.C. and A.E.; writing—review and editing, R.C., C.P., B.S. and F.G. All authors have read and agreed to the published version of the manuscript.

Funding: This research received no external funding.

Institutional Review Board Statement: The study was approved by the institutional ethical committee of Ulm University, Germany (89/20-FSt/TR, approved on 9 April 2020).

Informed Consent Statement: Informed consent was obtained from all subjects involved in the study.

Conflicts of Interest: The authors declare no conflict of interest.

References

1. Wall, L.B. Staying Out of Trouble Performing Intramedullary Nailing of Forearm Fractures. *J. Pediatr. Orthop.* **2016**, *36*, S71–S73. [CrossRef]
2. Bae, D.S. Pediatric Distal Radius and Forearm Fractures. *J. Hand. Surg.* **2008**, *33*, 1911–1923. [CrossRef] [PubMed]
3. Zionts, L.E.; Zalavras, C.G.; Gerhardt, M.B. Closed Treatment of Displaced Diaphyseal Both-Bone Forearm Fractures in Older Children and Adolescents. *J. Pediatr. Orthop.* **2005**, *25*, 507–512. [CrossRef]
4. Cheng, J.C.; Ng, B.K.W.; Ying, S.Y.; Lam, P.K.W. A 10-year study of the changes in the pattern and treatment of 6,493 fractures. *J. Pediatr. Orthop.* **1999**, *19*, 344–350. [CrossRef]
5. Kruppa, C.; Bunge, P.; Schildhauer, T.A.; Dudda, M. Low complication rate of elastic stable intramedullary nailing (ESIN) of pediatric forearm fractures: A retrospective study of 202 cases. *Medicine* **2017**, *96*, e6669. [CrossRef]
6. Smith, V.A.; Goodman, H.J.; Strongwater, A.; Smith, B. Treatment of Pediatric Both-Bone Forearm Fractures: A Comparison of Operative Techniques. *J. Pediatr. Orthop.* **2005**, *25*, 309–313. [CrossRef]
7. Shah, A.S.; Lesniak, B.P.; Wolter, T.D.; Caird, M.S.; Farley, F.A.; Vander Have, K.L. Stabilization of Adolescent Both-Bone Forearm Fractures: A Comparison of Intramedullary Nailing versus Open Reduction and Internal Fixation. *J. Orthop. Trauma* **2010**, *24*, 440–447. [CrossRef]
8. Cumming, D.; Mfula, N.; Jones, J.W.M. Paediatric forearm fractures: The increasing use of elastic stable intra-medullary nails. *Int. Orthop.* **2008**, *32*, 421–423. [CrossRef]
9. Parikh, S.N.; Jain, V.V.; Denning, J.; Tamai, J.; Mehlman, C.T.; McCarthy, J.J.; Wall, E.J.; Crawford, A.H. Complications of elastic stable intramedullary nailing in pediatric fracture management: AAOS exhibit selection. *J. Bone Jt. Surg. Am.* **2012**, *94*, e184. [CrossRef]
10. Gustilo, R.B.; Anderson, J.T. Prevention of infection in the treatment of one thousand and twenty-five open fractures of long bones: Retrospective and prospective analyses. *J. Bone Jt. Surg. Am.* **1976**, *58*, 453–458. [CrossRef]
11. Kang, K.W. History and Organizations for Radiological Protection. *J. Korean Med. Sci.* **2016**, *31* (Suppl. 1), S4–S5. [CrossRef] [PubMed]
12. Schmittenbecher, P.P. State-of-the-art treatment of forearm shaft fractures. *Injury* **2005**, *36* (Suppl. 1), A25–A34. [CrossRef] [PubMed]
13. Richter, D.; Ostermann, P.A.; Ekkernkamp, A.; Muhr, G.; Hahn, M.P. Elastic intramedullary nailing: A minimally invasive concept in the treatment of unstable forearm fractures in children. *J. Pediatr. Orthop.* **1998**, *18*, 457–461. [CrossRef]
14. Flynn, J.M.; Sarwark, J.F.; Waters, P.M.; Bae, D.S.; Lemke, L.P. The surgical management of pediatric fractures of the upper extremity. *Instr. Course Lect.* **2003**, *52*, 635–645. [PubMed]
15. Lyman, A.; Wenger, D.; Landin, L. Pediatric diaphyseal forearm fractures: Epidemiology and treatment in an urban population during a 10-year period, with special attention to titanium elastic nailing and its complications. *J. Pediatr. Orthop. B* **2016**, *25*, 439–446. [CrossRef] [PubMed]
16. Lascombes, P.; Prevot, J.; Ligier, J.N.; Metaizeau, J.P.; Poncelet, T. Elastic stable intramedullary nailing in forearm shaft fractures in children: 85 cases. *J. Pediatr. Orthop.* **1990**, *10*, 167–171. [CrossRef] [PubMed]
17. Fernandez, F.F.; Langendörfer, M.; Wirth, T.; Eberhardt, O. Failures and complications in intramedullary nailing of children's forearm fractures. *J. Child Orthop.* **2010**, *4*, 159–167. [CrossRef]
18. Murphy, H.A.; Jain, V.V.; Parikh, S.N.; Wall, E.J.; Cornwall, R.; Mehlman, C.T. Extensor Tendon Injury Associated With Dorsal Entry Flexible Nailing of Radial Shaft Fractures in Children: A Report of 5 New Cases and Review of the Literature. *J. Pediatr. Orthop.* **2019**, *39*, 163–168. [CrossRef] [PubMed]
19. Varga, M.; Gáti, N.; Kassai, T.; Papp, S.; Pintér, S. Intraoperative sonography may reduce the risk of extensor pollicis longus tendon injury during dorsal entry elastic intramedullary nailing of the radius in children. *Medicine* **2018**, *97*, e11769. [CrossRef] [PubMed]
20. Lee, A.K.; Beck, J.D.; Mirenda, W.M.; Klena, J.C. Incidence and Risk Factors for Extensor Pollicis Longus Rupture in Elastic Stable Intramedullary Nailing of Pediatric Forearm Shaft Fractures. *J. Pediatr. Orthop.* **2016**, *36*, 810–815. [CrossRef] [PubMed]
21. Schmittenbecher, P.P.; Dietz, H.G.; Linhart, W.E.; Slongo, T. Complications amd Problems in Intramedullary Nailing of Children's Fractures. *Eur. J. Trauma* **2000**, *26*, 287–293. [CrossRef]
22. Lieber, J.; Joeris, A.; Knorr, P.; Schalamon, J.; Schmittenbecher, P.P. ESIN in Forearm Fractures: Clear Indications, Often Used, but Some Avoidable Complications. *Eur. J. Trauma* **2005**, *31*, 3–11. [CrossRef]
23. Cullen, M.C.; Roy, D.R.; Giza, E.; Crawford, A.H. Complications of intramedullary fixation of pediatric forearm fractures. *J. Pediatr. Orthop.* **1998**, *18*, 14–21. [CrossRef] [PubMed]

24. Du, M.; Han, J. Antegrade elastic stable intramedullary nail fixation for paediatric distal radius diaphyseal metaphyseal junction fractures: A new operative approach. *Injury* **2019**, *50*, 598–601. [CrossRef]
25. Slongo, T.F.; Audigé, L. AO Pediatric Classification Group. Fracture and dislocation classification compendium for children: The AO pediatric comprehensive classification of long bone fractures (PCCF). *J. Orthop. Trauma* **2007**, *21* (Suppl. 10), S135–S160. [CrossRef]

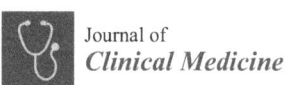

Article

Early Surgical Care of Anticoagulated Hip Fracture Patients Is Feasible—A Retrospective Chart Review of Hip Fracture Patients Treated with Hip Arthroplasty within 24 Hours

Carlos Pankratz *, Raffael Cintean, Dominik Boitin, Matti Hofmann, Christoph Dehner, Florian Gebhard and Konrad Schuetze *

Department of Trauma-, Hand-, and Reconstructive Surgery, Ulm University, Albert-Einstein-Allee 23, 89081 Ulm, Germany
* Correspondence: carlos.pankratz@uniklinik-ulm.de (C.P.); konrad.schuetze@uniklinik-ulm.de (K.S.)

Abstract: Anticoagulative medication such as antiplatelet drugs (PAI, acetylsalicylic acid and direct platelet aggregation inhibitors), vitamin-K-antagonist Warfarin (VKA) or direct oral anticoagulants (DOAC) are common among hip fracture patients, and the perioperative management of these patients is a rising challenge in orthopaedic trauma. Our objective was to determine the effect of oral anticoagulation in patients receiving early endoprosthetic treatment within 24 h after their admission. For the period from 2016 to 2020, a retrospective chart review of 221 patients (mean age 83 ± 7 years; 161 women and 60 men) who were treated either with hemi- (n = 209) or total hip arthroplasty (n = 12) within 24 h after their admission was performed. We identified 68 patients who took PAI, 34 who took DOAC and 9 who took VKA medications. The primary outcome measures were the transfusion rate and the pre- and postoperative haemoglobin (Hb) difference. The secondary outcome measures were the in-patient mortality and the rate of postoperative haematomas that needed operative treatment. A logistic/ordinal regression was performed considering the related variables to prevent cofounding occurring. The mean time to surgery was significantly longer for the DOAC and VKA groups when they were compared to the controls (none 14.7 ± 7.0 h; PAI 12.9 ± 6.7 h; DOAC 18.6 ± 6.3 h; VKA 19.4 ± 5.5 h; p < 0.05). There was no difference in the preoperative Hb level between the groups. Overall, 62 patients (28%) needed blood transfusions during the in-patient stay with an ASA classification (p = 0.022), but the type of anticoagulative medication was not a significant predictor in the logistic regression. Anticoagulation with DOAC and grouped surgery times were positive predictors for a higher Hb difference in the patients who did not undergo an intraoperative blood transfusion (n = 159). Postoperative haematomas only occurred in patients taking anticoagulative medication (four cases in PAI group, and three cases in DOAC group), but the logistic regression showed that the anticoagulative medication had no effect. The in-patient mortality was significantly influenced by a high ASA grade (p = 0.008), but not by the type of anticoagulative medication in patients who were treated within 24 h. We conclude that the early endoprosthetic treatment of the anticoagulated hip fracture patient is safe, and a delayed surgical treatment is no longer justifiable.

Keywords: hip fracture; anticoagulation; early surgical care; geriatric trauma

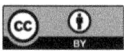

1. Introduction

The demographic changes that are occurring in developing countries is inevitably associated with a rising number of hip fractures [1]. Until the present day, hip fractures have been associated with a high morbidity and mortality, as the 1-year mortality rates reach up to 20% [2]. Hip fracture patients are often multimorbid and suffer from various medical conditions such as cardiovascular diseases [3], with the indication for an anticoagulative medication. In 2020, already over 40% of all hip fracture patients in Germany had an anticoagulant in their long-term medication [4,5]. Consequently, the surgical treatment of the anticoagulated patient is a rising challenge for attending physicians. Most common among these are platelet aggregation inhibitors (PAI) such as Clopidogrel, Ticagrelor or acetylsalicylic acid (ASS) after a myocardial infarction or a stent implantation. The effect of these drugs lasts up to 7 days [6]. In parallel, the intake of direct oral anticoagulants such as Rivaroxaban, Dabigatran and Apixaban (DOAC) are becoming more and more popular. DOAC show shorter lasting effects and half-life times of 8–15 h. However, due to the renal and hepatic metabolism there are a wide range of individual elimination rates, especially in the frail geriatric patient [7,8]. The usage of special antidotes such as idarucizumab for dabigatran or andexanet for factor Xa inhibitors rivaroxaban and apixaban are still not a part of common clinical practice [9]. In contrast, the established vitamin-K-antagonist Warfarin (VKA) can be antagonised by vitamin K administration or prothrombin complex concentrates.

By pausing the drug intake and degradation, over time, each anticoagulant loses its effect, but a delayed surgical treatment of hip fractures is widely accepted as a major factor for having an extended hospital stay [10,11], increased mortality [12–16] and an elevated risk for postoperative complications such as pulmonary embolism, infections, renal failure, decubitus ulcers, acute pulmonary edema or myocardial ischemia [17–19]. Hip fractures are surgical emergencies, and there are clear international recommendations for an early surgery [20,21]. For example, the current S2 level guideline of the German traumatology society recommends the treatment of hip and proximal femur fractures within 24 h [22], whereas the optimal window of opportunity for surgery remains a subject of scientific discourse, and the surgery of anticoagulated patients is often reported to be delayed [23,24], and attending physicians find themselves caught between avoiding the unnecessary delay of surgical treatment and preventing serious bleeding complications.

Here, we hypothesise that the urgent arthroplasty of the anticoagulated hip fracture patient is safe and does not go along with an increased rate of red blood cell transfusions (RBCT) or significant postoperative haemoglobin differences. For this purpose, we retrospectively evaluated hip fracture patients who have been treated within 24 h by hip arthroplasty to investigate the effects of different oral anticoagulants on bleeding complications.

2. Materials and Methods

All of the presented data were obtained retrospectively with permission from the local ethical committee, and they were stored anonymously. Between January 2016 and December 2020, 431 patients were treated for an acute hip fracture in our level 1 trauma centre. We subsequently excluded patients who did not undergo a following surgical treatment due to death or them having a conservative treatment, patients with haematological disorders and the regular periodic need of RBCT, patients with blood clotting disorders, patients with additional injuries in need of surgical care and patients who were not operated within 24 h after their admission. The main reasons for surgery being performed after 24 h were an acute medical condition that needed to be treated before surgery, and organisational reasons, such as a lack of operating room capacity. After applying the exclusion criteria, 329 patients were identified. From the patients who were treated within 24 h, 221 received hip arthroplasty surgery and 108 patients received joint-conserving surgery (DHS or FNS, Co. DePuy Synthes, West Chester, PA, USA). Ultimately, we included 221 patients in the study, and from these, 209 received a dual head prothesis (CORAIL® Hip System, SELF-CENTERING™ Bipolar head, Co. DePuy Synthes, West Chester, PA, USA) and 12 received a total endoprothesis (CORAIL® Hip System, PINNACLE® Acetabular Cup System, Co. DePuy Synthes, West Chester, PA, USA; Figure 1).

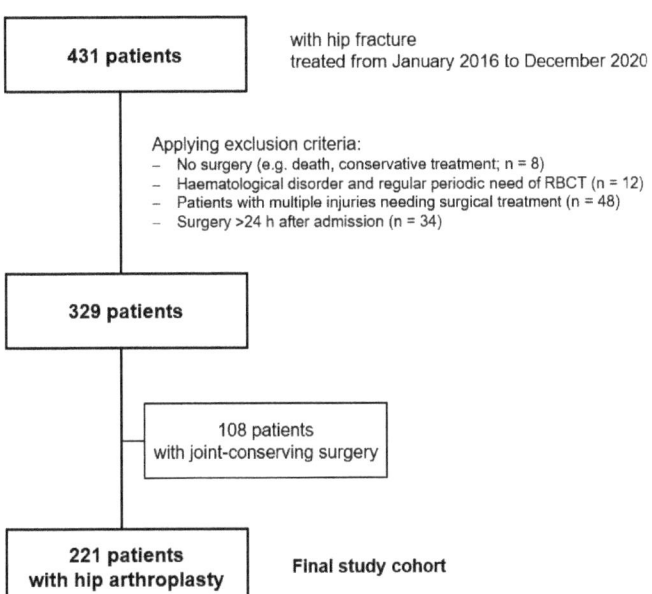

Figure 1. Study flow chart: a retrospective chart review.

The patients were operated on while they were in a supine position using the modified lateral hip approach. All of the surgery procedures were performed or supervised by experienced orthopaedic trauma surgeons. The PAI were administered perioperatively, and they were not paused. The DOAC were stopped and bridged from the first postoperative day depending on patient's specific thromboembolic risk with an intermediate-dose (enoxaparin 40 mg, 2 times a day) or high-dose (enoxaparin 1 mg/kg, 2 times a day) low-molecular-weight heparin. The VKA patients were treated with a vitamin K admission and had an INR control immediately before the surgery. If the INR was still over 1.5, prothrombin complex concentrates were administered. The VKA patients were postoperatively bridged depending on their INR and specific thromboembolic risk with an intermediate-dose or high-dose low-molecular-weight heparin. The DOAC and VKA treatments were resumed on postoperative day 8 if no bleeding complications had occurred.

We reviewed their clinical records—including the patient charts, blood values, anaesthesia protocols, surgery protocols and doctor's letters. The primary outcome parameters were the intraoperative blood transfusion rate, the pre- to postoperative Hb difference and the postoperative haematoma requiring surgical revision during the in-patient stay. The indication of blood transfusion was made individually for every patient based on the factors such as Hb value < 8g/dL with accompanying clinicals symptoms such as hypotension, tachycardia, or vertigo. Here, only the red blood cell transfusions were considered. The preoperative Hb was measured at the point of admission; the postoperative Hb was measured on the first postoperative day. The secondary outcome parameter was in-patient mortality.

The data analysis was performed using SPSS (v25.0, Co. IBM, Armonk, NY, USA). The demographic characteristics are described as mean, standard deviation and range for the continuous data, and absolute and relative frequencies for the categorical data. For the categorial outcome measures, an logistic/ordinal regression was performed considering the related variables to prevent cofounding. Additionally, for the continuous outcome measures, a regression was performed including all of the possibly confounding variables. A p-value < 0.05 was considered as statistically significant.

3. Results

3.1. Patient Population

We reviewed medical records of 221 patients. General parameters such as age, gender, the American Society of Anesthesiologists Classification (ASA) and the type of anticoagulation were recorded (Table 1). For the statistical analysis, age (<80 years; ≥80 years), surgery time (<60 min; 60–90 min; >90 min) and time to surgery (type of anticoagulation) were divided into subgroups. The study cohort had a mean age of 83.2 ± 7.46 years, with 72.9% of them being female patients. The perioperative parameters such as AO/OTA fracture and dislocation classification, grouped operating time, grouped time to surgery and blood transfusion are listed in Table 2.

Table 1. Patient population.

Variable	Mean/Count	SD/Percent
Age [years]	83.2	±7.5
<80	71	32.1%
≥80	150	67.9%
Gender		
male	60	27.1%
female	161	72.9%
ASA		
1	-	0%
2	22	10%
3	163	73.8%
4	36	16.3%
Type of anticoagulation		
none	110	49.8%
PAI	68	30.8%
VKA	9	4.1%
DOAC	34	15.4%

ASA: American Society of Anesthesiologists classification; PAI: Platelet aggregation inhibitors including acetylsalicylic acid; VKA: Vitamin-K-antagonist Warfarin; DOAC: Direct oral anticoagulants.

Table 2. Perioperative factors.

Variable	Count/Mean	%/Range
AO fracture classification		
31B1	37	16.7%
31B2	149	67.4%
31B3	35	15.8%
Operating time [min]	79	27–235
Grouped operating time		
<60 min	43	19.5%
60–90 min	119	53.8%
>90 min	59	26.7%
Time to surgery [min]	895	92–1438
none	879	92–1438
PAI	776	150–1437
VKA	1165	400–1436
DOAC	1115	191–1436
RBCT		
Yes	62	28.1%
No	159	71.9%

PAI: Platelet aggregation inhibitors including acetylsalicylic acid; VKA: Vitamin-K-antagonist Warfarin; DOAC: Direct oral anticoagulants; RBCT: red blood cell transfusion.

3.2. Time to Surgery

The overall mean time to surgery was 14.9 ± 7.0 h (Table 2). The anticoagulative treatment with DOAC (18.6 ± 6.3 h, n = 34) and VKA (19.4 ± 5.5 h, n = 9) increased the time to surgery when it was compared to the controls (14.7 ± 7.0 h, $n = 110$). In the case of the non-anticoagulated group which was compared to the PAI patient group (12.9 ± 6.7 h, $n = 68$), the differences were not statistically significant ($p = 0.42$; Figure 2).

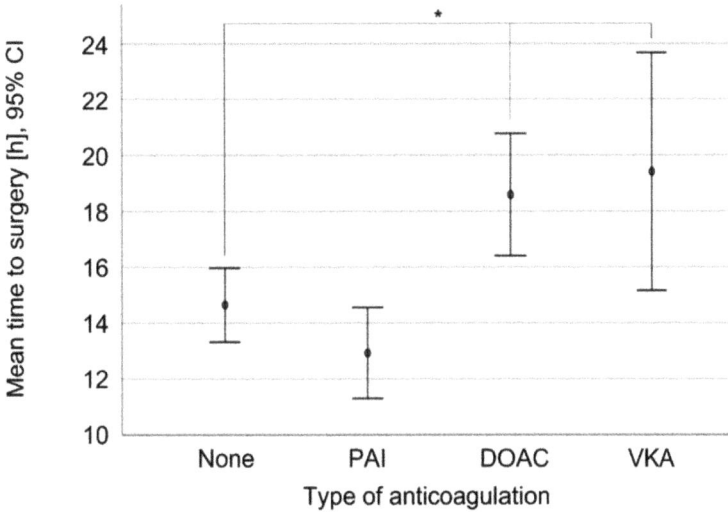

Figure 2. Mean time to surgery [h] depending on anticoagulative medication. PAI: Platelet aggregation inhibitors including acetylsalicylic acid; DOAC: Direct oral anticoagulants; VKA: Vitamin-K-antagonist Warfarin; $p < 0.05$ *.

3.3. Red Blood Cell Transfusion

Overall, 62 out of 221 patients, corresponding to 28%, received at least one RBCT (Table 2, Figure 3). The mean RBCT count was 0.55 ± 1.11 in the patients who did not take anticoagulative medication compared to 0.63 ± 1.03 in the PAI group, 0.82 ± 1.29 in the DOAC group and 0.33 ± 0.71 in the VKA group. A further analysis was performed by a logistic regression, which showed no dependency for the transfusion rate in relation to the type of anticoagulation, grouped age, AO fracture type or time to surgery. Only the ASA classification and the preoperative Hb level had a significant effect. In terms of the ASA, four patients had an increased risk for a red blood transfusion by a factor of 14.4 ($p = 0.022$). A lower preoperative Hb level significantly increased the risk for a red blood cell transfusion ($p < 0.001$).

3.4. Hb Level and Difference

There was no significant difference in the preoperative Hb levels in the patients who did and did not take anticoagulant medication (Figure 4). The postoperative Hb differences among the patients without the need for RBCT ($n = 159$) were investigated in dependence of their grouped age, AO fracture and dislocation classification, the type of anticoagulation, ASA classification, grouped surgery time and grouped time to surgery. The mean postoperative Hb difference in dependence of the anticoagulation treatment is shown in Table 3 and Figure 5. The logistic regression showed a significantly increased likelihood of higher Hb differences for the patients with higher preoperative Hb levels ($p < 0.001$), longer operating times ($p = 0.001$) and who took a DOAC treatment ($p = 0.020$). Without becoming statistically significant, the patients on VKA tended to a lower Hb difference when they were compared to the non-coagulated patients.

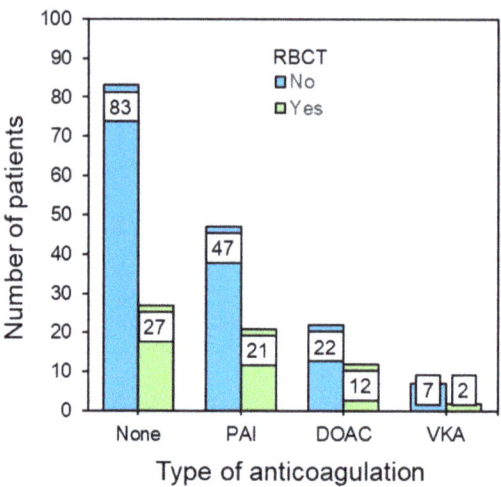

Figure 3. Red blood cell transfusion (RCBT) depending on anticoagulative medication. PAI: Platelet aggregation inhibitors including acetylsalicylic acid; DOAC: Direct oral anticoagulants; VKA: Vitamin-K-antagonist Warfarin.

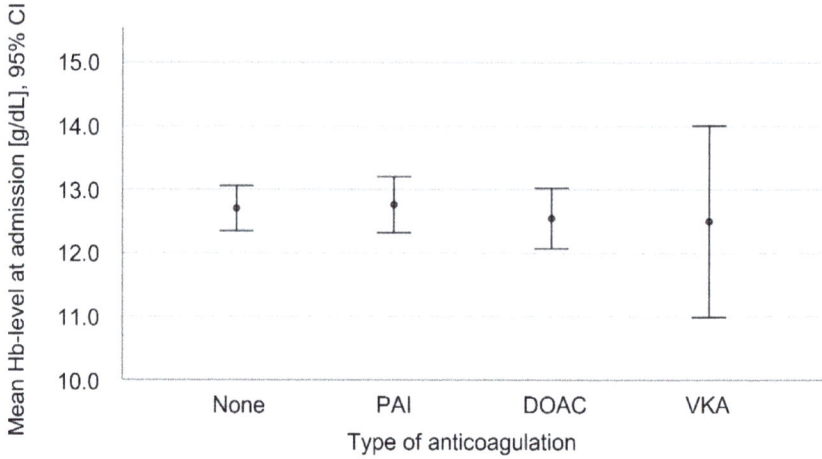

Figure 4. Hb levels at admission depending on anticoagulative medication. PAI: Platelet aggregation inhibitors including acetylsalicylic acid; DOAC: Direct oral anticoagulants; VKA: Vitamin-K-antagonist Warfarin.

Table 3. Postoperative Hb differences among patients who did not take RBCT ($n = 159$).

Variable	Mean	SD
Postoperative Hb differences [g/dL]	3.16	1.49
none	3.11	1.51
PAI	3.24	1.69
DOAC	3.52	0.87
VKA	2.14	0.81

PAI: Platelet aggregation inhibitors including acetylsalicylic acid; DOAC: Direct oral anticoagulants; VKA: Vitamin-K-antagonist Warfarin.

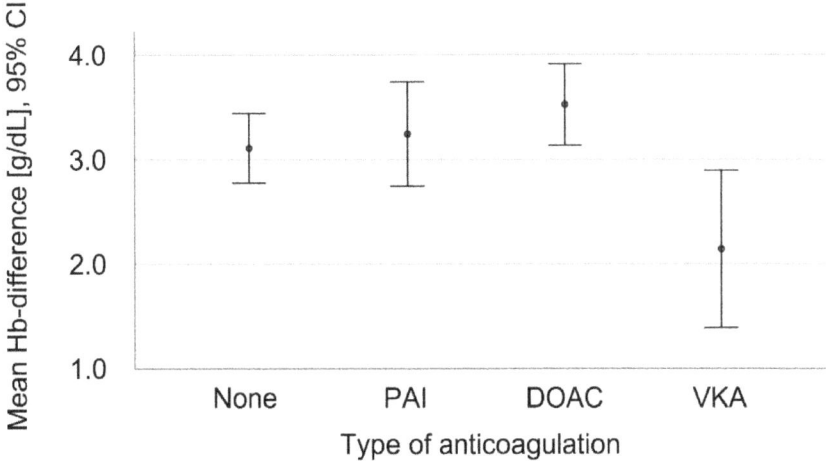

Figure 5. Mean postoperative Hb difference [g/dL] depending on different type of anticoagulation. Logistic regression showed only an increased risk for a higher Hb difference for patients taking DOAC. PAI: Platelet aggregation inhibitors including acetylsalicylic acid; DOAC: Direct oral anticoagulants; VKA: Vitamin-K-antagonist Warfarin.

3.5. Postoperative Haematoma

Out of two hundred and twenty-one included patients, seven of them needed surgical revision due to a postoperative haematoma. Four cases occurred in the group of patients who took PAI, and three cases occurred in the patients who took DOAC. Because of the low occurrence of postoperative haematomas, a statistical analysis was performed by merging the different types of anticoagulation into one group. A logistic regression using the factors of grouped age (<80 years; ≥80 years), AO classification, ASA classification, grouped surgery time (<60 min; 60–90 min; >90 min), time to surgery and type of anticoagulation showed that only the operating time had a statistical tendency to determine the occurrence of postoperative haematoma ($p = 0.086$).

3.6. In-Patient Mortality

Out of 221 patients, 17 of them, relating to 7.7%, died during their in-patient stay. Of those seventeen deaths, nine (53%) occurred in the non-anticoagulation group, five (29%) occurred in the PAI group, two (12%) occurred in the DOAC group, and one (6%) occurred in the VKA group. The logistic regression showed that a high ASA classification was significantly associated with a higher mortality risk ($p = 0.008$), and as well as this, rising age tended to increase the mortality ($p = 0.10$).

4. Discussion

A prolonged time to surgery is an independent risk factor of mortality after a hip fracture [25], and it is associated with higher patient morbidity and mortality [19,26]. An ageing population correlates with a rising number of patients requiring anticoagulant medication. For these patients, their time to surgery must be balanced with the risk of the bleeding complications. In presented study, more than 50% of the patients treated with hip arthroplasty within 24 h had an anticoagulative treatment in their long-term medication. Attending physicians face the challenge to ensure optimal conditions for surgery and the patients' safety regarding each type of anticoagulation therapy.

A treatment with PAI is the most common anticoagulative therapy. The mean wait until surgery in our PAI-study cohort was only 12.9 ± 6.7 h, and this did not differ among the non-coagulated patients. We could not observe an increased RBCT rate or Hb difference in the patients who were on PAI. These findings are in line with two meta-analyses examining the effect of clopidogrel [27,28]. Likewise, Collinge et al. reported no increased risk regarding the bleeding complication, transfusion rate and mortality after the surgical hip fracture treatment for patients on clopidogrel and ASS [29]. In all of the cited studies, the accepted delay until surgery was longer when it was compared to our mean time to surgery. Our results show that a surgical intervention should not be delayed in patients who are on PAI in terms of long-term medication.

The treatment with DOAC or VKA often expands the time to surgery for patients with an acute hip fracture [30–33]. Tran et al. reported a 40.0 h median time to surgery in patients who took DOAC or VKA compared to 26.2 h in the non-coagulated control group [24]. In our study, the mean time to surgery of patients on DOAC was 18.6 ± 6.3, and for patients on VKA, this was 19.4 ± 5.5 h. In contrast, the non-coagulated patients waited 14.7 ± 7.0 h until they underwent surgery. In our level I trauma department, acute hip fractures are treated as soon as possible regardless of the anticoagulation therapy. This study proves that there is still a delay to surgery for patients who are on DOAC and VKA. All of the patients were preoperatively prepared for intraoperative RBCT, and the patients on VKA were treated with vitamin K and prothrombin complex to achieve an INR that was less than 1.5. This preoperative coagulation optimisation might have further caused the observed prolonged time to surgery in patients who were on VKA.

The number of studies examining the complications and outcomes of anticoagulated patients receiving hip arthroplasty subsequent to experiencing an acute hip fracture is limited [34]. Overall, 28% of the patients in our study cohort needed at least one RBCT during or after surgery. However, we found no significant influence for the different types of anticoagulation on the RBCT rate. In accordance, Franklin et al., Schermann et al. as well as King et al. reported no difference in the blood transfusion rate and blood loss in the patients who were on DOAC who underwent early the surgical treatment of their hip fractures [30,31,35]. However, in all of the cited studies, the mean time to surgery for the anticoagulated patients outruns the critical 24 h mark after the patient's admission. Franklin et al. communicated a 28.9 ± 11.8 h mean time to surgery for the patients who were on DOAC, but they observed the study cohort needed a hemiarthroplasty as well as a cephalomedullary nailing treatment. Schermann et al. even reported a 42.3 ± 27.3 h average time to surgery for the patients who were on DOAC. For the patients without an RBCT, the intake of DOAC was a significant risk factor for higher postoperative Hb differences. This finding may be explained by the reported shorter time to surgery when they were compared to the mentioned studies.

In case of VKA, Cohn et al. showed no difference in the transfusion rate and blood loss in the VKA-treated patients when they were compared to the non-coagulated control group [32]. In our study, the patients on VKA showed even lower Hb differences when they were compared to the non-coagulated patients. Still, the number of VKA patients was low, and the VKA treatment showed no significant effect in the logistic regression, but there are similar observations in the literature in the course of proximal femur fractures [36]. In our department, the blood coagulation of all of the patients who are on VKA is laboratory controlled and antagonised with vitamin K or prothrombin complex concentrate if these are needed. This preoperative optimisation of the clotting might cause these findings. It remains unclear if the substitution of vitamin K or prothrombin complex concentrate might also reduce the blood loss in patients who do not undergo an anticoagulation therapy.

A high ASA grade was associated with a higher risk for RBCT and in-patient mortality. There is already some evidence that for patients with severe comorbidities and minor dislocated fractures, arthroplasty might not be the best line of treatment [37,38]. A prolonged operating time had a significant effect on the Hb difference and tended to increase the occurrence of postoperative haematoma. This underlines the importance and need of specialised orthopaedic trauma surgeons in the care of hip fracture patients.

Postoperative haematoma with the need of surgical intervention was observed in seven cases. All of the cases were associated with an anticoagulative therapy with either PAI ($n = 4$) or DOAC ($n = 3$) in terms of long-term medication. Still, anticoagulative medication showed no significant effect in the logistic regression which might be explained by the low frequency of haematomas. In contrast, in the case of ASS, Deveraux et al. demonstrated in a large, randomised trial that the perioperative intake of ASS had no significant effect on mortality and the rate of myocardial infarction, but it increased the risk of surgical bleeding complications [39]. Other recorded surgical complications such as thrombosis, pulmonary embolisms, cardiac infarctions, stroke, pneumonia, urinary tract infections, acute renal failure and deep tissue infections were not increased. Here, we observed an in-patient mortality of 7.7% that was in line with the values that have been reported elsewhere [2,40–42]. Thereby, mortality was significantly affected by the ASA classification but not by the anticoagulative therapy.

Elsewhere, in the course of proximal femur fractures, a significant lower Hb level at the point of admission and an increased blood transfusion rate for the patients on DOAC is reported [36]. Here, in accordance with Schermann et al., for hip fractures (AO type 31B), no differences in the Hb level at the point of admission was observed [31]. This may arise from different anatomical conditions, as proximal femur fractures are often associated with injuries of femoral circumflex arteries, while in hip fractures, intracapsular fracture bleeding is often self-limiting. These divergent findings may indicate that fracture morphology is an independent risk factor and might one day result in different guidelines.

Due to the retrospective design of it, our study has inevitably some limitations. The time to surgery included the time span from admission to surgical incision. Thereby, the exact time from trauma and admission could not be recorded. Additionally, because of different admission times, the blood draw interval varies as the Hb difference was calculated from the preoperative and postoperative Hb levels on the first postoperative day. Unfortunately, the one-year mortality rate could not be evaluated and was only recorded a small number of patients who had a later readmission to our hospital. A follow-up examination should be, therefore, part of further prospective studies. Finally, from a methodical point of view, only the patients who were operated within 24 h after their admission were included in the study which may have led to a certain selection bias.

Our study advocates for a short time to surgery as the mean time to surgery was only 14.9 ± 7.0 h. In almost all of the comparable studies, the mean time to surgery was clearly over 24 h. Therefore, to our knowledge this is the first study which focusing on anticoagulated patients with hip fractures that were treated by hemiarthroplasty within the first 24 h after their admission. Confounding variables such as fracture classification, surgery time, patient age and ASA classification have been considered. The evaluated parameters such as RBCT rate, pre- to postoperative Hb difference, postoperative haematoma and in-patient mortality are verifiable and of highly clinical relevance.

Our findings support the current guidelines recommending the urgent surgical treatment of hip fracture patients. As a consequence of this and a former work [36], we created an interdisciplinary standard operating procedure for our department in order to keep he time to surgery for all patients as low as possible despite their anticoagulation therapy type since the delayed surgical treatment of the anticoagulated hip fracture patient is no longer justifiable.

5. Conclusions

Using a standard operating procedure, the early surgical care of hip fractures in patients who take an anticoagulative therapy is proven to be safe, and this showed no increased bleeding risk in this retrospective study. All of the patients, regardless of their type of anticoagulative therapy, should be prepared preoperatively for possible intraoperative transfusions.

Author Contributions: Conceptualisation, C.P., R.C. and K.S.; data curation, D.B. and C.P.; formal analysis, K.S.; investigation, C.P. and D.B.; supervision, F.G. and C.D.; validation, F.G. and C.D.; visualisation, C.P.; writing—original draft, C.P. and K.S.; writing—review and editing, C.P., R.C. and M.H. All authors have read and agreed to the published version of the manuscript.

Funding: This research received no external funding.

Institutional Review Board Statement: The study was approved by the institutional ethics committee of Ulm University, Germany (89/20-FSt/TR, approved on 25 February 2021).

Informed Consent Statement: For this retrospective chart review informed consent was not required.

Data Availability Statement: The data presented in this study are available on reasonable request from the corresponding authors. The data are not publicly available due data protection reasons.

Conflicts of Interest: The authors declare no conflict of interest.

References

1. Veronese, N.; Maggi, S. Epidemiology and social costs of hip fracture. *Injury* **2018**, *49*, 1458–1460. [CrossRef] [PubMed]
2. Mahmood, A.; Thornton, L.; Whittam, D.G.; Maskell, P.; Hawkes, D.H.; Harrison, W.J. Pre-injury use of antiplatelet and anticoagulations therapy are associated with increased mortality in a cohort of 1038 hip fracture patients. *Injury* **2021**, *52*, 1473–1479. [CrossRef] [PubMed]
3. Lloyd, R.; Baker, G.; MacDonald, J.; Thompson, N.W. Co-morbidities in Patients with a Hip Fracture. *Ulster Med. J.* **2019**, *88*, 162–166. [PubMed]
4. IQTIG—Institut für Qualitätssicherung und Transparenz im Gesundheitswesen. *Bundesauswertung zum Erfassungsjahr 2020—Hüftgelenknahe Femurfraktur mit Osteosynthetischer Versorgung: Qualitätsindikatoren und Kennzahlen*; IQTIG: Berlin, Germany, 2021.
5. IQTIG—Institut für Qualitätssicherung und Transparenz im Gesundheitswesen. *Bundesauswertung zum Erfassungsjahr 2020—Hüftendoprothesenversorgung: Qualitätsindikatoren und Kennzahlen*; IQTIG: Berlin, Germany, 2021.
6. Weber, A.-A.; Braun, M.; Hohlfeld, T.; Schwippert, B.; Tschöpe, D.; Schrör, K. Recovery of platelet function after discontinuation of clopidogrel treatment in healthy volunteers. *Br. J. Clin. Pharmacol* **2001**, *52*, 333–336. [CrossRef]
7. Viktil, K.K.; Lehre, I.; Ranhoff, A.H.; Molden, E. Serum Concentrations and Elimination Rates of Direct-Acting Oral Anticoagulants (DOACs) in Older Hip Fracture Patients Hospitalized for Surgery: A Pilot Study. *Drugs Aging* **2018**, *36*, 65–71. [CrossRef]
8. Ingrasciotta, Y.; Crisafulli, S.; Pizzimenti, V.; Marcianò, I.; Mancuso, A.; Andò, G.; Corrao, S.; Capranzano, P.; Trifirò, G. Pharmacokinetics of new oral anticoagulants: Implications for use in routine care. *Expert Opin. Drug. Metab. Toxicol.* **2018**, *14*, 1057–1069. [CrossRef]
9. Godier, A.; Martin, A.C. Specific Antidotes for Direct Oral Anticoagulant Reversal: Case Closed or Cold Case? *Circulation* **2019**, *140*, 1445–1447. [CrossRef]
10. Siegmeth, A.W.; Gurusamy, K.; Parker, M.J. Delay to surgery prolongs hospital stay in patients with fractures of the proximal femur. *J. Bone Jt. Surg. Br.* **2005**, *87*, 1123–1126. [CrossRef]
11. Chechik, O.; Amar, E.; Khashan, M.; Kadar, A.; Rosenblatt, Y.; Maman, E. In Support of Early Surgery for Hip Fractures Sustained by Elderly Patients Taking Clopidogrel. *Drugs Aging* **2012**, *29*, 63–68. [CrossRef]
12. Lieten, S.; Herrtwich, A.; Bravenboer, B.; Scheerlinck, T.; van Laere, S.; Vanlauwe, J. Analysis of the effects of a delay of surgery in patients with hip fractures: Outcome and causes. *Osteoporos. Int.* **2021**, *32*, 2235–2245. [CrossRef]
13. Shiga, T.; Wajima, Z.'i.; Ohe, Y. Is operative delay associated with increased mortality of hip fracture patients? Systematic review, meta-analysis, and meta-regression. *Can. J. Anaesth.* **2008**, *55*, 146–154. [CrossRef] [PubMed]
14. Moran, C.G.; Wenn, R.T.; Sikand, M.; Taylor, A.M. Early Mortality After Hip Fracture: Is Delay Before Surgery Important? *J. Bone Joint Surg. Am.* **2005**, *87*, 483–489. [CrossRef] [PubMed]
15. Bottle, A.; Aylin, P. Mortality associated with delay in operation after hip fracture: Observational study. *BMJ* **2006**, *332*, 947–951. [CrossRef] [PubMed]
16. Pincus, D.; Ravi, B.; Wasserstein, D.; Huang, A.; Paterson, J.M.; Nathens, A.B.; Kreder, H.J.; Jenkinson, R.J.; Wodchis, W.P. Association Between Wait Time and 30-Day Mortality in Adults Undergoing Hip Fracture Surgery. *JAMA* **2017**, *318*, 1994–2003. [CrossRef]
17. Kostuj, T.; Smektala, R.; Schulze-Raestrup, U.; Müller-Mai, C. Einfluss des Operationszeitpunkts und -verfahrens auf Mortalität und Frühkomplikationen der Schenkelhalsfraktur. *Unfallchirurg* **2013**, *116*, 131–137. [CrossRef]
18. Lefaivre, K.A.; Macadam, S.A.; Davidson, D.J.; Gandhi, R.; Chan, H.; Broekhuyse, H.M. Length of stay, mortality, morbidity and delay to surgery in hip fractures. *J. Bone Jt. Surg. Br.* **2009**, *91*, 922–927. [CrossRef]
19. Simunovic, N.; Devereaux, P.J.; Sprague, S.; Guyatt, G.H.; Schemitsch, E.; DeBeer, J.; Bhandari, M. Effect of early surgery after hip fracture on mortality and complications: Systematic review and meta-analysis. *CMAJ* **2010**, *182*, 1609–1616. [CrossRef]
20. NICE. *Hip Fracture: Management: Clinical Guideline [CG124]*; National Institute for Health and Care Excellence: London, UK, 2017; ISBN 978-1-4731-2449-3.
21. NHS Scotland. Scottish Standards of Care for Hip Fracture Patients 2020. 2019. Available online: https://www.shfa.scot.nhs.uk/_docs/2020/Scottish-standards-of-care-for-hip-fracture-patients-2020.pdf (accessed on 17 October 2022).

22. Deutschen Gesellschaft für Unfallchirurgie e.V.; Österreichischen Gesellschaft für Unfallchirurgie. S2e-Leitlinie 012/001: Schenkelhalsfraktur des Erwachsenen: Leitlinien Unfallchirurgie—Überarbeitete Leitlinie ICD S-72.0. 2015. Available online: https://www.awmf.org/uploads/tx_szleitlinien/012-001l_S2e_Schenkelhalsfraktur_2015-10-abgelaufen_02.pdf (accessed on 17 October 2022).
23. Lawrence, J.E.; Fountain, D.M.; Cundall-Curry, D.J.; Carrothers, A.D. Do Patients Taking Warfarin Experience Delays to Theatre, Longer Hospital Stay, and Poorer Survival After Hip Fracture? *Clin. Orthop. Relat. Res.* **2017**, *475*, 273–279. [CrossRef]
24. Tran, T.; Delluc, A.; de Wit, C.; Petrcich, W.; Le Gal, G.; Carrier, M. The impact of oral anticoagulation on time to surgery in patients hospitalized with hip fracture. *Thromb. Res.* **2015**, *136*, 962–965. [CrossRef]
25. Chang, W.; Lv, H.; Feng, C.; Yuwen, P.; Wei, N.; Chen, W.; Zhang, Y. Preventable risk factors of mortality after hip fracture surgery: Systematic review and meta-analysis. *Int. J. Surg.* **2018**, *52*, 320–328. [CrossRef]
26. Ryan, D.J.; Yoshihara, H.; Yoneoka, D.; Egol, K.A.; Zuckerman, J.D. Delay in Hip Fracture Surgery: An Analysis of Patient-Specific and Hospital-Specific Risk Factors. *J. Orthop. Trauma* **2015**, *29*, 343–348. [CrossRef] [PubMed]
27. Soo, C.G.K.M.; Della Torre, P.K.; Yolland, T.J.; Shatwell, M.A. Clopidogrel and hip fractures, is it safe? A systematic review and meta-analysis. *BMC Musculoskelet. Disord.* **2016**, *17*, 136. [CrossRef] [PubMed]
28. Mattesi, L.; Noailles, T.; Rosencher, N.; Rouvillain, J.-L. Discontinuation of Plavix ®(clopidogrel) for hip fracture surgery. A systematic review of the literature. *Orthop. Traumatol. Surg. Res.* **2016**, *102*, 1097–1101. [CrossRef] [PubMed]
29. Collinge, C.A.; Kelly, K.C.; Little, B.; Weaver, T.; Schuster, R.D. The Effects of Clopidogrel (Plavix) and Other Oral Anticoagulants on Early Hip Fracture Surgery. *J. Orthop. Trauma* **2012**, *26*, 568–573. [CrossRef]
30. Franklin, N.A.; Ali, A.H.; Hurley, R.K.; Mir, H.R.; Beltran, M.J. Outcomes of early surgical intervention in geriatric proximal femur fractures among patients receiving direct oral anticoagulation. *J. Orthop. Trauma* **2018**, *32*, 269–273. [CrossRef]
31. Schermann, H.; Gurel, R.; Gold, A.; Maman, E.; Dolkart, O.; Steinberg, E.L.; Chechik, O. Safety of urgent hip fracture surgery protocol under influence of direct oral anticoagulation medications. *Injury* **2019**, *50*, 398–402. [CrossRef]
32. Cohn, M.R.; Levack, A.E.; Trivedi, N.N.; Villa, J.C.; Wellman, D.S.; Lyden, J.P.; Lorich, D.G.; Lane, J.M. The Hip Fracture Patient on Warfarin: Evaluating Blood Loss and Time to Surgery. *J. Orthop. Trauma* **2017**, *31*, 407–413. [CrossRef]
33. You, D.; Xu, Y.; Ponich, B.; Ronksley, P.; Skeith, L.; Korley, R.; Carrier, M.; Schneider, P.S. Effect of oral anticoagulant use on surgical delay and mortality in hip fracture. *Bone Jt. J.* **2021**, *103*, 222–233. [CrossRef]
34. Cheung, Z.B.; Xiao, R.; Forsh, D.A. Time to surgery and complications in hip fracture patients on novel oral anticoagulants: A systematic review. *Arch. Orthop. Trauma Surg.* **2021**, *142*, 633–640. [CrossRef]
35. King, K.; Polischuk, M.; Lynch, G.; Gergis, A.; Rajesh, A.; Shelfoon, C.; Kattar, N.; Sriselvakumar, S.; Cooke, C. Early Surgical Fixation for Hip Fractures in Patients Taking Direct Oral Anticoagulation: A Retrospective Cohort Study. *Geriatr. Orthop. Surg. Rehabil.* **2020**, *11*, 2151459320944854. [CrossRef]
36. Schuetze, K.; Eickhoff, A.; Dehner, C.; Gebhard, F.; Richter, P.H. Impact of oral anticoagulation on proximal femur fractures treated within 24 h—Retrospective chart review. *Injury* **2019**, *50*, 2040–2044. [CrossRef] [PubMed]
37. Cintean, R.; Pankratz, C.; Hofmann, M.; Gebhard, F.; Schütze, K. Early Results in Non-Displaced Femoral Neck Fractures Using the Femoral Neck System. *Geriatr. Orthop. Surg. Rehabil.* **2021**, *12*, 21514593211050153. [CrossRef] [PubMed]
38. Schuetze, K.; Eickhoff, A.; Rutetzki, K.-S.; Richter, P.H.; Gebhard, F.; Ehrnthaller, C. Geriatric patients with dementia show increased mortality and lack of functional recovery after hip fracture treated with hemiprosthesis. *Eur. J. Trauma Emerg. Surg.* **2020**, *48*, 1827–1833. [CrossRef]
39. Devereaux, P.J.; Mrkobrada, M.; Sessler, D.I.; Leslie, K.; Alonso-Coello, P.; Kurz, A.; Villar, J.C.; Sigamani, A.; Biccard, B.M.; Meyhoff, C.S.; et al. Aspirin in Patients Undergoing Noncardiac Surgery. *N. Engl. J. Med.* **2014**, *370*, 1494–1503. [CrossRef] [PubMed]
40. Mullins, B.; Akehurst, H.; Slattery, D.; Chesser, T. Should surgery be delayed in patients taking direct oral anticoagulants who suffer a hip fracture? A retrospective, case-controlled observational study at a UK major trauma centre. *BMJ Open* **2018**, *8*, e020625. [CrossRef]
41. Hoerlyck, C.; Ong, T.; Gregersen, M.; Damsgaard, E.M.; Borris, L.; Chia, J.K.; Yap, Y.Y.W.; Weerasuriya, N.; Sahota, O. Do anticoagulants affect outcomes of hip fracture surgery? A cross-sectional analysis. *Arch. Orthop. Trauma Surg.* **2020**, *140*, 171–176. [CrossRef]
42. Daugaard, C.; Pedersen, A.B.; Kristensen, N.R.; Johnsen, S.P. Preoperative antithrombotic therapy and risk of blood transfusion and mortality following hip fracture surgery: A Danish nationwide cohort study. *Osteoporos. Int.* **2019**, *30*, 583–591. [CrossRef]

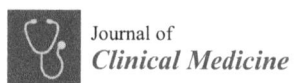

Journal of
Clinical Medicine

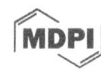

Article

Feasibility and Radiological Outcome of Minimally Invasive Locked Plating of Proximal Humeral Fractures in Geriatric Patients

Konrad Schuetze, Alexander Boehringer, Raffael Cintean, Florian Gebhard, Carlos Pankratz, Peter Hinnerk Richter, Michael Schneider and Alexander M. Eickhoff *

Center of Surgery, Department of Traumatology, Hand-, Plastic-, and Reconstructive Surgery, University of Ulm, 89075 Ulm, Germany
* Correspondence: alexander.eickhoff@uniklinik-ulm.de

Abstract: Background: Proximal humerus fractures are common injuries in the elderly. Locked plating showed high complication and reoperation rates at first. However, with second-generation implants and augmentation, minimally invasive locked plating might be a viable alternative to arthroplasty or conservative treatment. Material and Methods: A retrospective chart review was performed for all patients with proximal humerus fractures treated between 2014 and 2020 with locked plating. All patients over 60 years of age who underwent surgery for a proximal humerus fracture with plate osteosynthesis (NCB, Philos, or Philos with cement) during the specified period were included. Pathological fractures, intramedullary nailing, or arthroplasty were excluded. Primary outcome measurements included secondary displacement and surgical complications. Secondary outcomes comprised function and mortality within one year. Results: A total of 249 patients (mean age 75.6 +/− 8.9 years; 194 women and 55 men) were included in the study. No significant difference in the AO fracture classification could be found. Ninety-two patients were surgically treated with first-generation locked plating (NCB, Zimmer Biomet, Wayne Township, IN, USA), 113 patients with second-generation locked plating (Philos, Depuy Synthes, Wayne Township, IN, USA), and 44 patients with cement-augmented second-generation locked plating (Philos, Traumacem V+, Depuy Synthes). A 6-week radiological follow-up was completed for 189 patients. In all groups, X-rays were performed one day after surgery, and these showed no differences concerning the head shaft angle between the groups. The mean secondary varus dislocation (decrease of the head shaft angle) after six weeks for first-generation locked plating was 6.6 ± 12° (n = 72), for second-generation locked plating 4.4 ± 6.5 (n = 83), and for second-generation with augmentation 1.9 ± 3.7 (n = 35) with a significant difference between the groups (p = 0.012). Logistic regression showed a significant dependency for secondary dislocation for the type of treatment (p = 0.038), age (p = 0.01), and preoperative varus fracture displacement (p = 0.033). Significantly fewer surgical complications have been observed in the augmented second-generation locked plating group (NCB: 26.3%; Philos 21.5%; Philos-augmented 8.6%; p = 0.015). Range of motion was documented in 122 out of 209 patients after 3 months. In the Philos-augmented group, 50% of the patients achieved at least 90° anteversion and abduction, which was only about a third of the patients in the other 2 groups (NCB 34.8%, n = 46; Philos 35.8%, n = 56; augmented-Philos 50.0%, n = 20; p = 0.429). Conclusion: Minimally invasive locked plating is still a valuable treatment option for geriatric patients. With augmentation and modern implants, the complication rate is low and comparable to those of reverse shoulder arthroplasty reported in the literature, even in the challenging group of elderly patients.

Keywords: proximal humerus fractures; geriatric patients; cement augmentation; modern implant for proximal humerus; complications in proximal humerus fractures

Citation: Schuetze, K.; Boehringer, A.; Cintean, R.; Gebhard, F.; Pankratz, C.; Richter, P.H.; Schneider, M.; Eickhoff, A.M. Feasibility and Radiological Outcome of Minimally Invasive Locked Plating of Proximal Humeral Fractures in Geriatric Patients. *J. Clin. Med.* **2022**, *11*, 6751. https://doi.org/10.3390/jcm11226751

Academic Editor: Christian Carulli

Received: 9 October 2022
Accepted: 12 November 2022
Published: 15 November 2022

Publisher's Note: MDPI stays neutral with regard to jurisdictional claims in published maps and institutional affiliations.

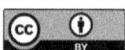

Copyright: © 2022 by the authors. Licensee MDPI, Basel, Switzerland. This article is an open access article distributed under the terms and conditions of the Creative Commons Attribution (CC BY) license (https://creativecommons.org/licenses/by/4.0/).

1. Introduction

Fractures of the proximal humerus are common injuries, especially in women above the age of 60. In an aging population, an even higher incidence of these fracture can be expected. Rupp et al. reported an increase of proximal humerus fractures of 10% between 2009 and 2019 in Germany. Reasons for this include a higher incidence of osteoporosis and the increasing number of falls [1,2]. Determining the best treatment for proximal humerus fractures remains a challenge. In the case of undisplaced or minimally displaced fractures, a non-operative procedure is favorable and the most common [3]. Even in displaced fractures, no significant difference in regards to function and quality of life could be found between an operative and non-operative treatment [4]. However, surgery is recommended for displaced and three- or four-part fractures. Depending on the fracture morphology, locked nailing, locked plating, or even shoulder arthroplasty with a reverse prosthesis are common options [5,6]. Locking nail systems do not appear to be an option for complex fractures involving a displacement of the tuberosities [6]. Primary reverse shoulder arthroplasty (RSA) is often chosen when a significant reduction and stable fixation are not achievable and the vascularity of the humeral head is damaged [7].

Compared to RSA, surgical complications in locking plates, such as the loss of reduction and cut outs, are common, with revision rates up to 32% [8,9]. However, similar functional results are shown one year after surgery [9], and high revision rates were observed in first-generation implants. Due to the high complication rate, various surgical options have been developed, such as inferomedial screws or fibula allograft augmentation [10]. Many studies are investigating complications and clinical results after conservative treatment, plating of proximal humerus fractures, and primary reverse shoulder arthroplasty, but only one clinical study is available evaluating complications and clinical results after screw tip augmentation [11]. The first hypothesis of this investigation argues that screw tip cement augmentation reduces the risk of the implant loosening in geriatric proximal humerus fractures. After cement augmentation, no influence on the one-year mortality figures is expected (second hypothesis).

2. Methods

The study was approved by the institutional ethical committee under the number, 169/20-FSt/TR. The study was a retrospective cohort study at a level one trauma center. All patients over the age of 60 years with a proximal humerus fracture treated between January 2014 and December 2020 were included in the study (Table 1).

Table 1. Inclusion and exclusion criteria.

Inclusion Criteria	Exclusion Criteria
- Proximal humerus fractures in patients over 60 years of age	- Patients under 60 years of age
- Plating with NCB®, Philos® and Philos® with cement	- Patients treated with intramedullary nailing or arthroplasty
	- Pathological fracture

Indications for surgery included the translation of the humerus shaft and a multifragmentary fracture morphology with displacement.

The type of osteosynthesis was chosen individually by availability, the personal preference of the surgeon (NCB vs. Philos), and subjective quality of the bone (Philos vs. Philos with screw tip augmentation).

Ninety-two patients were treated with first-generation locked plating (NCB Proximal humerus plating, Zimmer Biomet, Wayne Township, IN, USA) from 2014 to 2018, 113 with second-generation locked plating (Philos, Depuy Synthes, Wayne Township, IN, USA,

2014–2020) and 44 with augmented second-generation locked plating (Philos + Traumacem V+, Depuy Synthes, 2018–2020). Mean time to surgery was 3.9 +/− 4.4 days.

Surgery was performed in beach chair position and traction was applied with a Trimano Fortis (Arthrex, Port of Naples, FL, USA) fixed to the arm (Figure 1).

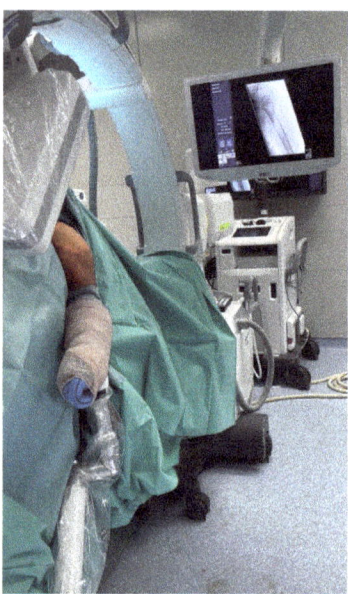

Figure 1. Patient positioning.

After a minimally invasive delta split procedure, traction sutures were applied through the rotator cuff. A reduction was achieved by the traction and manipulation of the sutures. In some cases, a reduction was achieved by the direct manipulation of the humeral head through the fracture. After a provisional fixation was achieved with 1.6 mm K-wires, the plate was placed and fixed with four to seven screws in the head and three screws in the diaphysis (Figure 2).

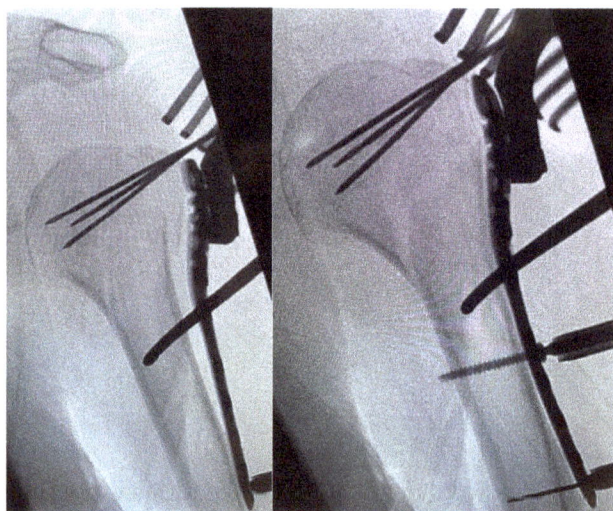

Figure 2. Plate placement, temporary fixation with K-wires and implantation of a cortex screw.

After fluoroscopic control of reduction and screw placement, a radiological contrast agent was injected prior to augmentation to prevent leakage into the joint. Afterwards, every screw was augmented with 0.5–1 mL of Traumacem V+ under fluoroscopic control (Figure 3).

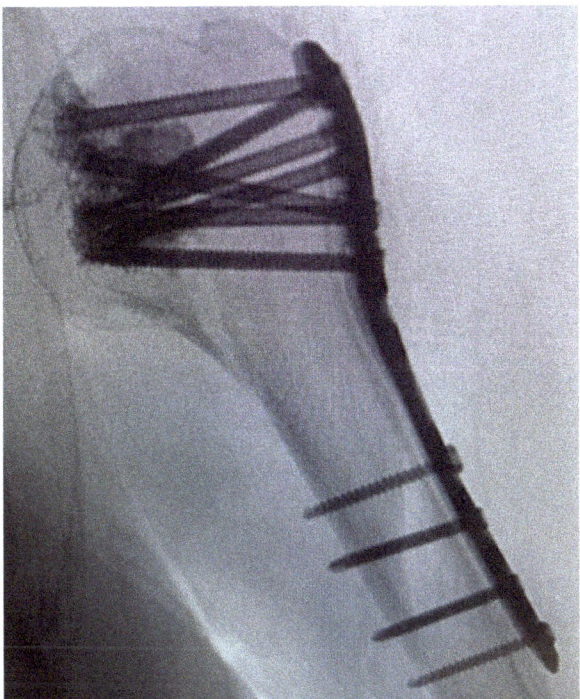

Figure 3. Fluoroscopic control after cement augmentation of the screws.

The arm was immobilized for 10 days after surgery. Physiotherapy with passive forward flexion and abduction up to 90° started on day 11. Lifting and free motion was allowed starting week 7 after surgery.

The head-shaft angle (HSA) was measured by a resident and a consultant radiologically preoperatively, postoperatively, and after 6 weeks in all fractures except A1 fractures (Figure 4). Primary outcome measures included secondary dislocation and surgical complications. Secondary outcome measures included function after 3 months, mortality, and discharge disposition. A one-year follow up to obtain information about the mortality and complications was performed by analyzing the electronic record of the patient. In the geriatric and partly immobilized collective, many patients were not seen as outpatients. In these cases, follow up was performed by phoning the patients.

Data analysis was performed with IBM SPSS Statistics (V21.0, SPSS Inc. Chicago, IL, USA) and Microsoft Excel (V16.3, Microsoft Cooperation, Redmond, WA, USA). Demographic characteristics are described as mean and standard deviation. Group comparisons via the chi-square test were used to compare secondary dislocations between the groups. For further analysis, a logistic regression was performed for all variables related to the secondary dislocation and surgical complications. Group comparisons via Chi-square test were performed for number of revision surgeries and rate of secondary arthroplasty.

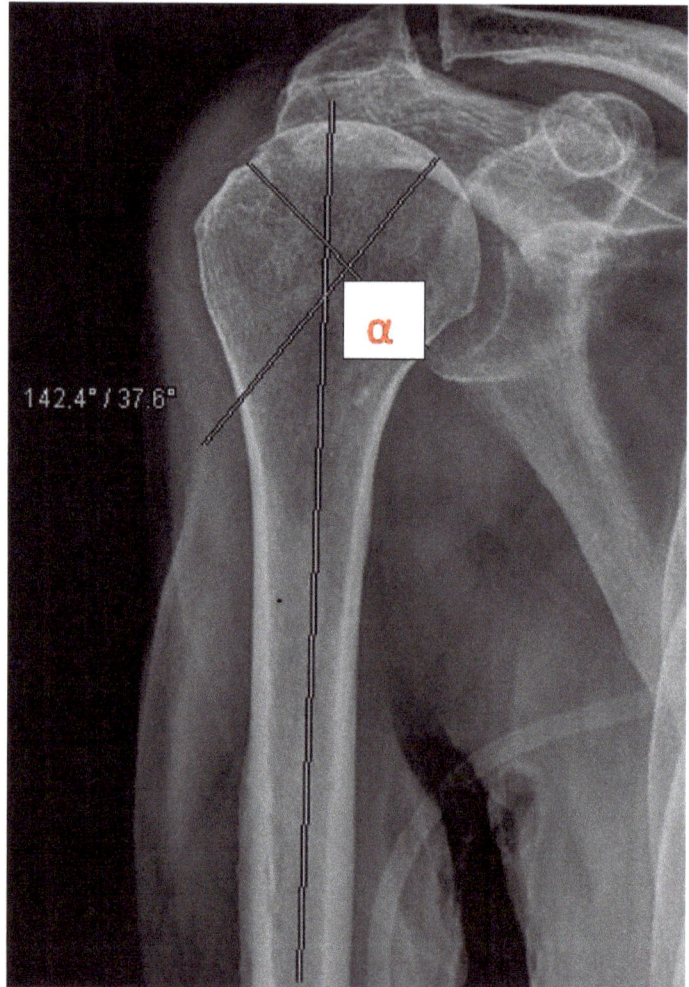

Figure 4. Measurement of the head shaft angle (HAS, e.g., 14.2°).

3. Results

3.1. Patient Population

For 249 patients, medical records were reviewed. Out of these 249 patients, 55 were male and 194 were female. The mean age was 75.6 +/− 8.9 years. Eight patients were classified as ASA I, 66 as ASA II, 154 as ASA III, and 21 as ASA IV. The mean time to surgery was 3.9 +/− 4.4 days, and the mean surgery time was 69.5 +/− 66.1 min. After the hospital discharge, 40 patients were lost to follow up, and the remaining 209 patients were followed up to one year. Twenty out of these 209 patients had a secondary dislocation within the first 6 weeks and were, therefore, excluded from the 6-week radiographical follow up. Overall, out of the 249 patients, radiological follow up was possible for 189 patients after 6 weeks.

3.2. Fracture Classification

All fractures were classified according to the AO-classification. Five fractures were classified as 11-A1, 50 as A2, 10 as A3, and 89 as B1. C1 fractures occurred in 17 and C3 fractures in 88 patients. Ninety-three patients showed a varus displacement with an HSA smaller than 135°, while 149 patients showed a valgus displacement with an HSA > 135°.

A1 fractures showed no varus/valgus dislocation. Fracture classification and type of treatment for all patients is shown in Figure 5.

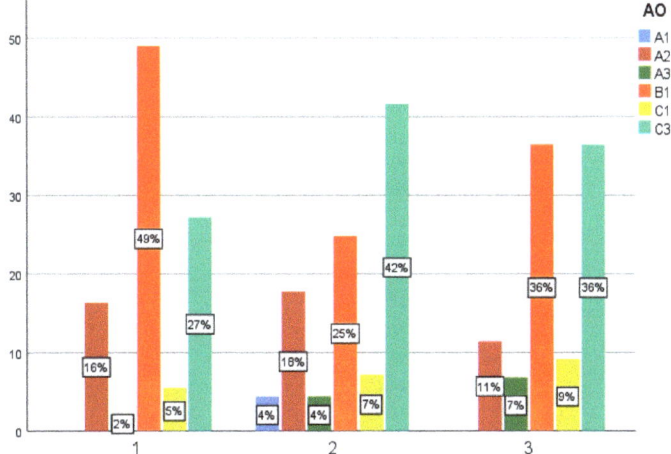

Figure 5. Different treatment options (1 = NCB, 2 = Philos, 3 = Philos-augmented) divided according to the AO classification (x axis) in percent (y axis).

3.3. Radiological Outcome

The mean postoperative HSA was 132.4 +/− 9.7°. One hundred and fifty-five cases had a mean postoperative varus HSA of 8.5 +/− 7.2°. Ninety-nine cases had a mean postoperative valgus HSA of 6.4 +/− 5.1°. There was no difference between the postoperative HSA between the 3 groups, showing a comparable quality of reduction. After 6 weeks, 189 patients had a radiological follow up. The mean secondary dislocation for first-generation locked plating was 6.6 +/− 12° (n = 72, 38%), for second-generation locked plating, 4.4 +/− 6.5° (n = 83, 43.9%), and for second-generation with augmentation, 1.9 +/− 3.7° (n = 35, 18.5%). The difference between the groups was significant (p = 0.012). Logistic regression showed a significant dependency for the secondary displacement for the type of treatment (p = 0.038), age (p = 0.01), and preoperative varus fracture displacement (p = 0.033). Varus displaced fractures had a 6-fold increased risk for secondary displacement. For every year above 60 years of age, the risk for secondary displacement increased by a factor of 1.1. The mean secondary displacement after 6 weeks is shown in Figure 6.

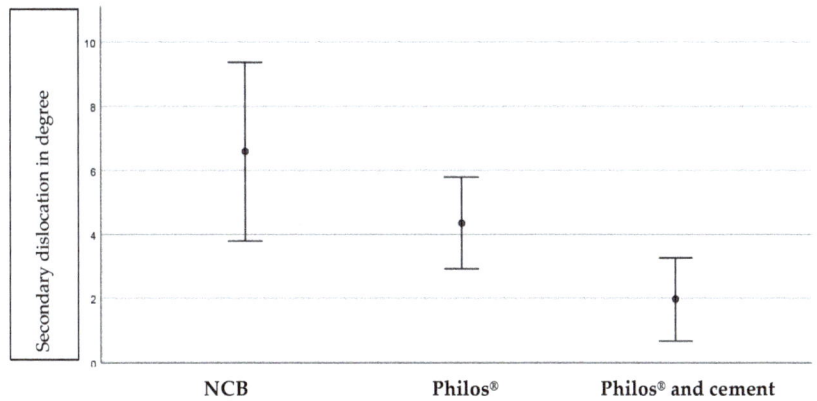

Figure 6. Secondary dislocation in degree (y axis) divided into the different type of treatments.

3.4. Complications

Surgical complications occurred in 44 (21%) out of 209 patients that could be followed up to one year. Varus collapse, defined as a varus displacement leading to surgery, occurred in 31 patients; 5 patients had other secondary displacements; 2 patients had implant related infections; and 6 patients had primary screw misplacements. Surgical complications occurred significantly less in the second-generation locked plating with augmentation group (NCB: 26.3%; Philos 21.5%; Philos-augmented 8.6%; $p = 0.015$). Logistic regression showed no dependency for age, AO-classification, or pre- or postoperative HSA. Severe cases of varus collapse were observed only in the NCB and Philos groups without cement augmentation. Twelve patients needed revision surgery with implant removal in 4 cases (NCB 2.5%; Philos 2.1%; $p = 0.102$) and reverse shoulder arthroplasty in 8 cases (NCB 6.3%; Philos 3.2%; $p = 0.345$), with no significant difference between the groups.

3.5. Discharge Disposition and Mortality

The mean hospital stay was 7.4 +/− 3.2 days. Overall, 86.7% ($n = 216$) of the patients could be discharged home or to inpatient rehabilitation. Thirty patients were discharged to a nursing home, and 3 patients died during the hospital stay. Eighteen out of 209 patients (8.6%) that were followed up for 1 year died within the first year after surgery.

3.6. Function

The range of motion was only documented in 122 out of 209 patients after 3 months. In the Philos-augmented group, 50% of the patients achieved at least 90° anteversion and abduction, which was only about a third of the patients in the other 2 groups (NCB 34.8%, $n = 46$; Philos 35.8%, $n = 56$; augmented-Philos 50.0%, $n = 20$; $p = 0.429$). There was no significant difference between the groups.

4. Discussion

Proximal humerus fractures are commonly treated conservatively. However, in complex fracture situations, surgery is necessary. Knowing of the adverse events after the plating of proximal humerus fractures, especially in geriatric patients, primary reverse arthroplasty is becoming more of a common treatment option, accompanied with a more invasive surgery [3]. The aim of this study was to prove the feasibility of minimally invasive, modern locked plating for the treatment of proximal humerus fractures in geriatric patients. For this purpose, two generations of locking plates with or without cement augmentation were compared. In this study, second-generation locked plating with cement augmentation was found to be superior to first-generation locked plating and second-generation without augmentation regarding the secondary displacements. An overall surgical complication rate of 21% was found, occurring significantly less frequen when the second-generation locked plate with augmentation was used (NCB: 26.3%; Philos 21.5%; Philos-augmented 8.6%; $p < 0.05$).

In surgery for proximal humerus fractures, an especially feared complication is the varus collapse, which occurred in 31 out of 209 patients in this study but only in the NCB and Philos groups.

The biomechanical studies of Unger et al., Röderer et al., and Scola et al. support the advantages of augmentation, particularly, a delayed varus collapse and significant more load cycles until failure [12–14]. There are only a few clinical studies for screw augmentation. Katthagen et al. investigated a smaller cohort of 24 patients after screw tip augmentation, reporting that augmentation reduces the risk of the loss of reduction and screw perforation significantly. In the present study, the complication rate for augmented plating was 8%, comparable to that in Katthagen et al. [14]. Foruria et al. investigated a much larger cohort using the deltopectoral approach. They reported a complication rate of 15% in the cemented group compared to 8.6% in this study. Furthermore, Foruria et al. observed avascular necrosis in 4.8% of the cases [15]. No case of avascular necrosis of the humeral head was observed. This could be due to different surgical approaches. In this study, we only used the minimally invasive delta-split approach. In addition, the surgical time was 34 min shorter in this study compared to that in the studies of Foruria et al., Katthagen et al., and Foruria et al., and this study proved that locked plating with augmentation is a reasonable option with good clinical outcomes and a low complication rate, especially when combined with screw augmentation. Low complication and secondary dislocation rates could even be achieved in AO C-type fractures, which represent 45% of augmented cases. In the literature, these fractures are typically treated with reverse arthroplasty. However, reverse arthroplasty is not without complications. Paras et al. reported tuberosity complications in 25.9% of cases, scapular notching in 18.6%, and heterotopic ossification in 13.2%, and an overall revision rate of 1.8% [16]. Köppe et al. showed that, compared to osteosynthesis, reverse arthroplasty resulted in more hospital adverse events and surgical complications [17].

In their study, Porschke et al. compared the plating of humerus fractures in 31 patients with arthroplasties in 29 patients. They showed that, with the same functional outcome, surgical complications were significantly more frequent after plate osteosynthesis (32.6%) than after arthroplasty (7.2%) [9]. In the present study, a complication rate of 8.6% in augmented locked plating was found and, therefore, comparable to arthroplasty. In addition, the length of stay was, on average, 6 days shorter, and 86.7% of all patients could be discharged either home or to inpatient rehabilitation.

The one-year mortality rate of 9.5% in this study coincides with Lander et al., which, after analysing 42,511 patients following proximal humerus fractures, concluded that surgery is associated with a lower mortality (9.1% vs. 19.9%) [18].

The authors of this study recommend a critical evaluation of all treatment options, especially for the vulnerable geriatric patient group.

In conclusion, minimally invasive modern locked plating with screw tip augmentation is a valuable treatment option for geriatric patients. Compared to the often-cited high complication rates associated with first-generation implants, these complication rates might be comparable to reverse arthroplasty. For this reason, augmented locked plating became the standard treatment of geriatric proximal humerus fractures at our institution.

One limitation of this study is the retrospective design, the postoperative function of which, in contrast to other investigations, was only determined 3 months after surgery and in only 122 of 209 cases, with the understanding that follow up is difficult in the elderly and the expectation that cement has no other influence on the function [9]. On the other hand, in geriatric patients, not only the range of motion but also the loading is important.

Another limitation is that no questionnaires were sent to the patients for follow up to gain additional information, such as that of their quality of life.

The long study period included many different attending surgeons, which may have resulted in some postoperative bias.

The study is also limited by the small number of cases. After screw tip cement augmentation, only 44 patients could be included. Nevertheless, this study is one of the biggest investigations on this issue.

5. Conclusions

Screw tip augmentation in osteoporotic proximal humerus fractures leads, in this investigation, to a significantly lower rate of implant-associated complications, especially regarding revision surgery. Therefore, the trend to default to reverse shoulder arthroplasty in geriatric patients with a poor general condition and complex fracture situation should be critically questioned, considering the comparable complication rates in the literature and a less invasive surgery. In these cases, plating might be an alternative to primary reverse shoulder arthroplasty, depending on the fracture morphology and the bone quality.

Author Contributions: Conceptualization, K.S.; Methodology, K.S.; Formal analysis, K.S.; Investigation, A.B., C.P., P.H.R. and M.S.; Writing—original draft, A.M.E.; Writing—review & editing, R.C. and A.M.E.; Supervision, F.G. All authors have read and agreed to the published version of the manuscript.

Funding: No author is affiliated to any of the supporting companies or has received or will receive any form of payment related to this study.

Institutional Review Board Statement: This retrospective chart review study involving human participants was in accordance with the ethical standards of the institutional and national research committee and with the 1964 Helsinki Declaration and its later amendments or comparable ethical standards. The Human Investigation Committee (IRB) of the University of Ulm approved this study.

Informed Consent Statement: In accordance with the ethics committee of the University of Ulm, due to the retrospective design, consent to participate and publication were not necessary.

Data Availability Statement: The study did not report any data.

Conflicts of Interest: The authors declare that there is no conflict of interest. No company had influence in the collection of data or contributed to or had influence on the conception, design, analysis, and writing of the study. No further funding was received.

References

1. Fjalestad, T.; Iversen, P.; Hole, M.; Smedsrud, M.; Madsen, J.E. Clinical investigation for displaced proximal humeral fractures in the elderly: A randomized study of two surgical treatments: Reverse total prosthetic replacement versus angular stable plate Philos (The DELPHI-trial). *BMC Musculoskelet. Disord.* **2014**, *15*, 323. [CrossRef] [PubMed]
2. Rupp, M.; Walter, N.; Pfeifer, C.; Lang, S.; Kerschbaum, M.; Krutsch, W.; Baumann, F.; Alt, V. The incidence of fractures among the adult population of Germany. *Dtsch. Arztebl. Int.* **2021**, *118*, 665–669. [CrossRef] [PubMed]
3. Han, R.J.; Sing, D.C.; Feeley, B.T.; Ma, C.B.; Zhang, A.L. Proximal humerus fragility fractures: Recent trends in nonoperative and operative treatment in the Medicare population. *J. Shoulder Elb. Surg.* **2016**, *25*, 256–261. [CrossRef] [PubMed]
4. Fjalestad, T.; Hole, M.; Jørgensen, J.; Strømsøe, K.; Kristiansen, I. Health and cost consequences of surgical versus conservative treatment for a comminuted proximal humeral fracture in elderly patients. *Injury* **2010**, *41*, 599–605. [CrossRef]
5. Plath, J.E.; Kerschbaum, C.; Seebauer, T.; Holz, R.; Henderson, D.J.H.; Förch, S.; Mayr, E. Locking nail versus locking plate for proximal humeral fracture fixation in an elderly population: A prospective randomised controlled trial. *BMC Musculoskelet. Disord.* **2019**, *20*, 20. [CrossRef] [PubMed]
6. Gallinet, D.; Clappaz, P.; Garbuio, P.; Tropet, Y.; Obert, L. Three or four parts complex proximal humerus fractures: Hemiarthroplasty versus reverse prosthesis: A comparative study of 40 cases. *Orthop. Traumatol. Surg. Res.* **2009**, *95*, 48–55. [CrossRef] [PubMed]
7. Maier, D.; Jäger, M.; Strohm, P.C.; Südkamp, N.P. Treatment of proximal humeral fractures—A review of current concepts enlightened by basic principles. *Acta Chir. Orthop. Traumatol. Cechoslov.* **2012**, *79*, 307–316.
8. Laux, C.J.; Grubhofer, F.; Werner, C.M.L.; Simmen, H.-P.; Osterhoff, G. Current concepts in locking plate fixation of proximal humerus fractures. *J. Orthop. Surg. Res.* **2017**, *12*, 137. [CrossRef] [PubMed]
9. Porschke, F.; Bockmeyer, J.; Nolte, P.-C.; Studier-Fischer, S.; Guehring, T.; Schnetzke, M. More Adverse Events after Osteosyntheses Compared to Arthroplasty in Geriatric Proximal Humeral Fractures Involving Anatomical Neck. *J. Clin. Med.* **2021**, *10*, 979. [CrossRef] [PubMed]
10. Kim, D.-S.; Lee, D.-H.; Chun, Y.-M.; Shin, S.-J. Which additional augmented fixation procedure decreases surgical failure after proximal humeral fracture with medial comminution: Fibular allograft or inferomedial screws? *J. Shoulder Elb. Surg.* **2018**, *27*, 1852–1858. [CrossRef] [PubMed]
11. Biermann, N.; Prall, W.C.; Böcker, W.; Mayr, H.O.; Haasters, F. Augmentation of plate osteosynthesis for proximal humeral fractures: A systematic review of current biomechanical and clinical studies. *Arch. Orthop. Trauma. Surg.* **2019**, *139*, 1075–1099. [CrossRef] [PubMed]
12. Unger, S.; Erhart, S.; Kralinger, F.; Blauth, M.; Schmoelz, W. The effect of in situ augmentation on implant anchorage in proximal humeral head fractures. *Injury* **2012**, *43*, 1759–1763. [CrossRef]
13. Röderer, G.; Scola, A.; Schmölz, W.; Gebhard, F.; Windolf, M.; Hofmann-Fliri, L. Biomechanical in vitro assessment of screw augmentation in locked plating of proximal humerus fractures. *Injury* **2013**, *44*, 1327–1332. [CrossRef]
14. Scola, A.; Gebhard, F.; Röderer, G. Augmentationstechnik am proximalen Humerus. *Der Unf.* **2015**, *118*, 749–754. [CrossRef] [PubMed]
15. Foruria, A.M.; Martinez-Catalan, N.; Valencia, M.; Morcillo, D.; Calvo, E. Proximal humeral fracture locking plate fixation with anatomic reduction, and a short-and-cemented-screws configuration, dramatically reduces the implant related failure rate in elderly patients. *JSES Int.* **2021**, *5*, 992–1000. [CrossRef] [PubMed]
16. Paras, T.; Raines, B.; Kohut, K.; Sabzevari, S.; Chang, Y.-F.; Yeung, M.; Li, R.; Tublin, J.; Baradaran, A.; Lin, A. Clinical Outcomes of Reverse Total Shoulder Arthroplasty for Elective Indications versus Acute Three and Four-Part Proximal Humerus Fractures: A Systematic Review and Meta-Analysis. *J. Shoulder Elb. Surg.* **2022**, *31*, e14–e21. [CrossRef]
17. Köppe, J.; Stolberg-Stolberg, J.; Rischen, R.; Faldum, A.; Raschke, M.J.; Katthagen, J.C. In-hospital Complications Are More Likely to Occur After Reverse Shoulder Arthroplasty Than After Locked Plating for Proximal Humeral Fractures. *Clin. Orthop. Relat. Res.* **2021**, *479*, 2284–2292. [CrossRef] [PubMed]
18. Lander, S.T.; Mahmood, B.; Maceroli, M.A.; Byrd, J.; Elfar, J.C.; Ketz, J.P.; Nikkel, L.E. Mortality Rates of Humerus Fractures in the Elderly: Does Surgical Treatment Matter? *J. Orthop. Trauma* **2019**, *33*, 361–365. [CrossRef] [PubMed]

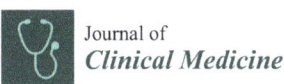

Article

Comparison of Prognostic Value of 10 Biochemical Indices at Admission for Prediction Postoperative Myocardial Injury and Hospital Mortality in Patients with Osteoporotic Hip Fracture

Alexander Fisher [1,2,3,*], Wichat Srikusalanukul [1], Leon Fisher [4] and Paul N. Smith [2,3]

1. Departments of Geriatric Medicine, The Canberra Hospital, ACT Health, Canberra 2605, Australia
2. Departments of Orthopaedic Surgery, The Canberra Hospital, ACT Health, Canberra 2605, Australia
3. Medical School, Australian National University, Canberra 2605, Australia
4. Department of Gastroenterology, Frankston Hospital, Peninsula Health, Melbourne 3199, Australia
* Correspondence: alex.fisher@act.gov.au

Citation: Fisher, A.; Srikusalanukul, W.; Fisher, L.; Smith, P.N. Comparison of Prognostic Value of 10 Biochemical Indices at Admission for Prediction Postoperative Myocardial Injury and Hospital Mortality in Patients with Osteoporotic Hip Fracture. *J. Clin. Med.* 2022, 11, 6784. https://doi.org/10.3390/jcm11226784

Academic Editor: Christian Ehrnthaller

Received: 27 October 2022
Accepted: 11 November 2022
Published: 16 November 2022

Publisher's Note: MDPI stays neutral with regard to jurisdictional claims in published maps and institutional affiliations.

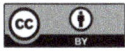

Copyright: © 2022 by the authors. Licensee MDPI, Basel, Switzerland. This article is an open access article distributed under the terms and conditions of the Creative Commons Attribution (CC BY) license (https://creativecommons.org/licenses/by/4.0/).

Abstract: Aim: To evaluate the prognostic impact at admission of 10 biochemical indices for prediction postoperative myocardial injury (PMI) and/or hospital death in hip fracture (HF) patients. Methods: In 1273 consecutive patients with HF (mean age 82.9 ± 8.7 years, 73.5% women), clinical and laboratory parameters were collected prospectively, and outcomes were recorded. Multiple logistic regression and receiver-operating characteristic analyses (the area under the curve, AUC) were preformed, the number needed to predict (NNP) outcome was calculated. Results: Age ≥ 80 years and IHD were the most prominent clinical factors associated with both PMI (with cardiac troponin I rise) and in-hospital death. PMI occurred in 555 (43.6%) patients and contributed to 80.3% (49/61) of all deaths (mortality rate 8.8% vs. 1.9% in non-PMI patients). The most accurate biochemical predictive markers were parathyroid hormone > 6.8 pmol/L, urea > 7.5 mmol/L, 25(OH)vitamin D < 25 nmol/L, albumin < 33 g/L, and ratios gamma-glutamyl transferase (GGT) to alanine aminotransferase > 2.5, urea/albumin ≥ 2.0 and GGT/albumin ≥ 7.0; the AUC for developing PMI ranged between 0.782 and 0.742 (NNP: 1.84–2.13), the AUC for fatal outcome ranged from 0.803 to 0.722, (NNP: 3.77–9.52). Conclusions: In HF patients, easily accessible biochemical indices at admission substantially improve prediction of hospital outcomes, especially in the aged >80 years with IHD.

Keywords: hip fracture; mortality; myocardial injury; biochemical markers; predictors

1. Introduction

Osteoporotic hip fracture (HF), one of the leading health problems in the geriatric population all over the world, is associated with serious postoperative complications and increased mortality (between 5.1% and 16.3% in the hospital, up to 36% within 1 year) [1–6]. Over the last four decades the mortality rates after HF surgery remain unchanged [7]. Cardiovascular diseases (CVDs), especially the ischaemic heart disease (IHD), are recognised as major contributors of poor outcome in patients undergoing major noncardiac surgery [8–16], including HF repair [17–25]. Perioperative cardiac complications substantially prolong hospitalisation and account between one third and one-half of all deaths [9,15,26–28]. Given the importance of perioperative evaluation, risk stratification and individualised management of patients undergoing non-cardiac surgery a set of clinical practice guidelines were developed by the Joint Task Force of the European Society of Cardiology (ESC) and European Society of Anaesthesiology (ESA) [8] and the American College of Cardiology (ACC) and the American Heart Association (AHH) [29].

Many prognostic models to estimate preoperatively the probability of developing in-hospital major adverse cardiac events (MACE) in patients undergoing noncardiac surgery have been proposed and the widely acknowledged: The American Society of Anaesthesiologists Physical Status [ASA-PS], The Revised Cardiac Risk Index [RCRI], The Universal

American College of Surgeons NSQIP surgical risk calculator [ACS NSQIP], Preoperative Score to Predict Postoperative Mortality (POSPOM), Clinical Frailty Scale [CFS]. However, some of these models rely on subjective clinician judgment (ASA score), other did not adjust for possible confounders, most of the scores require extensive information regarding comorbidities and laboratory data (e.g., 21 patient-specific variables for ACS NSQIP [30] and summarising the data on individual patients may be difficult (need use of calculators [31,32]). Most importantly, these prognostic models (based in total on 26 scores [33]), although effective on the population level [34], when applied to an individual patient quite often result in inconclusive predictions [35]. The RCRI score, for example, underestimated 50% of adverse events [36,37]. In non-cardiac surgery patients, the POSPOM showed good discriminatory performance, but poor calibration with an overestimation of in-hospital mortality as well as poor performance for prediction of postoperative complications [38,39].

The predictive value of several clinical scoring systems proposed for assessment outcome in HF patients is currently debated [5,40,41]; none of the existing models yielded excellent discrimination while some models had a lack of fit [42]. Despite extensive studies have been carried out the problem of risk stratification and predicting HF outcomes at admission is far from being solved. The vast majority of models predicting HF outcomes are based on demographics, comorbidities and rarely include few blood marker, the proposed preoperative patient risk scores remain imperfect [41] even when clinical, demographic and inflammatory indices are combined [43].

In recent years, a number of different biochemical dysregulations, come to light not only as conditions associated old age, systemic chronic diseases, including IHD, osteosarcopenia, falls and fractures, but as main factors contributing to postoperative complications and all-cause mortality. Converging evidence increasingly implicates that several serum biomarkers predict poor outcomes in different settings (such as surgery, trauma, sepsis, various cancers, etc.). However, research regarding biochemical predictors in HF is limited, only few studies have concentrated on 1–2 biomarkers of a single outcome and, not surprisingly, biochemical indices still are rarely used.

In this study we attempted to assess and compare the usefulness (incremental value) of measurement of routine biochemical parameters before HF surgery and identify which indices are best to predict postoperative myocardial injury (PMI) and/or in-hospital death. Among most often reported in the literature biochemical predictive indices we have chosen for evaluation 10 biomarkers focusing on easily obtained parameters known to be associated with chronic systemic diseases, in particular CVDs/IHD and osteoporosis, and being factors allowing modification. The battery of these serum biomarkers included: parathyroid hormone (PTH) [44–55], vitamin D [51,56–63], albumin, alanine aminotransferase (ALT), gamma-glutamyl transferase (GGT) [64–78], Urea [79–90], GGT/ALT ratio [51,91–95], GGT/Albumin ratio [96,97], Urea/Albumin ratio [98–102] and Platelets/Albumin ratio [103,104].

These biomarkers have not been systematically investigated to predict in HF patients at admission the risk of development postoperative myocardial injury (PMI) or death. No studies have compared the prognostic value of different indices, the proposed cut-off levels of which differed significantly, and the interpretation of the results was controversial (for example, ALT and mortality [76,105–108]). Thus, it remains to be established which on-admission biochemical indicators may be useful prognostic biomarkers in HF patients.

2. Patients and Methods
2.1. Participants

In total 1273 consecutive patients (older than 60 years) admitted with a low-trauma non-pathological HF (cervical or trochanteric) to the Department of Orthopaedic Surgery of the Canberra Hospital (tertiary university centre) between 2010 and 2019 and had operative fracture treatment were included in the study. Inclusion criteria were as follows: (1) a definite diagnosis of hip fracture (intracapsular [cervical] or trochanteric) by imaging, (2) surgical HF repair, (3) age $\geq$ 60 years, (4) complete clinical and laboratory data. Exclusion criteria were: (1) subtrochanteric fracture, (2) medium- or high- energy trauma fracture (fall from height, car accident, etc.); (3) multiple fractures or polytrauma, (4) pathological fracture (malignant tumour)" The mean age of patients was 82.9 ± 8.7 [SD] years, 73.5% were women, and 50.5% had a cervical fracture. All patients followed a similar postoperative protocol with mobilisation out of bed on day one and urinary catheter out on day two.

The validation cohort (n = 582, mean age 81.9 ± 9.13 years, 71.0% women, 52.9% with cervical fracture) included patients admitted after those in the derivation group; they had a similar to the main cohort profile of chronic comorbid diseases, admission laboratory characteristics and outcomes.

2.2. Data Collection

In all patients the previous hospital and general practitioners' medical case records were reviewed, data on socio-demographic (including pre-fracture residential status, use of walking aid), lifestyle factors (smoking status, alcohol use), clinical (12 chronic comorbidities, medications used) and laboratory parameters (21 variables) at admission and the hospital outcomes were prospectively recorded and analysed.

2.3. Laboratory Measurements

The routine laboratory tests included full blood count, serum electrolytes, creatinine, urea nitrogen, C-reactive protein (CRP), albumin and liver function tests, cardiac troponin I (cTnI), 25(OH) vitamin D (25(OH)D), intact PTH, thyroid stimulatory hormone (TSH), free thyroxine (T_4), vitamin B_{12}, folic acid, iron, ferritin, and transferrin. All these analyses were performed on the day of blood sampling (usually within 12–24 h after arrival at the Emergency Department) by standard automated laboratory methods. Serum calcium concentrations were corrected for serum albumin, glomerular filtration rate was estimated (eGFR). Serum cTnI and CRP levels were also assessed within 24 h post-operatively and then after if elevated and/or clinically indicated. All patients with elevated cTnI level of >20 ng/L or greater ("abnormal" laboratory threshold) were assessed for ischaemic features (ischaemic symptoms and 12-lead electrocardiogram).

2.4. Definitions

Chronic kidney disease (CKD) was defined as eGFR < 60 mL/min/1.73 m^2, which was calculated by the Modification of Diet in Renal Disease (MDRD) equation. Anaemia was defined as haemoglobin level < 130 g/L in men and <120 g/L in women. Vitamin D deficiency was defined as 25(OH) D < 25 nmol/L and hypovitaminosis D as < 50 nmol/L, hyperparathyroidism was defined as elevated serum PTH (>6.8 pmol/L, the upper limit of the laboratory reference range), hypoalbuminaemia—as <33 g/L (lower level of reference range). The cut-offs for other biochemical variables were as follows: for urea—7.5 mmol/L (upper limit of reference range), ALT ≥ 17 IU (median value), for GGT ≥ 26 IU (median value), for GGT/ALT > 2.5, for GGT/Albumin ≥ 7.0, for Urea/Albumin ≥ 2.0, for Platelets/Albumin ≥ 5.9. The robustness of the aforementioned cut-offs was validated in our prior studies [17,45,47,51,109,110].

2.5. Outcome Measures

These included: (1) postoperative myocardial injury (PMI) defined by cTnI rise (if at least one of postoperative cTnI measurement values was >20 ng/L on days 1–5 post surgery with or without associated ischemic symptoms); (2) high inflammatory response assessed by marked elevation of CRP (>100 mg/L after the 3rd postoperative day); (3) length of hospital stay (LOS); (4) all-cause in-hospital mortality.

Most HF patients are not candidates for and did not have a coronary angiogram and there are no general guidelines or thresholds for acceptable cTnI elevations after various non-cardiac surgical procedures [111]; therefore, in this study, postoperative new acute myocardial infarction (AMI) was defined by cTnI ≥ 500 ng/L (25 times above the upper limit of reference levels) accompanied by obvious ECG signs (Q-waves, ST-segment changes, T-wave inversion) indicative of myocardial infarct.

2.6. Ethical Approval

The study was performed in accordance with the Declaration of Helsinki (1964) and its later amendments (as revised in 2013). The study was approved by the Australian Capital Territory Research Ethics Committee (ETHLR.18.085; REGIS Reference 2020/ETH02069).

2.7. Statistical Analyses

Data analyses were carried out using Stata software version 16 (StataCorp, College Station, TX, USA). Continuous variables were reported as means ± SD and categorical variables as percentages. Comparisons between groups were performed using analysis of variance and Student's t-test for continuous variables and χ^2 test (Yates corrected) for categorical variables. Univariate and multivariate (both linear and logistic) regression analyses were used to determine the odds ratio (OR) and 95% confidence intervals (CI) for associations between an outcome (dependent variable) and different clinical and laboratory variables; all potential confounding variables with statistical significance ≤ 0.15 on univariate analyses were included in the final multivariate analyses. Receiver operating characteristic (ROC) curve analysis (the area under the ROC curve, AUC) was used to investigate the discriminatory power of preoperative indices to predict postoperative events. Sensitivity, specificity, accuracy, positive predictive value (PPV), negative predictive value (NPV), positive likelihood ratio (LP+), negative likelihood ratio (LP−) and number of patients needed to be examined for correct prediction (NNP [112,113]) were calculated to assess the discriminatory performance of the tests. The predictive performance of the models was further assessed using goodness-of-fit statistics for calibration by Hosmer-Lemeshow test. All tests were two-tailed; p-values < 0.05 were considered statistically significant.

3. Results

3.1. Baseline Characteristics and Outcomes

Of 1273 patients who underwent HF surgery during the study period, 361 (28.4%) have been previously diagnosed with IHD and 99 subjects (7.8% of the total cohort, 27.4% among IHD patients) had a history of AMI. Sociodemographic data, comorbidities, and outcomes in patients with and without IHD are presented in Table 1. The cohort was almost equally split with cervical (50.7%) and trochanteric (49.3%) HFs, and there was no significant difference between groups concerning surgery and anaesthesia. Patients with IHD were significantly older (+2.7 years on average), were less likely to be female and alcohol overusers, had a higher prevalence of hypertension, CKD, chronic obstructive pulmonary disease (COPD), cerebrovascular accident (CVA), type2 diabetes mellitus (T2DM) and Parkinson's disease (for two last diseases $p = 0.058$), and more often used walking aids. The percentage of ex-smokers, permanent residential care facilities (PRCF) residents and patients with dementia, anaemia and TIA did not differ in these two groups. The total all-cause in-hospital mortality was 4.8%, in patients without IHD—3.7%, with IHD—7.5% (contrast +3.8%, $p = 0.005$), and among those with previous AMI—11.8% (contrast +8.1%, $p < 0.001$). Patients with IHD, as would be expected, more often developed PMI (58.6% vs. 37.7%, $p < 0.001$), AMI (11.7% vs. 4.8%, $p < 0.001$), a high inflammatory response (CRP > 100 mg/L in 84.2% vs. 79.7%, $p = 0.037$) and had a prolonged hospital stay (LOS > 20 days in 25.8% vs. 20.4%, $p = 0.024$) compared with the non-IHD persons. IHD patients with a fatal outcome compared with survivors were older (+4.0 years: 88.6 ± 5.34 vs. 84.6 ± 7.23, $p = 0.006$), all but one > 80 years of age (96.3% vs. 75.1%, $p = 0.006$) and more often had CKD (70.4% vs. 44.0%, $p = 0.007$), while all other examined sociodemographic (including male sex prevalence: 9.1% vs. 6.8%, $p = 0.285$) and comorbid characteristics did not show statistical difference among the groups. In HF patients, presence of IHD increases the risk of a fatal outcome (after controlling for age, gender, HF type, preoperative residence, mobility status, comorbidities) by twofold (OR 2.1, 95% CI 1.24–3.51, $p = 0.005$), of developing PMI by 2.3-fold (OR 2.3, 95% CI 1.81–3.01, $p < 0.001$) and a postoperative AMI by 2.4-fold (OR 2.4, 95% CI 1.98–4.02, $p < 0.001$).

Table 1. Comparison of baseline clinical characteristics and outcomes in hip fracture patients with and without ischaemic heart disease (IHD).

Variable	Total Cohort (n = 1273)	With IHD (n = 361, 28.4%)	Without IHD (n = 912, 71.6%)	p Value
Age, mean ± SD, years	82.9 ± 8.68	84.9 ± 7.18	82.2 ± 9.10	<0.001
Aged > 80 years, %	70.6	76.7	68.2	0.001
Female, %	73.5	69.5	75.0	0.028
PRCF resident, %	32.8	30.9	31.6	0.090
HF type [trochanteric], %	49.3	51.5	48.5	0.178
History of AMI, %	7.8	27.7		
Hypertension, %	55.9	66.2	51.8	<0.001
CVA, %	10.8	15.0	9.1	0.002
TIA, %	10.1	11.6	9.4	0.141
CKD, %	34.0	46.1	29.2	<0.001
COPD, %	17.2	25.2	14.0	<0.001
Anaemia, %	41.8	44.3	40.8	0.138
T2 DM, %	19.7	23.0	18.3	0.058
Dementia, %	31.6	33.0	31.0	0.273
Parkinson's disease, %	5.0	3.3	5.6	0.058
Smoker, %	5.7	4.2	6.4	0.079
Ex-smoker, %	11.8	13.0	11.3	0.223
* Alcohol over-user, %	4.0	2.2	44.7	0.025
Walking aids user, %	37.3	41.0	35.8	0.048
In-hospital mortality, %	4.8	7.5	3.7	0.005
Myocardial injury, %	43.6	58.6	37.7	<0.001
Postoperative AMI, %	6.7	11.7	4.8	<0.001
LOS > 10 days, %	57.9	61.5	56.5	0.058
LOS > 20 days, %	22.0	25.8	20.4	0.024
CRP > 100 mg/L, %	80.9	84.2	79.7	0.037

Abbreviations: PRCF, permanent residential care facility; IHD, ischaemic heart disease; AMI, acute myocardial infarction; CKD, chronic kidney disease (estimated glomerular filtration rate < 60 mL/min/1.73 m^2); CVA, cerebrovascular accident (stroke); TIA, transient ischaemic attack; COPD, chronic obstructive airway disease; T2DM, type 2 diabetes mellitus; LOS, length of hospital stay; CRP, C-reactive protein; * ≥3 times per week.

PMI occurred in 555(43.6%) patients (Table 2). Compared to the rest of the cohort, patients with PMI, not surprisingly, were older (+5.3 years), more often >80 years of age (85.2% vs. 60.4%, $p < 0.001$), males (28.9% vs. 24.6%, $p = 0.054$), PRCF residents (38.7% vs. 28.4%, $p < 001$), more frequently had a history of IHD (37.7% vs. 20.6%, $p < 0.001$), AMI (11.1% vs. 5.2%, $p = 001$), hypertension (60.2% vs. 51.4%, $p = 0.001$), TIA (12.6% vs. 8.3%, $p = 0.009$), anaemia (46.0% vs. 38.4%, $p = 0.005$) and dementia (38.5% vs. 26.2%, $p < 0.001$), but less likely were alcohol over-users (1.9% vs. 5.4%, $p = 0.025$), current smokers (4.1% vs. 6.5%, $p = 0.068$) or suffered from Parkinson's disease (3.8% vs. 5.9%, $p = 0.052$); history of stroke, COPD, T2DM, ex-smoking and use of walking aids were not associated with PMI. Patients who developed PMI (irrespective of IHD history) had a significantly higher mortality rate (8.8% vs. 1.9%, contrast +6.9%, $p < 0.001$); in the PMI group the proportion of individuals with high inflammatory responses (CRP > 150 mg/L in 69.2% vs. 55.1%, $p < 0.001$) and LOS > 10 days (61.4% vs. 54.9%, $p = 0.013$) was also markedly higher. Postoperative AMI experienced in total 6.7% of patients, including 11.7% with previously known IHD and 4.8% without IHD. Notable, PMI was observed most often in the first

1–3 days after surgery (when patients were receiving analgesic medications that can mask ischaemic symptoms) and was asymptomatic in 97.8% of these patients, symptomatic only in 15 individuals, including 9 with postoperative AMI; the injury probably would have gone undetected without routine cTnI measurements. Rise of cTnI occurred in 58.6% of patients with IHD (hospital mortality 12.9%), and in 62.1% of patients with a history of AMI (mortality 15.8%). Both IHD and PMI were also associated with a high inflammatory response and prolonged hospital stay (Tables 1 and 2).

Table 2. Clinical characteristics and outcomes in hip fracture patients with and without postoperative myocardial injury (PMI).

Variable	With PMI (n = 555, 43.6%)	Without PMI (n = 718, 56.4%)	p Value
Age, mean ± SD, years	86.1 ± 6.82	80.8 ± 8.91	<0.001
Aged > 80 years, %	85.2	60.4	<0.001
Male, %	28.9	24.6	0.054
PRCF resident, %	38.7	28.4	<0.001
Trochanteric HF, %	48.2	49.6	0.341
History of IHD, %	37.7	20.6	<0.001
History of AMI, %	11.1	5.2	0.001
Hypertension, %	60.2	51.4	0.001
CVA, %	11.8	9.6	0.119
TIA, %	12.6	8.3	0.009
CKD, %	44.3	26.1	<0.001
COPD, %	16.5	17.5	0.347
Anaemia, %	46.0	38.4	0.005
T2DM, %	20.8	18.8	0.524
Dementia, %	38.5	26.2	<0.001
Parkinson's disease, %	3.8	5.9	0.052
Smoker, %	4.1	6.5	0.068
Ex-smoker, %	13.0	11.7	0.286
* Alcohol over-user, %	1.9	5.4	0.001
Walking aids user, %	38.7	36.0	0.341
In-hospital mortality, %	8.8	1.9	<0.001
LOS > 10 days, %	61.4	54.9	0.013
LOS > 20 days, %	22.1	21.0	0.645
CRP > 100 mg/L, %	88.0	77.3	<0.001
CRP > 150 mg/L, %	69.2	55.1	<0.001

Abbreviations: PRCF, permanent residential care facility; IHD, ischaemic heart disease; AMI, acute myocardial infarction; CKD, chronic kidney disease (estimated glomerular filtration rate < 60 mL/min/1.73 m^2); CVA, cerebrovascular accident (stroke); TIA, transient ischaemic attack; COPD, chronic obstructive airway disease; T2DM, type 2 diabetes mellitus; LOS, length of hospital stay; CRP, C-reactive protein; * ≥3 times per week.

Clearly, in HF patients, both advanced age (>80 years) and presence of IHD are strong indicators of worse in-hospital outcomes, in particular, PMI and mortality which are interconnected. Among patients who died 56 (91.8%) were aged >80 years, 27(42.3%) had a history of IHD (including previous AMI in 9 [33.3%]), and 48 (78.7%) experienced PMI. In the group who developed PMI, 37.7% of patients were previously diagnosed with IHD and most were aged >80 years (85.2%). As shown in Table 3, in HF patients, the risk of a fatal outcome is about 5-fold higher among the aged >80 years (OR 4.9 (1.95–12.33), twice as great in subjects with a history of IHD compared with those without IHD (OR 2.1, 95% CI 1.24–3.51, p = 0.005), and 5-fold higher among patients who developed PMI (OR 5.0, 95% CI 2.70–9.41, p < 0.001). Furthermore, in subjects aged >80 years with a history of IHD the risk of PMI is 8.3 times higher (OR 8.3, 95% CI 5.58–12.36, p < 0.001) and risk of a lethal outcome is 7.4 time higher (OR 7.4, 95% CI 2.55–21.51, p < 0.001) compared with HF patients without such characteristics.

Table 3. Prognostic value of age, presence of IHD and specific biochemical characteristics at admission for predicting in-hospital death and postoperative myocardial injury.

Variable	[1] Total Cohort (n = 1273)		[2] IHD (n = 361)		[3] IHD > 80 Years of Age (n = 277)	
	OR (95% CI)	p Value	OR (95% CI)	p Value	OR (95% CI)	p Value
In-hospital Mortality						
Age > 80 years	4.9 (1.95–12.33)	0.001	5.0 (1.96–12.62)	0.001		
IHD	2.1 (1.24–3.51)	0.005			7.4 (2.55–21.51)	<0.001
PTH > 6.8 pmol/L	1.9 (1.06–3.25)	0.031	3.7 (1.85–7.27)	<0.001	11.8 (2.71–51.19)	0.001
25(OH)D < 25 nmol/L	2.4 (1.25–4.68)	0.009	8.0 (3.46–18.28)	<0.001	23.6 (6.73–82.54)	<0.001
25(OH)D < 50 nmol/L	1.2 (0.71–2.11)	0.473	2.7 (1.43–5.24)	0.002	8.4 (2.72–25.89)	<0.001
Albumin < 33 g/L	1.2 (0.64–2.23)	0.573	3.3 (1.46–7.64)	0.004	15.2 (3.87–59.53)	<0.001
Urea > 7.5 mmol/L	2.2 (1.34–3.95)	0.007	5.1 (2.48–1066)	<0.001	9.5 (2.8–32.47)	<0.001
GGT ≥ 26 IU	1.7 (1.01–2.94)	0.047	1.7 (0.98–2.89)	0.057	7.7 (1.72–34.33)	0.008
GGT/Albumin ratio ≥ 7	2.1 (1.21–3.69)	0.008	4.0 (1.85–8.78)	<0.001	16.5 (2.16–126.33)	0.007
GG/ALT ratio > 2.5	1.3 (0.74–2.23)	0.372	2.6 (1.129–5.44)	0.008	8.5 (2.30–31.15)	0.001
Urea/Albumin ratio ≥ 2.0	2.2 (1.22–4.07)	0.009	5.2 (2.50–11.03)	<0.001	9.2 (2.70–31.44)	<0.001
Plt/Albumin ratio ≥ 5.9	1.8 (1.05–3.16)	0.032	4.0 (1.83–8.55)	<0.001	21.8 (2.85–166.99)	<0.001
ALT ≥ 17 IU	1.1 (0.64–1.85)	0.751	1.7 (0.73–4.14)	0.216	2.42 (0.71–8.29)	0.158
Postoperative Myocardial Injury						
Age > 80 years	3.8 (2.83–4.99)	<0.001	3.9 (2.92–5.27)	<0.001		
IHD	2.3 (1.81–3.01)	<0.001			8.3 (5.58–12.36)	<0.001
PTH > 6.8 pmol/L	1.3 (1.02–1.68)	0.032	3.1 (2.20–4.35)	<0.001	8.3 (5.01–13.73)	<0.001
25(OH)D < 25 nmol/L	0.97 (0.65–1.44)	0.869	3.9 (1.92–8.03)	<0.001	18.0 (7.00–46.26)	<0.001
25(OH)D < 50 nmol/L	1.04 (0.80–1.35)	0.768	2.3 (1.55–3.33)	<0.001	10.4 (5.78–18.83)	<0.001
Albumin < 33 g/L	0.8 (0.59–1.09)	0.162	1.8 (1.07–3.02)	0.026	6.6 (3.37–13.08)	<0.001
Urea ≥ 7.5 mmol/L	1.5 (1.21–1.99)	0.001	4.4 (3.12–6.36)	<0.001	12.8 (7.71–21.31)	<0.001
GGT ≥ 26 IU	0.98 (0.76–1.25)	0.861	2.5 (1.74–3.64)	<0.001	9.1 (5.07–16.16)	<0.001
GGT/Albumin ratio ≥ 7.0	1.04 (0.81–1.33)	0.753	2.4 (1.66–3.33)	<0.001	9.9 (5.51–17.62)	<0.001
GG/ALT ratio ≥ 2.5	0.99 (0.761.30)	0.965	2.1 (1.44–3.14)	<0.001	11.4 (6.25–20.71)	<0.001
Urea/Albumin ratio ≥ 2.0	1.50 (1.19–1.96)	0.001	4.5 (3.18–6.39)	<0.001	12.6 (7.62–20.89)	<0.001
Plt/Albumin ratio ≥ 5.9	0.89 (0.70–1.14)	0.351	2.1 (1.45–3.10)	<0.001	6.1 (3.50–10.53)	<0.001
ALT ≥ 17 IU	0.95 (0.74–1.21)	0.661	2.8 (1.96–3.88)	<0.001	7.5 (4.05–13.77)	<0.001

Abbreviations: OR, odds ratio; CI, confidence interval; IHD, ischaemic heart disease; PTH, parathyroid hormone; 25(OH)D, 25 hydroxy vitamin D; GGT, gamma-glutamyl transferase; ALT, alanine aminotransferase; Plt, platelets. [1] adjusted for age, gender and all clinical variables which were significantly associated with hospital mortality on univariate analyses; [2] comparison IHD patients with the rest of the cohort, adjusted for age (as a continues variable), gender and clinical variables significantly associated with hospital mortality or postoperative myocardial injury on univariate analyses (Tables 1 and 2); [3] comparison of IHD patients aged >80 years and younger than 80 years with and without the analysed characteristic.

These findings, which are in line with intuitive expectations and in accordance with results of previous studies, once again underscore the importance and utility of advanced age, history of IHD and developing PMI for elucidating the prognosis and identifying the highest risk groups. On the other hand, it should be emphasised that most of aged HF

Whereas IHD and advanced age alone demonstrated a fair prognostic ability for mortality and PMI, the on-admission biochemical parameters add net benefit showing clinical usefulness, especially when patients were stratified into groups representing IHD and aged > 80 years. For example, PTH > 6.8 pmol/L at admission increased the risk of a fatal outcome in the total HF cohort by 1.9-fold, the risk of developing PMI by 1.3-fold, in patients with IHD by 3.7- and 3.1-fold, respectively, and among individuals with IHD aged > 80 years by 11.8- and 8.3-fold, respectively. Similarly, admission urea > 7.5 mmol/L indicated a 2.2-fold higher risk of lethal outcome in the total HF cohort, 5.1-fold higher risk among IHD patients and 9.5-fold higher risk in the aged IHD group (Table 3). Some biomarkers (25(OH)D < 50 mmol/L, Albumin < 33 g/L, and GGT/ALT > 2.5) did not show prognostic value when analysed in the total HF cohort but demonstrated a significant prognostic effect in IHD patients (ORs of 2.7, 3.3 and 2.6, respectively), especially in the aged with IHD (OR of 8.4, 15.2 and 8.5, respectively). These observations indicate that metabolic parameters even prognostically not significant for the total HF cohort are useful when clinical characteristics are taken into account. It is worth to note that in our study most preoperative biochemical variables and their ratios were in the "normal range" or only mildly elevated and commonly have been considered as non-diagnostic and non-prognostic. It appears that in aged HF patients with IHD presence on arrival at least one of abovementioned biomarkers increases the risk of a fatal outcome or PMI by 3–4 times.

3.3. Predicting Performance of Biochemical Indices at Admission

In the total HF population, multivariate logistic regression model (included all variables associated with in-hospital death on univariate analysis) revealed as significant independent predictors of mortality at admission the following: age > 80 years, PTH > 6.8 pmol/L, urea > 7.5 mmol/L and GGT/Albumin $\geq$ 7.0; this model yielded AUC of 0.725 (95% CI 0.663–0.788). The multivariate logistic regression for hospital death based on the same approach and development of PMI (postoperative cTnI rise) demonstrated in addition to abovementioned characteristics as independent predictors also vitamin D < 25 mmol/L and PMI; this model improved the prediction a fatal outcome and yielded AUC of 0.767 (95% CI 0.710–0.824). The independent preoperative predictors of PMI (in the total HF cohort) were history of IHD, age > 80 years, PTH > 6.8 pmol/L, urea > 7.5 mmol/L and male sex, AUC 0.700 (95% CI 0.671–0.730).

Next, we evaluated the predictive performance of the biochemical parameters at admission for in-hospital mortality or/and developing PMI. Table 4 provides the summary of discrimination ability (AUC and related characteristics) and calibration of the tests for IHD patients aged >80 years, the group with the highest risk of poor outcomes. Although in this group all evaluated biomarkers demonstrated an increased OR for mortality or/and PMI, not all of them had a reasonable predictive performance.

For predicting mortality, models based on the clinical characteristics (age > 80 years, presence of IHD), or GGT $\geq$ 26 IU, or ALT $\geq$ 17 IU, or combination of these variables demonstrated low-modest values for AUC (0.591–0.700), while in other tests/models AUC ranged from 0.803 to 0.722. Metabolic indicators when added to two clinical characteristics (IHD, age > 80 years) significantly improved the prediction of postoperative mortality: AUC increased from 0.591 (for IHD) or 0.637 (for age > 80 years) to 0.803 (if 25(OH)D < 25 mmol/L), to 0.789 (if Albumin < 33 g/L), to 0.742 (if GGT/ALT > 2.5), to 0.729 (if Urea > 7.5 mmol/L) and to 0.725 (if PTH > 6.8 pmol/L). The sensitivity and specificity as well as PPV, NPV and other performance parameters of different biomarkers varied broadly (as expected, less-sensitive variables being more specific). Four tests have a very good sensitivity above 90% (90.9% to 94.1%), and 5 other tests have sensitivity of 80% and above (80.0–88.2%). On the contrary, the majority of tested models (7) have a specificity slightly above 50% (50.6–58.7%), in 3 tests it ranged from 68.6% to 72.4%, one variable (age > 80 years) was not specific (30%), and only two indices—albumin < 33 g/L and 25(OH)D < 25 mmol/L- have a specificity of 84.6% and 90.3%, respectively. Accordingly, the positive predictive values (PPV) of the tests were quite low (ranging from 6.2% to 28.1%)

but the negative predictive values (NPV) were very good (96.8%-99.3%). All models, except one (with 25(OH)D < 50 mmol/L), showed appropriate calibration: Hosmer-Lemeshow goodness-of-fit test consisted of 0.17–14.82 (p value ranged between 0.1908 and 0.9941), in the poorly calibrated model it was 20.39 (p = 0.0401). In our cohort, the predictive performance of three ratios—GGT/Albumin, Urea/Albumin and Platelet/Albumin ratio was not superior (or even slightly lower) to that of serum albumin (<33 mg/L) and Urea (>7.5 mmol/L) alone.

A helpful and practical criterion to compare the prediction validity (robustness) of the studied models is the number of patients with a given condition (s) who need to be examined in order to detect/correctly predict one person with a certain outcome (number needed to predict, NNP). The NNP a fatal outcome in HF patients based only on the presence of IHD was 26.3, based only on age > 80 years was 20.4, and on combination of both characteristics was 12.5. The NNP decreased dramatically when biochemical parameters at admission were taken into account: 25(OH)D < 25 mmol/L (NNP = 3.8), GGT/ALT > 2.5 (NNP = 4.8), Platelets/Albumin ≥ 5.9 (NNP = 5.2), albumin < 33 g/L(NNP = 6.8), and 25(OH)D < 50 mmol/L (NNP = 7.1); use of other biochemical markers showed NNP between 9.2 and 10.6. These data further confirm the prognostic usefulness of biochemical characteristics at admission.

To sum, for predicting at admission in-hospital mortality in HF patients with IHD aged >80 years the best values showed five models (based on vitamin D deficiency/insufficiency or Albumin < 33 g/L or GGT/ALT > 2.5 or Urea > 7.5 mmol/L or PTH > 6.8 pmol/L). Presence of vitamin D deficiency (25(OH)D < 25 mmol/L) had the largest AUC (0.803), the highest predictive accuracy (90.3%), NPV (98.4%), LR+ (7.946), LR− (0.337) and the lowest NNP (3.8). A high discrimination performance demonstrated also four other models comprised of Albumin < 33 g/L (AUC 0.789, accuracy 84.6%, NPV 98.8%, NNP 6.8), or GGT/ALT > 2.5 (AUC 0.742, accuracy 70.2%, NPV 98.4%, NNP 4.8), or urea > 7.5 mmol/L (AUC 0.729, accuracy 60.4%, NPV 98.5%, NNP 9.5), or PTH > 6.8 pmol/L (AUC 0.725, accuracy 56.4%, NPV 98.9%, NNP 9.2). In terms of sensitivity three biomarkers (25(OH)D < 25 mmol/L [69.2%], Albumin < 33 g/L [72.7%], GGT/ALT > 2.5 [78.6%]) are inferior to PTH > 6.8 pmol/L [90.9%] but have higher specificity (91.3%, 85.1%, 69.8%, vs. 54.1%, respectively). These indicate that in the heterogeneous HF cohort different biomarkers possible identify subgroups of patients with specific or more pronounced metabolic changes; therefore, using simultaneously different indices would further benefit the prediction decision.

Of 61 patents who died in the hospital, 56 (91.8%) subjects at admission had at least one of these five indicators, 48 (78.7%) patients (96.3% among IHD patients) had two or more and 26 (42.6%) had three or more biomarkers, while only in 5 (8.2%) patients, including one (3.7%) with IHD, none of these biomarkers was found. In other words, the on-admission prediction by biochemical characteristics for a fatal outcome in the total cohort of HF patients was consistent with the actual observation.

Regarding the preoperative prediction of PMI, 5 tests at admission (urea > 7.5 mmol/L; Urea/Albumin ≥ 2.0, GGT/ALT > 2.5, 25(OH)D < 50 mmol/L and GGT/Albumin ≥ 7.0) showed a good discriminative performance with values for AUC ranging between 0.782 and 0.755, and 5 more tests have modest AUC values (between 0.742 and 0.711). Sensitivity above 80% (80.7–87.7%) demonstrated 4 tests, between 70% and 80% (71.0–79.2%) other 5 tests, whereas 2 tests (25(OH)D < 25 mmol/L and IHD) showed low sensitivity (36.1% and 37.7%, respectively). Specificity above 90% exhibited 2 tests (25(OH)D < 25 mmol/L [97.0%] and albumin < 33 g/L [90.7%]), between 80% and 90%—2 tests, and between 70% and 80%—9 tests, while age > 80 years was not specific (39.6%). A PPV above 70% have only 2 tests, and the NPV was above 80% in 11 tests. Values for the likelihood (LR+) of PMI to be predicted by these biomarkers were high (range 11.9–2.5) suggesting balance in favour of wright conclusion over misdiagnosis. All models were well calibrated. Of note, urea alone had a slighter larger AUC compared with the Urea/Albumin ratio (0.782 vs. 0.780), the AUC for GGT/ALT ratio (0.760) was larger than that for GGT/Albumin ratio

(0.755) but the Platelet/Albumin ratio was inferior to that of IHD in aged >80 years (0.711 vs. 0.741).

As shown in Table 4, the NNP the development of PMI based only on IHD history was 4.8, based on advanced age was 3.4, on both characteristics was 2.2. The NNP decreased below 2.0 by adding one of the following biochemical parameters: urea > 7.5 mmol/L (NNP = 1.6), 25(OH)D < 25 mmol/L (NNP = 1.6), GGT $\geq$ 26 IU (NNP = 1.8), Urea/Albumin $\geq$ 2.0 (NNP = 1.8), GGT/ALT > 2.5 (NNP = 1.9), 25(OH)D < 50 mmol/L (NNP = 1.96).

The first 5 places in terms of the weight of the pre-operative prediction PMI in the aged IHD patients (the greatest AUCs) occupied the models with the following indices: Urea > 7.5 mmol/L (AUC 0.782, accuracy 82.2%, NPV 91.3%, NNP 1.6), Urea/Albumin $\geq$ 2.0 (AUC 0.780, accuracy 77.8%, NPV 84.5%, NNP 1.8), GGT/ALT > 2.5 (AUC 0.760, accuracy 79.0%, NPV 84.2%, NNP 1.9), 25(OH)D < 50 mmol/L (AUC 0.757, accuracy 77.7%, NPV 83.0%, NNP 1.96), and PTH > 6.8 pmol/L (AUC 0.742, accuracy 73.7%, NPV 81.3%, NNP 2.1).

These biomarkers demonstrated also high predictive performance for PMI in the total HF cohort. Among 555 patients who developed PMI, 500 (90.1%) had at least one of the abovementioned five biomarkers, 396 (71.4%) patients had two or more such characteristics including 235 (42.3%) subjects with $\geq$3 biomarkers; only in 55 (9.9%) of patients with PMI none of the five biomarkers presented at admission; these 5 biomarkers were able to predict PMI in most cases (in 500 among 555 actually observed).

Notable, four on-admission biomarkers—GGT/ALT > 2.5, PTH > 6.8 pmol/L, vitamin D deficiency/insufficiency, and Urea > 7.5 mmol/L—were the best at admission predictors for both PMI and hospital death, confirming, as would be expected, commonality of risk factors and underlying pathophysiological mechanisms.

Next it was important to determine which (if any) preoperative factors increase the risk of death among individuals who developed PMI (regardless history of IHD). Our analysis revealed that in the group with PMI, most likely to progress to a lethal outcome were patients with the following on-admission characteristics: urea > 7.5 mmol/L (74.5% vs. 53.6%, $p = 0.006$), PTH > 6.8 pmol/L (71.7% vs. 52.6%, $p = 0.013$), urea/albumin $\geq$ 2.0 (78.7% vs. 56.8%, $p = 0.004$), Platelets/albumin $\geq$ 5.9 (67.4% vs. 45.3%, $p = 0.004$), GGT/Albumin $\geq$ 7.0 (63.8% vs. 48.4%, $p = 0.044$), 25(OH)D < 25 mmol/L (15.8% vs. 10.0%, $p = 0.039$) and CKD (59.6% vs. 42.8%, $p = 0.027$). These observations emphasise the role of shared physiological pathways and biochemical dysregulations as factors underlying adverse postoperative outcomes in HF patients.

Taken together, our results demonstrated that preoperative biochemical indices are helpful and can significantly improve the discrimination capability of the clinical factors (e.g., advanced age, IHD, CKD) for predicting worse hospital outcomes. For example, if a HF patient with IHD had at admission vitamin D deficiency the risk for developing PMI or hospital death was 3.9 and 8.0 times higher, respectively, than in those without such characteristics, and if this subject was >80 years old the corresponding figures were 18.0 and 23.6. Similarly, the risks of PMI or/and death in HF patients with IHD and Urea > 7.5 mmol/L at admission were 4.4- and 5.1-fold higher, respectively, compared with individuals without these features, whereas in the IHD patients $\geq$ 80 year these risks were 12.8 and 9.5 times higher, respectively. Understandable, indices with high sensitivity and low specificity should be used for identifying patients with a high probability of poor outcomes, while tests with low sensitivity and high specificity may be considered as indicators for excluding poor outcomes (a poor outcome is unlikely).

In the total HF cohort, at arrival at least one of the 5 strongest predictive biochemical indices was observed in 91.8% of all subjects with a fatal outcome and in 90.1% of all patients who developed PMI. In patients with IHD, presence of these biochemical parameters at admission increased the risk of PMI and/or death by 2–3.5-fold. Neither presence of IHD, no age > 80 years per se are predictive of PMI and/or a fatal outcome if these clinical characteristics are not combined with at least one of the following metabolic abnormalities: vitamin D insufficiency/deficiency, hypoalbuminaemia, hyperparathyroidism,

GGT/ALT > 2.5, Urea > 7.5 mmol/l, or Urea/Albumin ≥ 2.0. In other words, these factors associated with coexisting chronic diseases reflect significant pathophysiological conditions contributing to adverse outcomes and, therefore, may be complementary for prediction decisions in HF.

Importantly, the abovementioned metabolic dysregulations, are not only strongly indicative of poor outcomes in HF patients but are potentially modifiable and, therefore, should be diagnosed and addressed before a fracture occur. Can perioperative interventions aimed to normalise these metabolic disturbances improve HF outcomes need to be investigated.

3.4. Internal Validation

In the validation cohort, sociodemographic characteristics and the comorbidity profile, including the proportion of patients with IHD (28.3%), were not significantly different from that in the derivation group, PMI was observed in 44.1%, and the all-cause mortality rate was 4.1%. The on-admission biochemical parameters in both cohorts produced, in general, similar prognostic and predictive values. For example, risk of hospital death in IHD patients aged >80 years with Urea > 7.5 mmol/L was 9.2 (95% CI 1.89–14.82) times higher than in patients without such signs, AUC = 0.749 (95% CI 0.614–0.884), NNP 8.7; in subjects with GGT/ALT > 2.5 the corresponding figures were: OR 10.2 (95% CI 1.03–17.47), AUC 0.761 (95% CI 0.514–1.000), NNP 11.5; in case of Albumin < 33 g/L the corresponding figures were: OR 16.3 (95% CI 1.62–16.67), AUC 0.797 (95% CI 0.551–1.000), NNP 7.0; and if 25(OH)D was <50 mmol/L the corresponding figures were: OR 27.4(3.22–33.65), AUC 0.836 (95% CI 0.708–0.964), NNP 4.7. The AUC for prediction a lethal outcome by the 5 strongest biochemical indices ranged between 0.803 and 0.725 in the derivation, and between 0.836 and 0.749 in the validation cohort. All patents who died in the hospital had at admission at least one of the five indicators mentioned in derivation cohort, 82.6% subjects had two or more, and 47.8% had three or more such biomarkers. The Hosmer-Lemeshow statistic confirmed a good calibration of the models. In the validation cohort there were no lethal cases among the non-IHD group younger than 80 years with a normal PTH level, and there were no cases of PMI among individuals with GGT/Albumin ratio < 7 at admission.

The tested biochemical indices showed also a reasonable/good predictive performance for developing PMI, and the calibration was acceptable. As an example, in patients aged > 80 years and elevated PTH compared with subjects without these characteristics, the risk of PMI was 8.9-fold higher (95% CI 3.92–20.50), AUC 0.749 (95% CI 0.672–0.826), NNP 2.17; for Urea > 7.5 mmol/L the corresponding figures were: OR 10.2 (95% CI 4.33–24.14), AUC 0.756 (95% CI 0.672–0.841), NNP 2.24; for GGT/ALT > 2.5 the corresponding figures were: OR 9.0 (95% CI3.52–23.12), AUC 0.689 (95% CI 0.608–0.770), NNP 2.01. For the prediction of PMI, the AUC of the 5 best indicators ranged between 0.782 and 0.742 in the main cohort, and between 0.756 and 0.689 in validation cohort. In the group of patients who developed PMI, 88.6% had at least one of the five strongest biomarkers described in the derivation cohort, 58.2% patients had two or more such characteristics and in 34.7% subjects ≥ 3 biomarkers were found; however, in 11.4% of patients who experienced PMI none of these five biomarkers have been presented at admission suggesting an important role of some other factors responsible for this complication.

Taken together, internal validation showed satisfactorily calibrated prediction models, capable of predicting PMI and/or hospital death; these data confirm the prognostic usefulness (discrimination accuracy) and certainty of evidence based on consideration of abovementioned biochemical characteristics at admission.

4. Discussion

4.1. Main Findings

In HF patients, measurement of routine biochemical parameters at admission can significantly improve prognostication, risk stratification and individualised care, especially in persons of advanced age (>80 years) and/or with IHD, groups who are at the highest risk of poor outcomes (Figure 1). Among 10 biochemical indices evaluated and internally validated the best performance for predicting PMI and/or hospital death showed the following: GGT/ALT > 2.5, PTH > 6.8 pmol/L, Urea > 7.5 mmol/L, vitamin D deficiency (25(OH)D < 25 nmol/L) or insufficiency (25(OH)D < 50 nmol/L), Albumin < 33 g/L (for a fatal outcome) and Urea/Albumin $\geq$ 2.0 (for PMI). To the best of our knowledge, to date, no comprehensive comparative analysis of predictive values of biochemical indices at admission in HF patients has been performed, and none of the earlier studies have investigated any of these biomarkers to predict risk of development PMI.

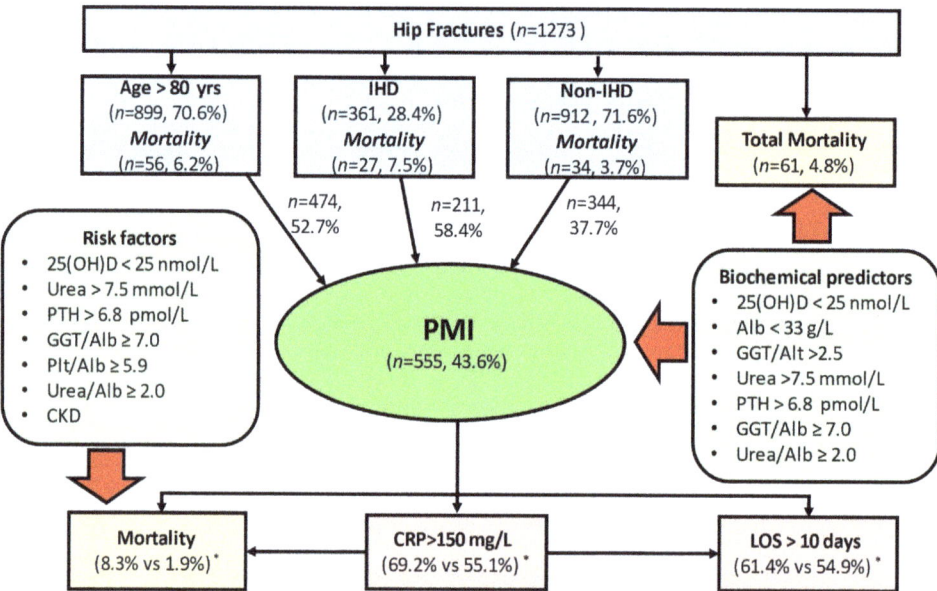

Figure 1. Relationships between ischaemic heart disease (IHD), postoperative myocardial injury (PMI), other adverse hospital outcomes and predictive biomarkers at admission in patients with hip fracture (HF). Among HF patients 70.6% were aged >80 years (mortality 6.2%), 28.4% have been diagnosed with IHD pre-fracture (mortality 7.5% vs. 3.7% in the non-IHD group); the total all-cause mortality 4.8%. PMI occurred in 43.6% of patients: in 58.6% among subjects with previously diagnosed IHD (11.1% had a history of AMI) and 37.7% in the non-IHD group. PMI developed in 52.7% of patients aged >80 years, in 58.4% of patients with pre-fracture known IHD, and in 37.7% of patients without IHD. PMI contributed to 80.3% (49 of 61 patients) of all deaths (mortality rate (8.8% vs. 1.9% in non-PMI) and was associated with a higher frequency of a high postoperative inflammatory response (CRP > 150 mg/L after the 3rd postoperative day: 69.2% vs. 55.1%) and prolonged hospital stay (LOS > 10 days: 61.4% vs. 54.9%). On-admission biochemical predictors of PMI and/or a fatal outcome are shown in the box on the right. Factors at admission that significantly (1.3–1.6-times) increase the risk of a lethal outcome in patients who developed PMI are listed in the left box. * Comparison with non-PMI patients.

This study suggested 4 important facts critical to osteoporotic HF management.

First, it confirmed that both age > 80 years and history of IHD are the strongest clinical factors indicative of worse short-term outcomes, namely, developing PMI and hospital death. Individuals aged >80 years accounted for 70.6% of the HF cohort, 76.7% among the IHD patients, 85.2% among subjects who developed PMI, and 91.8% in the fatal group. Patients with IHD accounted for 28.4% of the total HF cohort and 44.3% of all hospital deaths (mortality rate 7.5% vs. 3.7% among non- IHD subjects). PMI occurred (typically without chest pain or any ischemic symptoms) in 43.6% of HF patients (in 58.6% of individuals with IHD and in 37.7% without IHD). PMI was observed in 80.3% [49/61] of all deaths; the mortality rate among patients with PMI was approximately 4.6-fold higher than in patients without such complication (8.8% vs. 1.9%). PMI was also associated with high inflammatory responses and prolonged LOS. PMI (diagnosed by even minor troponin elevations), which is multifactorial (perioperative stress, blood loss, hypoxaemia, release of various inflammatory cytokines, arrhythmia, vascular endothelial cell injury, etc.) and often occurs in patients without previously known IHD (62.0% in our cohort), is currently recognised as a specific and sensitive indicator of perioperative complications and mortality in patients undergoing noncardiac surgery including orthopaedic surgery [7,13,35,114] and HF repair [7,24,114–119]. Therefore, it is important to have a sufficiently high index of suspicion for PMI, to consider its risk and timely predict in subjects with and without history of IHD.

Second. Although the prognostic role of advance age, presence of IHD and developing PMI is unquestionable, these factors, however, are not sufficient for individual predictions (i.e., identification of patients imminent for poor outcomes). In fact, only a small proportion of the "high-risk patients" demonstrated poor outcomes after HF: the majority of aged (>90%) or subjects with IHD (92.5%) or who developed PMI (91.2%) survived. Therefore, the crucial questions originated—how to determine at time of admission which aged HF patient, especially with IHD, is really at the highest risk of an adverse outcome (e.g., PMI and/or in-hospital death), in whom PMI (irrespective of presence underlying chronic diseases) should be expected and preventive measures applied. Obviously, the answers to these questions are enormously difficult because the pathogenesis of poor outcomes in HF is complex and multicausative. The outcomes are influenced by numerous interacting patient-related (age, gender, comorbidities), pre-, intra- (type of procedure, blood loss, hypotension, etc.) and postoperative (PMI, infection, delirium, acute kidney failure, etc.) factors—all of which may naturally increase the risks. In an attempt to come closer to a practical solution of the problem we evaluated 10 biochemical indices potential for predicting the occurrence of adverse postoperative events, focusing on factors allowing modification. We found that despite significant complexity and heterogeneity in clinical profile of HFs simple preoperative metabolic indices (even in supposedly "normal" range) provide significant prognostic information, substantially improving prediction of adverse outcomes, particularly among aged patients with IHD (the groups at the highest risks), and, possibly, may serve as important clues for treatment to reduce poor outcomes. Metabolic indicators integrate various genetic, lifestyle and environmental effects, reflect ongoing physiological processes in multiple organs, and, therefore, provide an insight into disease pathophysiology acting as powerful characteristics of an individual's health status. Metabolic dysregulations are implicated in the pathogenesis and severity of numerous human pathologies, including osteoporosis, atherosclerosis, IHD (reflecting systemic connectivities), and, consequently, underly the adverse outcomes in HF patients. In HF patients, alterations in biochemical indices, IHD and advanced age interact to increase risks of developing PMI, new AMI, high inflammatory response, prolonged LOS and mortality above the effect of each individual condition, as demonstrated in this and our previous studies [17,45,51,110,120–122].

Our findings that on-arrival insufficient 25(OH)D levels and/or elevated PTH predict PMI and/or death are in line with long-standing evidence that the physiological effects of vitamin D and PTH extend beyond calcium homeostasis and bone mineralisation and consistent with many previous reports [17,123–126]. Hypovitaminosis D is also known to correlate with higher inflammatory response [124,127–132], which together with increased PTH levels (a factor associated with multiple postoperative complications in HF patients [45,133] and/or PMI significantly increases the risk of poor outcomes.

Third, comparison of predictive performance of 10 different biomarkers revealed 6 indices with the strongest discriminant ability. The most significant net benefit in predicting both developing PMI and/or in-hospital mortality demonstrated preoperative GGT/ALT ratio > 2.5, elevated urea (>7.5 mmol/L), hyperparathyroidism (PTH > 6.8 pmol/L) and abnormal vitamin D status (deficiency or insufficiency); preoperative Urea/Albumin ≥ 2.0 strongly indicated risk of PMI, and hypoalbuminaemia (<33 g/L)—a high risk of a lethal outcome.

The presented data clearly demonstrated that the long-held belief that IHD (even history of AMI) are significant risk factors for poor outcomes in HF patients is true predominantly when IHD is accompanied by metabolic disturbances such as elevated PTH, urea, GGT/ALT ratio, low albumin or 25(OH)D levels. Indeed, these biochemical characteristics were not presented only in 1 of 27 patients with IHD who died and in 50 (9.0%) of 555 patients who developed PMI. In other words, the prognostic performance of IHD depends on the underlying biochemical status. Certainly, risk stratification at admission, preventive and therapeutic interventions would be more precise if based not only on the history of IHD per se, but also considered the clinically silent metabolic profile, a key player in the development of comorbidities and worse outcomes. As mentioned above (Introduction) most of the routinely used in clinical practice approaches for predicting the risk of MACE in patients undergoing noncardiac surgery do not include biochemical parameters (except for serum creatinine) and are imperfect on individual level [36,37].

Reports on predictive capacity of several existing cardiac risk indices [134–136], RCRI scores in HF patients are scarce and often controversial [35,137]. Our data show that biochemical indices at admission may help to identify patients at high risk of cardiac events during and after surgery as well as to avoid unnecessary preoperative cardiac assessment. The concept that all IHD patents with HF have the same high risk of poor outcome appears no longer viable; predictions and therapies to be efficacious should address specific (including metabolic) risk factors of individual patients. The results presented here add new insights regarding the prognostic usefulness of preoperative biochemical indices and (if externally validated) may allow preoperative estimation of cardiac risk independent of direct risks caused by surgical and post-surgical complications. These appear as one step towards the patient-level precision to predict/prevent adverse outcomes early, an ideal goal which currently remains unmet.

Our simple models (based on three variables—IHD, age > 80 years and one biochemical index) for prediction a fatal outcome (AUCs: 0.803–0.722 in the main cohort and 0.836–0.749 in the validation cohort) or developing PMI (AUCs: 0.782–0.742 in the main cohort and 0.756–0.689 in the validation cohort) performed better than the model which included all independent variables in the total HF cohort (AUCs 0.725 and 0.700, respectively). Moreover, the simplified on-admission models for predicting hospital mortality after HF performed as well as or even better than most of earlier proposed models based on multiple variables (usually between 7 and 29) often including intra- and postoperative characteristics. To name for comparison a few with the highest discrimination ability: (1) 29 variables, AUC 0.91 [138]; (2) 29 variables, AUC 0.895 and 0.797 in training and testing datasets, respectively [139]; (3) >60 variables, AUC 0.83 (for 30 day mortality) and AUC 0.75 (for 1-year mortality) [140]; (4) 9 predictors, AUC 0.81 and 0.79 in the development and validation cohorts, respectively [141]; (5) 13 variables, AUC 0.82 [142]; (6) 7 variables, AUC 0.82 [143]; (7) 9 variables (Sernbo score), AUC 0.79 (for 1-year mortality) [144]; (8) >30 variables, AUC 0.76 [32]; (9) 29 variables, AUC 0.74 [145]; (10) 22 variables, AUC 0.71; (11) 7 variables AUC 0.71 (UK National Hip Fracture Database)-0.70 (Nottingham model) [146]; (12) 10 variables, AUC 0.702 [31]; (13) 9 variables (Sernbo score), AUC 0.79 (for 1-year mortality) [144]; (14) Charlson comorbidity index, AUC 0.682 (for in-hospital mortality [147], AUC 0.769 [148]–0.607 [149] (for 1-year mortality). A recent systematic review of prediction models for osteoporotic fractures (68 studies) found that in 69 of 70 models AUC ranged from 0.60 to 0.91 including only two models (3%) with AUC > 0.90 and 9 (13%) with AUC 0.8–0.9 [150].

Furthermore, in HF patients aged >80 years with a history of IHD, for correct prediction at admission of one PMI biochemical indices need to be assessed in 2 patients, and for correct prediction of one fatal outcome 4–7 subjects (using different indices) need to be screened. These observations indicate that the proposed widely applicable, routine, quick, easily interpreted biochemical characteristics on arrival which are currently rarely used, add significant information over standard clinical markers and may be helpful in day-to day clinical practice. When interpreting the utility of individual biochemical parameters as predictors of outcomes it should be taken into account that: (1) the presented models indicate the number of subjects with specific characteristics in which adverse outcomes may be expected, it is not an individual/personalised prediction for each patient (any person may have non-measured by the models or not known characteristics which may modify the individual risk; the preoperative signs alone may be insufficient for predicting multifactorial outcomes; the intra- and postoperative quality of care has obviously a substantial impact on the patient's postoperative course), and (2) highly sensitive tests with low NNP are preferable to identify most cases (minimal false negatives, despite consequent risk of false positives) but tests with high specificity outweigh low NNP if the goal is to exclude most false positives (non-cases). Analysis of 2–3 tests together gives a better understanding of their prognostic gain for prediction a specific outcome; therefore, it is desirable to assess different biochemical indices as they may be complementary for prediction decisions.

In summary, the presented here simple prediction models fulfill three main criteria—acceptable discrimination power, calibration and decreased NNP. While the clinical approach to preoperative prediction may be subjective, variable among clinicians and prone to error, assessment of biochemical indices at admission provides significant objective prognostic information and improves prediction.

Furthermore, the data on prognostic value of the analysed circulating biochemical parameters all of which reflect reversible/modifiable conditions provide important knowledge regarding possible areas accessible for interventions—perioperative as well as pre-fracture. The clinical implications of considering metabolic derangements are threefold: to optimise prognostication in HF patients and avoid unnecessary perioperative assessment (i.e., cardiac), to improve clinical outcomes and to select appropriate patients for intervention prior fracture occurred.

To identify the most vulnerable HF patients at risk of an adverse outcome at admission our study focuses on two clinical characteristics (age, history of IHD) and simple biochemical indices; this approach provides useful prediction information to guide and support the shared (doctors-patient/carer) decision-making process (including selection which patient may benefit from arthroplasty surgery, internal fixation or nonoperative management) and might improve outcomes by early introducing appropriate individualised medical treatment aimed at controllable risk factors including abovementioned biochemical abnormalities. Given that developing PMI accounted for 80.3% of in-hospital mortality and was associated with elevated inflammatory response and prolonged LOS, predicting and targeting subjects with a high probability of this complication is reasonable.

Currently there is no consensus regarding perioperative management of HF patients at risk of PMI, the available data are scarce, and recommendations are controversial. Numerous studies on benefits and risks of beta-blockers in patients undergoing non-cardiac surgery, including HF, yielded controversial results [151–162]. However, reduction in cardiac complications has often been reported in patients with risk factors indicating that perioperative beta-blocker management should be individualised [163]. Similarly, perioperative use, continuation or discontinuation of antiplatelet (especially dual) therapy [164–169], antihypertensive drugs, renin-angiotensin-aldosterone system inhibitors, diuretics [170–172] remain debatable issues. It was reported that prophylactic nitrates [26,173], as well as alpha-2 adrenergic agonists [174] do not prevent death and cardiac complications in non-cardiac surgery. Statins are recommended preoperatively in patients with atherosclerotic CVD [12]. In patients who suffer PMI, risk-adjusted observational data suggest that aspirin and a statin can reduce the risk of 30-day mortality [175,176] and PMI, but the risk of perioperative bleeding should be fully considered before using antiplatelet and anticoagulant drugs. Obviously, the treatment decision should be discussed in a multidisciplinary way and based on patient-specific conditions (e.g., documented IHD, coronary stents, CABGs, AF, recent thromboembolic disease, inherited coagulopathy, etc.) to balance risks of possible drug-related ischemic-bleeding complications, prevent stroke, avoid intra- and postoperative hypotension, bradycardia and/or fluid overload; lower doses should be considered.

Clearly, attention to biochemical characteristics (e.g., vitamin D status, hyperparathyroidism, hypoalbuminaemia, liver function indices, etc.) should drive the much need individualised preventive management in persons at high risk of osteoporotic fracture long before the fracture occurred. Our observations on prevalence among older HF patients of alterations in serum vitamin D [51,124,126,133,177–179], PTH [44–51,53,133,180], albumin levels [16,51,53,54,58,80,181–189] and liver function [76,77,107,110,190–196] are consistent with reported in the literature. These data strongly suggest that these metabolic dysregulations known to be linked to osteoporosis, falls, factures and to many chronic diseases are often not remedied with standard treatment. Attempts to identify and address metabolic alterations prior to the onset of disease(s) and end-organ complications should be an important part of preventive management of osteoporotic fractures across disciplines; such approach will increase the effectiveness and quality of patient care and may reduce health care costs in the ageing population.

Our findings are particularly noteworthy in the context of current demographic and epidemiological trends. Due to increase in life expectancy (ageing population), the number of patients with osteoporosis, sarcopenia, CVD/IHD, other chronic conditions and, consequently, geriatric low energy/fragility fractures with worse prognosis after orthopaedic surgery will increase. Physicians and orthopaedic surgeons can utilise biochemical indices to predict timely adverse events. Given that metabolic alterations often present for years before becoming clinically apparent and effective interventions are usually available earlier identification of individuals at risk is particularly important.

4.2. Strength and Limitations

Strengths of the study include the relatively large sample of patients with any type of surgery for HF, simultaneous testing of 10 different biomarkers making direct comparisons of predictive performance of all tested indices possible, robust statistical methods used, and internal validation of the proposed models. To the best of our knowledge, this is the first study to evaluate and compare in HF patients the predictive value at admission of a wide range of commonly available different biochemical indices.

Several limitations of this study deserve comment. As it was an observational single-centre study, selective bias cannot be rule out and cause–effect relationships cannot be fully inferred from it; the data are limited to HF surgeries and may not reflect outcomes for other orthopaedic or non-cardiac surgeries. The number of deaths was relatively low. The set of biochemical indices included form only a fraction of all available metabolic variables (other characteristics may also be predictive) and no comparison with haematologic parameters of known predictive value (e.g., anaemia [197–199], or lymphocyte-neutrophil ratio [51,200,201], or red blood cell distribution width [202,203]) has been done. Our findings need external validation. The patients were predominantly white and of European descent, which may limit the generalisability of our results. However, the sociodemographic, clinical and laboratory characteristics, type and incidence of hospital outcomes in our cohort seems representative of the average HF population; the findings could therefore be applied at least to the whole Caucasian HF population; further studies are needed to determine whether the findings extend to other racial/ethnic groups.

In conclusion, we identified main clinical and several biochemical parameters that carry a high prognostic potential for preoperative prediction of hospital outcomes in patients with HF. The most important clinical characteristics in guiding short-term prognosis, predicting PMI and/or death include age > 80 years and history of IHD. The proposed routine easily accessible biochemical indices at admission substantially improve prognostic accuracy and prediction of outcomes and may be useful for early risk stratification and identification of the most vulnerable patients (especially among the aged >80 years with IHD) in whom appropriate treatment focused on factors allowing modification might reduce poor outcomes and improve survival.

Author Contributions: Conceptualisation, A.F. and L.F.; Data curation, A.F.; Methodology, A.F., L.F. and W.S.; Statistical analysis, W.S. and A.F.; Visualisation. W.S. and A.F.; Supervision, A.F. and P.N.S.; Validation, A.F. and W.S.; Writing—original draft preparation, L.F. and A.F.; Writing—review and editing, L.F., A.F. and P.N.S. All authors have read and agreed to the published version of the manuscript.

Funding: This research received no external funding.

Informed Consent Statement: Not applicable. This study does not contain individual or personal data in any form (including individual details, images, or videos).

Data Availability Statement: All data analysed as part of the study are included.

Conflicts of Interest: The authors declare no competing interest.

Abbreviations

IHD, ischaemic heart disease; PMI, postoperative myocardial injury; CKD, chronic kidney disease; PTH, parathyroid hormone; Plt, platelets; GGT, *gamma-glutamyl transferase*; 25(OH)D, 25-hydroxy vitamin D; CRP, C-reactive protein; LOS, length of hospital stay.

References

1. Hietala, P.; Strandberg, M.; Strandberg, N.; Gullichsen, E.; Airaksinen, K.E. Perioperative myocardial infarctions are common and often unrecognized in patients undergoing hip fracture surgery. *J. Trauma Acute Care Surg.* **2013**, *74*, 1087–1091. [CrossRef] [PubMed]
2. Mohd-Tahir, N.A.; Li, S.C. Economic burden of osteoporosis-related hip fracture in Asia: A systematic review. *Osteoporos. Int.* **2017**, *28*, 2035–2044. [CrossRef] [PubMed]
3. Downey, C.; Kelly, M.; Quinlan, J.F. Changing trends in the mortality rate at 1-year post hip fracture—A systematic review. *World J. Orthop.* **2019**, *10*, 166–175. [CrossRef] [PubMed]
4. Smeets, S.J.M.; van Wunnik, B.P.W.; Poeze, M.; Slooter, G.D.; Verbruggen, J. Cardiac overscreening hip fracture patients. *Arch. Orthop. Trauma Surg.* **2020**, *140*, 33–41. [CrossRef]
5. Nelson, M.J.; Scott, J.; Sivalingam, P. Evaluation of Nottingham Hip Fracture Score, Age-Adjusted Charlson Comorbidity Index and the Physiological and Operative Severity Score for the enumeration of Mortality and morbidity as predictors of mortality in elderly neck of femur fracture patients. *SAGE Open Med.* **2020**, *8*, 2050312120918268. [CrossRef]
6. Bergh, C.; Moller, M.; Ekelund, J.; Brisby, H. Mortality after Sustaining Skeletal Fractures in Relation to Age. *J. Clin. Med.* **2022**, *11*, 2313. [CrossRef]
7. Vacheron, C.H.; Hentzen, J.; Fauvernier, M.; Fessy, M.; Chaudier, P.; Landel, V.; David, J.S.; Incagnoli, P.; Piriou, V.; Friggeri, A. Association between Short-, Intermediate-, and Long-term Mortality and Myocardial Injury after Noncardiac Surgery after Hip Fracture Surgery: A Retrospective Cohort. *Anesth. Analg.* **2021**, *133*, 915–923. [CrossRef]
8. Kristensen, S.D.; Knuuti, J.; Saraste, A.; Anker, S.; Botker, H.E.; Hert, S.D.; Ford, I.; Gonzalez-Juanatey, J.R.; Gorenek, B.; Heyndrickx, G.R.; et al. 2014 ESC/ESA Guidelines on non-cardiac surgery: Cardiovascular assessment and management: The Joint Task Force on non-cardiac surgery: Cardiovascular assessment and management of the European Society of Cardiology (ESC) and the European Society of Anaesthesiology (ESA). *Eur. Heart J.* **2014**, *35*, 2383–2431.
9. Devereaux, P.J.; Sessler, D.I. Cardiac Complications in Patients Undergoing Major Noncardiac Surgery. *N. Engl. J. Med.* **2015**, *373*, 2258–2269. [CrossRef]
10. Mauermann, E.; Bolliger, D.; Seeberger, E.; Puelacher, C.; Corbiere, S.; Filipovic, M.; Seeberger, M.; Mueller, C.; Lurati Buse, G. Incremental Value of Preoperative Copeptin for Predicting Myocardial Injury. *Anesth. Analg.* **2016**, *123*, 1363–1371. [CrossRef]
11. De Hert, S.; Staender, S.; Fritsch, G.; Hinkelbein, J.; Afshari, A.; Bettelli, G.; Bock, M.; Chew, M.S.; Coburn, M.; De Robertis, E.; et al. Pre-operative evaluation of adults undergoing elective noncardiac surgery: Updated guideline from the European Society of Anaesthesiology. *Eur. J. Anaesthesiol.* **2018**, *35*, 407–465. [CrossRef] [PubMed]
12. Smilowitz, N.R.; Berger, J.S. Perioperative Cardiovascular Risk Assessment and Management for Noncardiac Surgery: A Review. *JAMA* **2020**, *324*, 279–290. [CrossRef] [PubMed]
13. Thomas, S.; Borges, F.; Bhandari, M.; De Beer, J.; Urrutia Cuchi, G.; Adili, A.; Winemaker, M.; Avram, V.; Chan, M.T.V.; Lamas, C.; et al. Association Between Myocardial Injury and Cardiovascular Outcomes of Orthopaedic Surgery: A Vascular Events in Noncardiac Surgery Patients Cohort Evaluation (VISION) Substudy. *J. Bone Jt. Surg. Am.* **2020**, *102*, 880–888. [CrossRef] [PubMed]
14. Qamar, A.; Bangalore, S. Biomarkers to Personalize Preoperative Cardiovascular Risk Stratification: Ready for Prime Time? *Ann. Intern. Med.* **2020**, *172*, 149–150. [CrossRef] [PubMed]
15. Banco, D.; Dodson, J.A.; Berger, J.S.; Smilowitz, N.R. Perioperative cardiovascular outcomes among older adults undergoing in-hospital noncardiac surgery. *J. Am. Geriatr. Soc.* **2021**, *69*, 2821–2830. [CrossRef] [PubMed]

16. Bass, A.R.; Levin, L.F. Should All Orthopaedic Patients Undergo Postoperative Troponin Testing?: Commentary on an article by Sabu Thomas, MD, MSc; et al.: "Association Between Myocardial Injury and Cardiovascular Outcomes of Orthopaedic Surgery. A Vascular Events in Noncardiac Surgery Patients Cohort Evaluation (VISION) Substudy". *J. Bone Jt. Surg. Am.* **2020**, *102*, e46.
17. Fisher, A.A.; Southcott, E.K.; Srikusalanukul, W.; Davis, M.W.; Hickman, P.E.; Potter, J.M.; Smith, P.N. Relationships between myocardial injury, all-cause mortality, vitamin D, PTH, and biochemical bone turnover markers in older patients with hip fractures. *Ann. Clin. Lab. Sci.* **2007**, *37*, 222–232.
18. Fisher, A.A.; Southcott, E.N.; Goh, S.L.; Srikusalanukul, W.; Hickman, P.E.; Davis, M.W.; Potter, J.M.; Budge, M.M.; Smith, P.N. Elevated serum cardiac troponin I in older patients with hip fracture: Incidence and prognostic significance. *Arch. Orthop. Trauma Surg.* **2008**, *128*, 1073–1079. [CrossRef]
19. Nordling, P.; Kiviniemi, T.; Strandberg, M.; Strandberg, N.; Airaksinen, J. Predicting the outcome of hip fracture patients by using N-terminal fragment of pro-B-type natriuretic peptide. *BMJ Open* **2016**, *6*, e009416. [CrossRef]
20. Urban, M.K.; Wolfe, S.W.; Sanghavi, N.M.; Fields, K.; Magid, S.K. The Incidence of Perioperative Cardiac Events after Orthopedic Surgery: A Single Institutional Experience of Cases Performed over One Year. *HSS J.* **2017**, *13*, 248–254. [CrossRef]
21. Cha, Y.H.; Lee, Y.K.; Koo, K.H.; Wi, C.; Lee, K.H. Difference in Mortality Rate by Type of Anticoagulant in Elderly Patients with Cardiovascular Disease after Hip Fractures. *Clin. Orthop. Surg.* **2019**, *11*, 15–20. [CrossRef] [PubMed]
22. Norring-Agerskov, D.; Madsen, C.M.; Bathum, L.; Pedersen, O.B.; Lauritzen, J.B.; Jorgensen, N.R.; Jorgensen, H.L. History of cardiovascular disease and cardiovascular biomarkers are associated with 30-day mortality in patients with hip fracture. *Osteoporos. Int.* **2019**, *30*, 1767–1778. [CrossRef] [PubMed]
23. Rostagno, C.; Cartei, A.; Rubbieri, G.; Ceccofiglio, A.; Magni, A.; Forni, S.; Civinini, R.; Boccaccini, A. Perioperative Myocardial Infarction/Myocardial Injury Is Associated with High Hospital Mortality in Elderly Patients Undergoing Hip Fracture Surgery. *J. Clin. Med.* **2020**, *9*, 4043. [CrossRef] [PubMed]
24. Wang, L.; Cai, M.; Li, X.; Deng, X.; Xue, Q.; Zhou, L.; Yang, M. Association of Acute Perioperative Myocardial Injury With All-Cause Mortality Within 90 Days After Hip Fracture Repair in the Elderly: A Prospective Study. *Geriatr. Orthop. Surg. Rehabil.* **2022**, *13*, 21514593211070129. [CrossRef] [PubMed]
25. Katsanos, S.; Sioutis, S.; Reppas, L.; Mitsiokapa, E.; Tsatsaragkou, A.; Mastrokalos, D.; Koulalis, D.; Mavrogenis, A.F. What do hip fracture patients die from? *Eur. J. Orthop. Surg. Traumatol.* **2022**; in press. [CrossRef]
26. Pannell, L.M.; Reyes, E.M.; Underwood, S.R. Cardiac risk assessment before non-cardiac surgery. *Eur. Heart J. Cardiovasc. Imaging* **2013**, *14*, 316–322. [CrossRef]
27. Writing Committee for the VISION Study Investigators; Devereaux, P.J.; Biccard, B.M.; Sigamani, A.; Xavier, D.; Chan, M.T.V.; Srinathan, S.K.; Walsh, M.; Abraham, V.; Pearse, R.; et al. Association of Postoperative High-Sensitivity Troponin Levels With Myocardial Injury and 30-Day Mortality Among Patients Undergoing Noncardiac Surgery. *JAMA* **2017**, *317*, 1642–1651.
28. Lobo, S.A.; Fischer, S. Cardiac Risk Assessment. In *StatPearls*; StatPearls: Treasure Island, FL, USA, 2022.
29. Fleisher, L.A.; Fleischmann, K.E.; Auerbach, A.D.; Barnason, S.A.; Beckman, J.A.; Bozkurt, B.; Davila-Roman, V.G.; Gerhard-Herman, M.D.; Holly, T.A.; Kane, G.C.; et al. 2014 ACC/AHA guideline on perioperative cardiovascular evaluation and management of patients undergoing noncardiac surgery: A report of the American College of Cardiology/American Heart Association Task Force on practice guidelines. *J. Am. Coll. Cardiol.* **2014**, *64*, e77–e137. [CrossRef]
30. Bilimoria, K.Y.; Liu, Y.; Paruch, J.L.; Zhou, L.; Kmiecik, T.E.; Ko, C.Y.; Cohen, M.E. Development and evaluation of the universal ACS NSQIP surgical risk calculator: A decision aid and informed consent tool for patients and surgeons. *J. Am. Coll. Surg.* **2013**, *217*, 833–842.e1-3. [CrossRef]
31. Pugely, A.J.; Martin, C.T.; Gao, Y.; Klocke, N.F.; Callaghan, J.J.; Marsh, J.L. A risk calculator for short-term morbidity and mortality after hip fracture surgery. *J. Orthop. Trauma.* **2014**, *28*, 63–69. [CrossRef]
32. Harris, A.H.S.; Trickey, A.W.; Eddington, H.S.; Seib, C.D.; Kamal, R.N.; Kuo, A.C.; Ding, Q.; Giori, N.J. A Tool to Estimate Risk of 30-day Mortality and Complications after Hip Fracture Surgery: Accurate Enough for Some but Not All Purposes? A Study from the ACS-NSQIP Database. *Clin. Orthop. Relat. Res.* **2022**; in press. [CrossRef] [PubMed]
33. Kivrak, S.; Haller, G. Scores for preoperative risk evaluation of postoperative mortality. *Best. Pract. Res. Clin. Anaesthesiol.* **2021**, *35*, 115–134. [CrossRef] [PubMed]
34. Markovic, D.; Jevtovic-Stoimenov, T.; Stojanovic, M.; Vukovic, A.; Dinic, V.; Markovic-Zivkovic, B.; Jankovic, R.J. Addition of clinical risk scores improves prediction performance of American Society of Anesthesiologists (ASA) physical status classification for postoperative mortality in older patients: A pilot study. *Eur. Geriatr. Med.* **2018**, *9*, 51–59. [CrossRef]
35. Vernooij, L.M.; van Klei, W.A.; Moons, K.G.; Takada, T.; van Waes, J.; Damen, J.A. The comparative and added prognostic value of biomarkers to the Revised Cardiac Risk Index for preoperative prediction of major adverse cardiac events and all-cause mortality in patients who undergo noncardiac surgery. *Cochrane Database Syst. Rev.* **2021**, *12*, CD013139.
36. Davis, C.; Tait, G.; Carroll, J.; Wijeysundera, D.N.; Beattie, W.S. The Revised Cardiac Risk Index in the new millennium: A single-centre prospective cohort re-evaluation of the original variables in 9,519 consecutive elective surgical patients. *Can. J. Anaesth.* **2013**, *60*, 855–863. [CrossRef] [PubMed]
37. Vascular Events In Noncardiac Surgery Patients Cohort Evaluation (VISION) Study Investigators; Devereaux, P.J.; Chan, M.T.; Alonso-Coello, P.; Walsh, M.; Berwanger, O.; Villar, J.C.; Wang, C.Y.; Garutti, R.I.; Jacka, M.J.; et al. Association between postoperative troponin levels and 30-day mortality among patients undergoing noncardiac surgery. *JAMA* **2012**, *307*, 2295–2304. [PubMed]

38. Stolze, A.; van de Garde, E.M.W.; Posthuma, L.M.; Hollmann, M.W.; de Korte-de Boer, D.; Smit-Fun, V.M.; Buhre, W.; Boer, C.; Noordzij, P.G.; TRACE Study Investigators. Validation of the PreOperative Score to predict Post-Operative Mortality (POSPOM) in Dutch non-cardiac surgery patients. *BMC Anesthesiol.* **2022**, *22*, 58. [CrossRef] [PubMed]
39. Menzenbach, J.; Layer, Y.C.; Layer, Y.L.; Mayr, A.; Coburn, M.; Wittmann, M.; Hilbert, T. The level of postoperative care influences mortality prediction by the POSPOM score: A retrospective cohort analysis. *PLoS ONE* **2021**, *16*, e0257829. [CrossRef]
40. Wanjiang, F.; Xiaobo, Z.; Xin, W.; Ye, M.; Lihua, H.; Jianlong, W. Application of POSSUM and P-POSSUM scores in the risk assessment of elderly hip fracture surgery: Systematic review and meta-analysis. *J. Orthop. Surg. Res.* **2022**, *17*, 255. [CrossRef]
41. Yang, L.; Yang, H.; Chen, Q.; Shen, H.; Wang, Z. Analysis of risk factors for 90-day mortality after surgery in elderly patients with intertrochanteric fractures and a history of cardiovascular disease. *Ann. Palliat. Med.* **2022**, *11*, 155–162. [CrossRef]
42. Karres, J.; Heesakkers, N.A.; Ultee, J.M.; Vrouenraets, B.C. Predicting 30-day mortality following hip fracture surgery: Evaluation of six risk prediction models. *Injury* **2015**, *46*, 371–377. [CrossRef] [PubMed]
43. Niessen, R.; Bihin, B.; Gourdin, M.; Yombi, J.C.; Cornu, O.; Forget, P. Prediction of postoperative mortality in elderly patient with hip fractures: A single-centre, retrospective cohort study. *BMC Anesthesiol.* **2018**, *18*, 183. [CrossRef] [PubMed]
44. Danese, M.D.; Kim, J.; Doan, Q.V.; Dylan, M.; Griffiths, R.; Chertow, G.M. PTH and the risks for hip, vertebral, and pelvic fractures among patients on dialysis. *Am. J. Kidney Dis.* **2006**, *47*, 149–156. [CrossRef]
45. Fisher, A.; Goh, S.; Srikusalanukul, W.; Davis, M. Elevated serum PTH is independently associated with poor outcomes in older patients with hip fracture and vitamin D inadequacy. *Calcif. Tissue Int.* **2009**, *85*, 301–309. [CrossRef] [PubMed]
46. Hosking, D.; Alonso, C.G.; Brandi, M.L. Management of osteoporosis with PTH: Treatment and prescription patterns in Europe. *Curr. Med. Res. Opin.* **2009**, *25*, 263–270. [CrossRef]
47. Fisher, A.; Srikusalanukul, W.; Davis, M.; Smith, P. Hip fracture type: Important role of parathyroid hormone (PTH) response to hypovitaminosis D. *Bone* **2010**, *47*, 400–407. [CrossRef]
48. Madsen, C.M.; Jorgensen, H.L.; Lind, B.; Ogarrio, H.W.; Riis, T.; Schwarz, P.; Duus, B.R.; Lauritzen, J.B. Secondary hyperparathyroidism and mortality in hip fracture patients compared to a control group from general practice. *Injury* **2012**, *43*, 1052–1057. [CrossRef]
49. Van Ballegooijen, A.J.; Reinders, I.; Visser, M.; Brouwer, I.A. Parathyroid hormone and cardiovascular disease events: A systematic review and meta-analysis of prospective studies. *Am. Heart J.* **2013**, *165*, 655–664, 664 e1-5. [CrossRef]
50. Domiciano, D.S.; Machado, L.G.; Lopes, J.B.; Figueiredo, C.P.; Caparbo, V.F.; Oliveira, R.M.; Scazufca, M.; McClung, M.R.; Pereira, R.M. Bone Mineral Density and Parathyroid Hormone as Independent Risk Factors for Mortality in Community-Dwelling Older Adults: A Population-Based Prospective Cohort Study in Brazil. The Sao Paulo Ageing & Health (SPAH) Study. *J. Bone Miner. Res.* **2016**, *31*, 1146–1157.
51. Fisher, A.; Fisher, L.; Srikusalanukul, W.; Smith, P.N. Usefulness of simple biomarkers at admission as independent indicators and predictors of in-hospital mortality in older hip fracture patients. *Injury* **2018**, *49*, 829–840. [CrossRef]
52. Gambardella, J.; De Rosa, M.; Sorriento, D.; Prevete, N.; Fiordelisi, A.; Ciccarelli, M.; Trimarco, B.; De Luca, N.; Iaccarino, G. Parathyroid Hormone Causes Endothelial Dysfunction by Inducing Mitochondrial ROS and Specific Oxidative Signal Transduction Modifications. *Oxid. Med. Cell. Longev.* **2018**, *2018*, 9582319. [CrossRef] [PubMed]
53. Baggio, M.; Oliveira, D.T.; Locks, R. Evaluation of the Laboratorial Profile of Elderlies with Proximal Femur Fracture by Low Energy Mechanism. *Rev. Bras. Ortop.* **2019**, *54*, 382–386.
54. Lizaur-Utrilla, A.; Gonzalez-Navarro, B.; Vizcaya-Moreno, M.F.; Lopez-Prats, F.A. Altered seric levels of albumin, sodium and parathyroid hormone may predict early mortality following hip fracture surgery in elderly. *Int. Orthop.* **2019**, *43*, 2825–2829. [CrossRef] [PubMed]
55. Gutierrez-Landaluce, C.; Acena, A.; Pello, A.; Martinez-Milla, J.; Gonzalez-Lorenzo, O.; Tarin, N.; Cristobal, C.; Blanco-Colio, L.M.; Martin-Ventura, J.L.; Huelmos, A.; et al. Parathormone levels add prognostic ability to N-terminal pro-brain natriuretic peptide in stable coronary patients. *ESC Heart Fail.* **2021**, *8*, 2713–2722. [CrossRef] [PubMed]
56. Kestenbaum, B.; Katz, R.; de Boer, I.; Hoofnagle, A.; Sarnak, M.J.; Shlipak, M.G.; Jenny, N.S.; Siscovick, D.S. Vitamin D, parathyroid hormone, and cardiovascular events among older adults. *J. Am. Coll. Cardiol.* **2011**, *58*, 1433–1441. [CrossRef]
57. Dadra, A.; Aggarwal, S.; Kumar, P.; Kumar, V.; Dibar, D.P.; Bhadada, S.K. High prevalence of vitamin D deficiency and osteoporosis in patients with fragility fractures of hip: A pilot study. *J. Clin. Orthop. Trauma* **2019**, *10*, 1097–1100. [CrossRef]
58. Lee, K.C.; Lee, I.O. Preoperative laboratory testing in elderly patients. *Curr. Opin. Anaesthesiol.* **2021**, *34*, 409–414. [CrossRef]
59. Meng, X.; Li, X.; Timofeeva, M.N.; He, Y.; Spiliopoulou, A.; Wei, W.Q.; Gifford, A.; Wu, H.; Varley, T.; Joshi, P.; et al. Phenome-wide Mendelian-randomization study of genetically determined vitamin D on multiple health outcomes using the UK Biobank study. *Int. J. Epidemiol.* **2019**, *48*, 1425–1434. [CrossRef]
60. Cosentino, N.; Campodonico, J.; Milazzo, V.; De Metrio, M.; Brambilla, M.; Camera, M.; Marenzi, G. Vitamin D and Cardiovascular Disease: Current Evidence and Future Perspectives. *Nutrients* **2021**, *13*, 3603. [CrossRef]
61. Navale, S.S.; Mulugeta, A.; Zhou, A.; Llewellyn, D.J.; Hypponen, E. Vitamin D and brain health: An observational and Mendelian randomization study. *Am. J. Clin. Nutr.* **2022**, *116*, 531–540. [CrossRef]
62. Thiele, K.; Cornelissen, A.; Florescu, R.; Kneizeh, K.; Brandenburg, V.M.; Witte, K.; Marx, N.; Schuh, A.; Stohr, R. The Role of Vitamin D3 as an Independent Predicting Marker for One-Year Mortality in Patients with Acute Heart Failure. *J. Clin. Med.* **2022**, *11*, 2733. [CrossRef] [PubMed]

63. Acharya, P.; Safarova, M.S.; Dalia, T.; Bharati, R.; Ranka, S.; Vindhyal, M.; Jiwani, S.; Barua, R.S. Effects of Vitamin D Supplementation and 25-Hydroxyvitamin D Levels on the Risk of Atrial Fibrillation. *Am. J. Cardiol.* **2022**, *173*, 56–63. [CrossRef] [PubMed]
64. Ruttmann, E.; Brant, L.J.; Concin, H.; Diem, G.; Rapp, K.; Ulmer, H.; Vorarlberg Health, M.; Promotion Program Study, G. Gamma-glutamyltransferase as a risk factor for cardiovascular disease mortality: An epidemiological investigation in a cohort of 163,944 Austrian adults. *Circulation* **2005**, *112*, 2130–2137. [CrossRef] [PubMed]
65. Lee, D.S.; Evans, J.C.; Robins, S.J.; Wilson, P.W.; Albano, I.; Fox, C.S.; Wang, T.J.; Benjamin, E.J.; D'Agostino, R.B.; Vasan, R.S. Gamma glutamyl transferase and metabolic syndrome, cardiovascular disease, and mortality risk: The Framingham Heart Study. *Arterioscler. Thromb. Vasc. Biol.* **2007**, *27*, 127–133. [CrossRef] [PubMed]
66. Ruhl, C.E.; Everhart, J.E. Elevated serum alanine aminotransferase and gamma-glutamyltransferase and mortality in the United States population. *Gastroenterology* **2009**, *136*, 477–485.e11. [CrossRef]
67. Targher, G. Elevated serum gamma-glutamyltransferase activity is associated with increased risk of mortality, incident type 2 diabetes, cardiovascular events, chronic kidney disease and cancer—A narrative review. *Clin. Chem. Lab. Med.* **2010**, *48*, 147–157. [CrossRef]
68. Dogan, A.; Icli, A.; Aksoy, F.; Varol, E.; Erdogan, D.; Ozaydin, M.; Kocyigit, S. Gamma-glutamyltransferase in acute coronary syndrome patients without ST elevation and its association with stenotic lesion and cardiac events. *Coron. Artery Dis.* **2012**, *23*, 39–44. [CrossRef]
69. Koenig, G.; Seneff, S. Gamma-Glutamyltransferase: A Predictive Biomarker of Cellular Antioxidant Inadequacy and Disease Risk. *Dis. Markers* **2015**, *2015*, 818570. [CrossRef]
70. Kunutsor, S.K. Gamma-glutamyltransferase-friend or foe within? *Liver Int.* **2016**, *36*, 1723–1734. [CrossRef]
71. Demirelli, S.; Firtina, S.; Askin, L.; Akgol Gur, S.T.; Tanrikulu, C.S.; Ermis, E.; Ipek, E.; Kalkan, K.; Yildirim, E.; Kiziltunc, A. Utility of gamma-Glutamyl Transferase in Predicting Troponin Elevation in Emergency Departments. *Angiology* **2016**, *67*, 737–741. [CrossRef]
72. Valjevac, A.; Rebic, D.; Hamzic-Mehmedbasic, A.; Sokolovic, E.; Horozic, D.; Vanis, N.; Hadzovic-Dzuvo, A. The value of gamma glutamyltransferase in predicting myocardial infarction in patients with acute coronary syndrome. *Future Cardiol.* **2018**, *14*, 37–45. [CrossRef] [PubMed]
73. Sun, D.; Liu, H.; Ouyang, Y.; Liu, X.; Xu, Y. Serum Levels of Gamma-Glutamyltransferase during Stable and Acute Exacerbations of Chronic Obstructive Pulmonary Disease. *Med. Sci. Monit.* **2020**, *26*, e927771. [CrossRef] [PubMed]
74. Danikiewicz, A.; Hudzik, B.; Nowak, J.; Kowalska, J.; Zielen-Zynek, I.; Szkodzinski, J.; Naung Tun, H.; Zubelewicz-Szkodzinska, B. Serum Gamma Glutamyltransferase Is Associated with 25-Hydroxyvitamin D Status in Elderly Patients with Stable Coronary Artery Disease. *Int. J. Environ. Res. Public Health* **2020**, *17*, 8980. [CrossRef] [PubMed]
75. Xing, Y.; Chen, J.; Liu, J.; Ma, H. Associations between GGT/HDL and MAFLD: A Cross-Sectional Study. *Diabetes Metab. Syndr. Obes.* **2022**, *15*, 383–394. [CrossRef] [PubMed]
76. Demirel, E.; Sahin, A. Predictive Value of Blood Parameters and Comorbidities on Three-Month Mortality in Elderly Patients with Hip Fracture. *Cureus* **2021**, *13*, e18634. [CrossRef] [PubMed]
77. Brozek, W.; Ulmer, H.; Pompella, A.; Nagel, G.; Leiherer, A.; Preyer, O.; Concin, H.; Zitt, E. Gamma-glutamyl-transferase is associated with incident hip fractures in women and men >/= 50 years: A large population-based cohort study. *Osteoporos. Int.* **2022**, *33*, 1295–1307. [CrossRef]
78. Takemura, K.; Yuasa, T.; Inamura, K.; Amori, G.; Koga, F.; Board, P.G.; Yonese, J. Impact of Serum gamma-Glutamyltransferase on Overall Survival in Patients with Metastatic Renal Cell Carcinoma in the Era of Targeted Therapy. *Target Oncol.* **2020**, *15*, 347–356. [CrossRef]
79. Lewis, J.R.; Hassan, S.K.; Wenn, R.T.; Moran, C.G. Mortality and serum urea and electrolytes on admission for hip fracture patients. *Injury* **2006**, *37*, 698–704. [CrossRef]
80. Turgut, N.; Unal, A.M. Standard and Newly Defined Prognostic Factors Affecting Early Mortality after Hip Fractures. *Cureus* **2022**, *14*, e21464. [CrossRef]
81. Kirtane, A.J.; Leder, D.M.; Waikar, S.S.; Chertow, G.M.; Ray, K.K.; Pinto, D.S.; Karmpaliotis, D.; Burger, A.J.; Murphy, S.A.; Cannon, C.P.; et al. Serum blood urea nitrogen as an independent marker of subsequent mortality among patients with acute coronary syndromes and normal to mildly reduced glomerular filtration rates. *J. Am. Coll. Cardiol.* **2005**, *45*, 1781–1786. [CrossRef]
82. Aronson, D.; Hammerman, H.; Beyar, R.; Yalonetsky, S.; Kapeliovich, M.; Markiewicz, W.; Goldberg, A. Serum blood urea nitrogen and long-term mortality in acute ST-elevation myocardial infarction. *Int. J. Cardiol.* **2008**, *127*, 380–385. [CrossRef] [PubMed]
83. Seyedi, H.R.; Mahdian, M.; Khosravi, G.; Bidgoli, M.S.; Mousavi, S.G.; Razavizadeh, M.R.; Mahdian, S.; Mohammadzadeh, M. Prediction of mortality in hip fracture patients: Role of routine blood tests. *Arch. Bone Jt. Surg.* **2015**, *3*, 51–55. [PubMed]
84. Horiuchi, Y.; Aoki, J.; Tanabe, K.; Nakao, K.; Ozaki, Y.; Kimura, K.; Ako, J.; Yasuda, S.; Noguchi, T.; Suwa, S.; et al. A High Level of Blood Urea Nitrogen Is a Significant Predictor for In-hospital Mortality in Patients with Acute Myocardial Infarction. *Int. Heart J.* **2018**, *59*, 263–271. [CrossRef] [PubMed]
85. Richter, B.; Sulzgruber, P.; Koller, L.; Steininger, M.; El-Hamid, F.; Rothgerber, D.J.; Forster, S.; Goliasch, G.; Silbert, B.I.; Meyer, E.L.; et al. Blood urea nitrogen has additive value beyond estimated glomerular filtration rate for prediction of long-term mortality in patients with acute myocardial infarction. *Eur. J. Intern. Med.* **2019**, *59*, 84–90. [CrossRef]

86. Liu, E.Q.; Zeng, C.L. Blood Urea Nitrogen and In-Hospital Mortality in Critically Ill Patients with Cardiogenic Shock: Analysis of the MIMIC-III Database. *Biomed. Res. Int.* **2021**, *2021*, 5948636. [CrossRef]
87. Adnan, M.; Hashmat, N.; Rahat, T.; Burki, A. Prognostic value of five serum markers predicting in-hospital mortality among adults with community acquired pneumonia. *J. Infect. Dev. Ctries.* **2022**, *16*, 166–172. [CrossRef]
88. Chen, L.; Chen, L.; Zheng, H.; Wu, S.; Wang, S. The association of blood urea nitrogen levels upon emergency admission with mortality in acute exacerbation of chronic obstructive pulmonary disease. *Chron. Respir. Dis.* **2021**, *18*, 14799731211060051. [CrossRef]
89. Wernly, B.; Lichtenauer, M.; Vellinga, N.A.R.; Boerma, E.C.; Ince, C.; Kelm, M.; Jung, C. Blood urea nitrogen (BUN) independently predicts mortality in critically ill patients admitted to ICU: A multicenter study. *Clin. Hemorheol. Microcirc.* **2018**, *69*, 123–131. [CrossRef]
90. Arihan, O.; Wernly, B.; Lichtenauer, M.; Franz, M.; Kabisch, B.; Muessig, J.; Masyuk, M.; Lauten, A.; Schulze, P.C.; Hoppe, U.C.; et al. Blood Urea Nitrogen (BUN) is independently associated with mortality in critically ill patients admitted to ICU. *PLoS ONE* **2018**, *13*, e0191697. [CrossRef]
91. Ebeling, F.; Lappalainen, M.; Vuoristo, M.; Nuutinen, H.; Leino, R.; Karvonen, A.L.; Lehtola, J.; Julkunen, R.; Pohjanpelto, P.; Farkkila, M. Factors predicting interferon treatment response in patients with chronic hepatitis c: Late viral clearance does not preclude a sustained response. *Am. J. Gastroenterol.* **2001**, *96*, 1237–1242. [CrossRef]
92. Ju, M.J.; Qiu, S.J.; Fan, J.; Zhou, J.; Gao, Q.; Cai, M.Y.; Li, Y.W.; Tang, Z.Y. Preoperative serum gamma-glutamyl transferase to alanine aminotransferase ratio is a convenient prognostic marker for Child-Pugh A hepatocellular carcinoma after operation. *J. Gastroenterol.* **2009**, *44*, 635–642. [CrossRef] [PubMed]
93. Zhou, X.; Wang, L.; Wang, G.; Cheng, X.; Hu, S.; Ke, W.; Li, M.; Zhang, Y.; Song, Z.; Zheng, Q. A new plasma biomarker enhance the clinical prediction of postoperative acute kidney injury in patients with hepatocellular carcinoma. *Clin. Chim. Acta* **2017**, *475*, 128–136. [CrossRef] [PubMed]
94. Zhang, Q.; Jiao, X. LDH and GGT/ALT Ratio as Novel Prognostic Biomarkers in Hepatocellular Carcinoma Patients after Liver Transplantation. *Comput. Math. Methods Med.* **2021**, *2021*, 9809990. [CrossRef] [PubMed]
95. Zhao, Z.; Zhu, Y.; Ni, X.; Lin, J.; Li, H.; Zheng, L.; Zhang, C.; Qi, X.; Huo, H.; Lou, X.; et al. Serum GGT/ALT ratio predicts vascular invasion in HBV-related HCC. *Cancer Cell. Int.* **2021**, *21*, 517. [CrossRef]
96. Zheng, Y.Y.; Wu, T.T.; Chen, Y.; Hou, X.G.; Yang, Y.; Ma, X.; Ma, Y.T.; Zhang, J.Y.; Xie, X. Gamma-glutamyl transferase to albumin ratio as a novel predictor of bleeding events and mortality in patients after percutaneous coronary intervention: A retrospective cohort study. *Catheter. Cardiovasc. Interv.* **2020**, *95* (Suppl. 1), 572–578. [CrossRef]
97. Li, H.; Liu, R.; Li, J.; Li, J.; Wu, H.; Wang, G.; Li, Z.; Li, D. Prognostic significance of gamma-glutamyl transpeptidase to albumin ratio in patients with intrahepatic cholangiocarcinoma after hepatectomy. *J. Cell. Mol. Med.* **2022**, *26*, 3196–3202. [CrossRef]
98. Zhao, D.; Chen, S.; Liu, Y.; Xu, Z.; Shen, H.; Zhang, S.; Li, Y.; Zhang, H.; Zou, C.; Ma, X. Blood Urea Nitrogen-to-Albumin Ratio in Predicting Long-Term Mortality in Patients Following Coronary Artery Bypass Grafting: An Analysis of the MIMIC-III Database. *Front. Surg.* **2022**, *9*, 801708. [CrossRef]
99. Xia, B.; Song, B.; Zhang, J.; Zhu, T.; Hu, H. Prognostic value of blood urea nitrogen-to-serum albumin ratio for mortality of pneumonia in patients receiving glucocorticoids: Secondary analysis based on a retrospective cohort study. *J. Infect. Chemother.* **2022**, *28*, 767–773. [CrossRef]
100. Milas, G.P.; Issaris, V.; Papavasileiou, V. Blood urea nitrogen to albumin ratio as a predictive factor for pneumonia: A meta-analysis. *Respir. Med. Res.* **2022**, *81*, 100886. [CrossRef]
101. He, T.; Li, G.; Xu, S.; Guo, L.; Tang, B. Blood Urea Nitrogen to Serum Albumin Ratio in the Prediction of Acute Kidney Injury of Patients with Rib Fracture in Intensive Care Unit. *Int. J. Gen. Med.* **2022**, *15*, 965–974. [CrossRef]
102. Ye, L.; Shi, H.; Wang, X.; Duan, Q.; Ge, P.; Shao, Y. Elevated Blood Urea Nitrogen to Serum Albumin Ratio Is an Adverse Prognostic Predictor for Patients Undergoing Cardiac Surgery. *Front. Cardiovasc. Med.* **2022**, *9*, 888736. [CrossRef] [PubMed]
103. Ma, C.; Li, R.; Yu, R.; Guo, J.; Xu, J.; Yuan, X.; Guo, J. Predictive value of preoperative platelet-to-albumin ratio and apolipoprotein B-to-apolipoprotein A1 ratio for osteosarcoma in children and adolescents: A retrospective study of 118 cases. *BMC Cancer* **2022**, *22*, 113. [CrossRef] [PubMed]
104. Yang, Y.; Yuan, J.; Liu, L.; Qie, S.; Yang, L.; Yan, Z. Platelet-to-albumin ratio: A risk factor associated with technique failure and mortality in peritoneal dialysis patients. *Ren. Fail.* **2021**, *43*, 1359–1367. [CrossRef] [PubMed]
105. Talsnes, O.; Hjelmstedt, F.; Dahl, O.E.; Pripp, A.H.; Reikeras, O. Biochemical lung, liver and kidney markers and early death among elderly following hip fracture. *Arch. Orthop. Trauma Surg.* **2012**, *132*, 1753–1758. [CrossRef] [PubMed]
106. Yardeni, D.; Toledano, R.; Novack, V.; Shalev, A.; Wolak, A.; Rotman, Y.; Etzion, O. The Association of Alanine Aminotransferase Levels with Myocardial Perfusion Imaging and Cardiovascular Morbidity. *J. Cardiovasc. Pharmacol. Ther.* **2022**, *27*, 10742484221074585. [CrossRef] [PubMed]
107. Kashkosh, R.; Gringauz, I.; Weissmann, J.; Segal, G.; Swartzon, M.; Adunsky, A.; Justo, D. Prerehabilitation alanine aminotransferase blood levels and one-year mortality rates in older adults following hip fracture. *Int. J. Rehabil. Res.* **2020**, *43*, 214–218. [CrossRef]
108. Kawamoto, R.; Kikuchi, A.; Akase, T.; Ninomiya, D.; Tokumoto, Y.; Kumagi, T. Association between alanine aminotransferase and all-cause mortality rate: Findings from a study on Japanese community-dwelling individuals. *J. Clin. Lab. Anal.* **2022**, *36*, e24445. [CrossRef]

109. Fisher, A.A.; Srikusalanukul, W.; Davis, M.W.; Smith, P.N. Clinical profiles and risk factors for outcomes in older patients with cervical and trochanteric hip fracture: Similarities and differences. *J. Trauma Manag. Outcomes* **2012**, *6*, 2. [CrossRef]
110. Fisher, L.; Srikusalanukul, W.; Fisher, A.; Smith, P. Liver function parameters in hip fracture patients: Relations to age, adipokines, comorbidities and outcomes. *Int. J. Med. Sci.* **2015**, *12*, 100–115. [CrossRef]
111. Devereaux, P.J.; Sessler, D.; Lalu, M. Myocardial injury after noncardiac surgery. *Can. J. Anaesth.* **2022**, *69*, 561–567. [CrossRef]
112. Linn, S.; Grunau, P.D. New patient-oriented summary measure of net total gain in certainty for dichotomous diagnostic tests. *Epidemiol. Perspect. Innov.* **2006**, *3*, 11. [CrossRef] [PubMed]
113. Larner, A.J. Number Needed to Diagnose, Predict, or Misdiagnose: Useful Metrics for Non-Canonical Signs of Cognitive Status? *Dement. Geriatr. Cogn. Dis. Extra* **2018**, *8*, 321–327. [CrossRef] [PubMed]
114. Hu, W.; Chen, Y.; Zhao, K.; Wang, J.; Zheng, M.; Zhao, Y.; Han, H.; Zhao, Q.; Zhao, X. Association of Perioperative Myocardial Injury with 30-Day and Long-Term Mortality in Older Adult Patients Undergoing Orthopedic Surgery in China. *Med. Sci. Monit.* **2021**, *27*, e932036. [CrossRef] [PubMed]
115. Sa-Ngasoongsong, P.; Thamyongkit, S.; Kulachote, N.; Luksameearunothai, K.; Ngamukos, T.; Suphachatwong, C. Usefulness of Serum Cardiac Biomarkers for Predicting In-Hospital Cardiac Complications in Acute Hip Fracture: A Prospective Cohort in 20 High Surgical Risk patients with Age over 55 Years. *Biomed. Res. Int.* **2018**, *2018*, 3453652. [CrossRef] [PubMed]
116. Chuang, A.M.; Nguyen, M.T.; Khan, E.; Jones, D.; Horsfall, M.; Lehman, S.; Smilowitz, N.R.; Lambrakis, K.; Than, M.; Vaile, J.; et al. Troponin elevation pattern and subsequent cardiac and non-cardiac outcomes: Implementing the Fourth Universal Definition of Myocardial Infarction and high-sensitivity troponin at a population level. *PLoS ONE* **2021**, *16*, e0248289. [CrossRef] [PubMed]
117. Sazgary, L.; Puelacher, C.; Lurati Buse, G.; Glarner, N.; Lampart, A.; Bolliger, D.; Steiner, L.; Gurke, L.; Wolff, T.; Mujagic, E.; et al. Incidence of major adverse cardiac events following non-cardiac surgery. *Eur. Heart J. Acute Cardiovasc. Care* **2020**, *10*, 550–558. [CrossRef]
118. Costa, M.; Furtado, M.V.; Borges, F.K.; Ziegelmann, P.K.; Suzumura, E.A.; Berwanger, O.; Devereaux, P.J.; Polanczyk, C.A. Perioperative Troponin Screening Identifies Patients at Higher Risk for Major Cardiovascular Events in Noncardiac Surgery. *Curr. Probl. Cardiol.* **2021**, *46*, 100429. [CrossRef]
119. Liu, J.; Huang, L.; Shi, X.; Gu, C.; Xu, H.; Liu, S. Clinical Parameters and Metabolomic Biomarkers That Predict Inhospital Outcomes in Patients With ST-Segment Elevated Myocardial Infarctions. *Front. Physiol.* **2021**, *12*, 820240. [CrossRef]
120. Fisher, A.A.; Goh, S.L.; Srikusalankul, W.; Southcott, E.N.; Davis, M.W. Serum leptin levels in older patients with hip fracture—Impact on peri-operative myocardial injury. *Am. Heart Hosp. J.* **2009**, *7*, 9–16. [CrossRef]
121. Fisher, A.; Srikusalanukul, W.; Davis, M.; Smith, P. Interactions between Serum Adipokines and Osteocalcin in Older Patients with Hip Fracture. *Int. J. Endocrinol.* **2012**, *2012*, 684323. [CrossRef]
122. Fisher, A.; Srikusalanukul, W.; Davis, M.; Smith, P. Cardiovascular diseases in older patients with osteoporotic hip fracture: Prevalence, disturbances in mineral and bone metabolism, and bidirectional links. *Clin. Interv. Aging* **2013**, *8*, 239–256. [CrossRef] [PubMed]
123. Nurmi-Luthje, I.; Luthje, P.; Kaukonen, J.P.; Kataja, M. Positive Effects of a Sufficient Pre-fracture Serum Vitamin D Level on the Long-Term Survival of Hip Fracture Patients in Finland: A Minimum 11-Year Follow-Up. *Drugs Aging* **2015**, *32*, 477–486. [CrossRef] [PubMed]
124. Fakler, J.K.; Grafe, A.; Dinger, J.; Josten, C.; Aust, G. Perioperative risk factors in patients with a femoral neck fracture—Influence of 25-hydroxyvitamin D and C-reactive protein on postoperative medical complications and 1-year mortality. *BMC Musculoskelet. Disord.* **2016**, *17*, 51. [CrossRef]
125. Grubler, M.R.; Marz, W.; Pilz, S.; Grammer, T.B.; Trummer, C.; Mullner, C.; Schwetz, V.; Pandis, M.; Verheyen, N.; Tomaschitz, A.; et al. Vitamin-D concentrations, cardiovascular risk and events—A review of epidemiological evidence. *Rev. Endocr. Metab. Disord.* **2017**, *18*, 259–272. [CrossRef]
126. Cher, E.W.L.; Allen, J.C.; Moo, I.H.; Lo, E.C.; Peh, B.; Howe, T.S.; Koh, J.S.B. Sub-optimal serum 25-hydroxyvitamin D level affects 2-year survival after hip fracture surgery. *J. Bone Miner. Metab.* **2020**, *38*, 555–562. [CrossRef]
127. Pilz, S.; Tomaschitz, A.; Marz, W.; Drechsler, C.; Ritz, E.; Zittermann, A.; Cavalier, E.; Pieber, T.R.; Lappe, J.M.; Grant, W.B.; et al. Vitamin D, cardiovascular disease and mortality. *Clin. Endocrinol.* **2011**, *75*, 575–584. [CrossRef]
128. Boccardi, V.; Lapenna, M.; Gaggi, L.; Garaffa, F.M.; Croce, M.F.; Baroni, M.; Ercolani, S.; Mecocci, P.; Ruggiero, C. Hypovitaminosis D: A Disease Marker in Hospitalized Very Old Persons at Risk of Malnutrition. *Nutrients.* **2019**, *11*, 128. [CrossRef] [PubMed]
129. Ismailova, A.; White, J.H. Vitamin D, infections and immunity. *Rev. Endocr. Metab. Disord.* **2022**, *23*, 265–277. [CrossRef] [PubMed]
130. Dong, C.; Hu, X.; Tripathi, A.S. A brief review of vitamin D as a potential target for the regulation of blood glucose and inflammation in diabetes-associated periodontitis. *Mol. Cell. Biochem.* **2022**, *477*, 2257–2268. [CrossRef] [PubMed]
131. Matta Reddy, A.; Iqbal, M.; Chopra, H.; Urmi, S.; Junapudi, S.; Bibi, S.; Kumar Gupta, S.; Nirmala Pangi, V.; Singh, I.; Abdel-Daim, M.M. Pivotal role of vitamin D in mitochondrial health, cardiac function, and human reproduction. *EXCLI J.* **2022**, *21*, 967–990.
132. Mohd Ghozali, N.; Giribabu, N.; Salleh, N. Mechanisms Linking Vitamin D Deficiency to Impaired Metabolism: An Overview. *Int. J. Endocrinol.* **2022**, *2022*, 6453882. [CrossRef] [PubMed]
133. Alarcon, T.; Gonzalez-Montalvo, J.I.; Hoyos, R.; Diez-Sebastian, J.; Otero, A.; Mauleon, J.L. Parathyroid hormone response to two levels of vitamin D deficiency is associated with high risk of medical problems during hospitalization in patients with hip fracture. *J. Endocrinol. Investig.* **2015**, *38*, 1129–1135. [CrossRef] [PubMed]

134. Goldman, L.; Caldera, D.L.; Nussbaum, S.R.; Southwick, F.S.; Krogstad, D.; Murray, B.; Burke, D.S.; O'Malley, T.A.; Goroll, A.H.; Caplan, C.H.; et al. Multifactorial index of cardiac risk in noncardiac surgical procedures. *N. Engl. J. Med.* **1977**, *297*, 845–850. [CrossRef] [PubMed]
135. Detsky, A.S.; Abrams, H.B.; Forbath, N.; Scott, J.G.; Hilliard, J.R. Cardiac assessment for patients undergoing noncardiac surgery. A multifactorial clinical risk index. *Arch. Intern. Med.* **1986**, *146*, 2131–2134. [CrossRef] [PubMed]
136. Lee, T.H.; Marcantonio, E.R.; Mangione, C.M.; Thomas, E.J.; Polanczyk, C.A.; Cook, E.F.; Sugarbaker, D.J.; Donaldson, M.C.; Poss, R.; Ho, K.K.; et al. Derivation and prospective validation of a simple index for prediction of cardiac risk of major noncardiac surgery. *Circulation* **1999**, *100*, 1043–1049. [CrossRef] [PubMed]
137. Azevedo, P.S.; Gumieiro, D.N.; Polegato, B.F.; Pereira, G.J.; Silva, I.A.; Pio, S.M.; Junior, C.P.; Junior, E.L.; de Paiva, S.A.; Minicucci, M.F.; et al. Goldman score, but not Detsky or Lee indices, predicts mortality 6 months after hip fracture. *BMC Musculoskelet. Disord.* **2017**, *18*, 134. [CrossRef]
138. Wu, H.H.L.; Van Mierlo, R.; McLauchlan, G.; Challen, K.; Mitra, S.; Dhaygude, A.P.; Nixon, A.C. Prognostic performance of clinical assessment tools following hip fracture in patients with chronic kidney disease. *Int. Urol. Nephrol.* **2021**, *53*, 2359–2367. [CrossRef]
139. Xing, F.; Luo, R.; Liu, M.; Zhou, Z.; Xiang, Z.; Duan, X. A New Random Forest Algorithm-Based Prediction Model of Post-operative Mortality in Geriatric Patients With Hip Fractures. *Front. Med.* **2022**, *9*, 829977. [CrossRef]
140. Li, Y.; Chen, M.; Lv, H.; Yin, P.; Zhang, L.; Tang, P. A novel machine-learning algorithm for predicting mortality risk after hip fracture surgery. *Injury* **2021**, *52*, 1487–1493. [CrossRef]
141. Karres, J.; Kieviet, N.; Eerenberg, J.P.; Vrouenraets, B.C. Predicting Early Mortality after Hip Fracture Surgery: The Hip Fracture Estimator of Mortality Amsterdam. *J. Orthop. Trauma* **2018**, *32*, 27–33. [CrossRef]
142. Jiang, H.X.; Majumdar, S.R.; Dick, D.A.; Moreau, M.; Raso, J.; Otto, D.D.; Johnston, D.W. Development and initial validation of a risk score for predicting in-hospital and 1-year mortality in patients with hip fractures. *J. Bone Miner. Res.* **2005**, *20*, 494–500. [CrossRef] [PubMed]
143. Nijmeijer, W.S.; Folbert, E.C.; Vermeer, M.; Slaets, J.P.; Hegeman, J.H. Prediction of early mortality following hip fracture surgery in frail elderly: The Almelo Hip Fracture Score (AHFS). *Injury* **2016**, *47*, 2138–2143. [CrossRef] [PubMed]
144. Mellner, C.; Eisler, T.; Borsbo, J.; Broden, C.; Morberg, P.; Mukka, S. The Sernbo score predicts 1-year mortality after displaced femoral neck fractures treated with a hip arthroplasty. *Acta Orthop.* **2017**, *88*, 402–406. [CrossRef]
145. Hjelholt, T.J.; Johnsen, S.P.; Brynningsen, P.K.; Knudsen, J.S.; Prieto-Alhambra, D.; Pedersen, A.B. Development and validation of a model for predicting mortality in patients with hip fracture. *Age Ageing* **2022**, *51*, afab233. [CrossRef] [PubMed]
146. Tsang, C.; Boulton, C.; Burgon, V.; Johansen, A.; Wakeman, R.; Cromwell, D.A. Predicting 30-day mortality after hip fracture surgery: Evaluation of the National Hip Fracture Database case-mix adjustment model. *Bone Jt. Res.* **2017**, *6*, 550–556. [CrossRef] [PubMed]
147. Tang, P.L.; Lin, H.S.; Hsu, C.J. Predicting in-hospital mortality for dementia patients after hip fracture surgery—A comparison between the Charlson Comorbidity Index (CCI) and the Elixhauser Comorbidity Index. *J. Orthop. Sci.* **2021**, *26*, 396–402. [CrossRef]
148. Varady, N.H.; Gillinov, S.M.; Yeung, C.M.; Rudisill, S.S.; Chen, A.F. The Charlson and Elixhauser Scores Outperform the American Society of Anesthesiologists Score in Assessing 1-year Mortality Risk After Hip Fracture Surgery. *Clin. Orthop. Relat. Res.* **2021**, *479*, 1970–1979. [CrossRef]
149. Quach, L.H.; Jayamaha, S.; Whitehouse, S.L.; Crawford, R.; Pulle, C.R.; Bell, J.J. Comparison of the Charlson Comorbidity Index with the ASA score for predicting 12-month mortality in acute hip fracture. *Injury* **2020**, *51*, 1004–1010. [CrossRef]
150. Sun, X.; Chen, Y.; Gao, Y.; Zhang, Z.; Qin, L.; Song, J.; Wang, H.; Wu, I.X. Prediction Models for Osteoporotic Fractures Risk: A Systematic Review and Critical Appraisal. *Aging Dis.* **2022**, *13*, 1215–1238. [CrossRef]
151. Kaafarani, H.M.; Atluri, P.V.; Thornby, J.; Itani, K.M. beta-Blockade in noncardiac surgery: Outcome at all levels of cardiac risk. *Arch. Surg.* **2008**, *143*, 940–944; discussion 944. [CrossRef]
152. Auerbach, A.D.; Goldman, L. beta-Blockers and reduction of cardiac events in noncardiac surgery: Scientific review. *JAMA* **2002**, *287*, 1435–1444. [PubMed]
153. Talati, R.; Reinhart, K.M.; White, C.M.; Phung, O.J.; Sedrakyan, A.; Kluger, J.; Coleman, C.I. Outcomes of perioperative beta-blockade in patients undergoing noncardiac surgery: A meta-analysis. *Ann. Pharmacother.* **2009**, *43*, 1181–1188. [CrossRef] [PubMed]
154. Priebe, H.J. Perioperative use of beta-blockers. *F1000 Med. Rep.* **2009**, *1*, 77. [CrossRef] [PubMed]
155. Van Klei, W.A.; Bryson, G.L.; Yang, H.; Forster, A.J. Effect of beta-blocker prescription on the incidence of postoperative myocardial infarction after hip and knee arthroplasty. *Anesthesiology* **2009**, *111*, 717–724. [CrossRef]
156. Angeli, F.; Verdecchia, P.; Karthikeyan, G.; Mazzotta, G.; Gentile, G.; Reboldi, G. ss-Blockers reduce mortality in patients undergoing high-risk non-cardiac surgery. *Am. J. Cardiovasc. Drugs* **2010**, *10*, 247–259. [CrossRef]
157. Koniari, I.; Hahalis, G. Perioperative B-blockers in non-cardiac surgery: Actual situation. *Curr. Pharm. Des.* **2013**, *19*, 3946–3962. [CrossRef]
158. Andersson, C.; Merie, C.; Jorgensen, M.; Gislason, G.H.; Torp-Pedersen, C.; Overgaard, C.; Kober, L.; Jensen, P.F.; Hlatky, M.A. Association of beta-blocker therapy with risks of adverse cardiovascular events and deaths in patients with ischemic heart disease undergoing noncardiac surgery: A Danish nationwide cohort study. *JAMA Intern. Med.* **2014**, *174*, 336–344. [CrossRef]

159. Dimmitt, S.B.; Stampfer, H.G.; Warren, J.B.; Paech, M.J. Hazards of perioperative beta-blockers are likely to be dose related. *Br. J. Anaesth.* **2015**, *115*, 944. [CrossRef]
160. Mostafaie, K.; Bedenis, R.; Harrington, D. Beta-adrenergic blockers for perioperative cardiac risk reduction in people undergoing vascular surgery. *Cochrane Database Syst. Rev.* **2015**, *1*, CD006342. [CrossRef]
161. Blessberger, H.; Lewis, S.R.; Pritchard, M.W.; Fawcett, L.J.; Domanovits, H.; Schlager, O.; Wildner, B.; Kammler, J.; Steinwender, C. Perioperative beta-blockers for preventing surgery-related mortality and morbidity in adults undergoing non-cardiac surgery. *Cochrane Database Syst. Rev.* **2019**, *9*, CD013438. [CrossRef]
162. Wongcharoen, W.; Chotayaporn, T.; Chutikhongchalermroj, K.; Tantraworasin, A.; Saeteng, S.; Arworn, S.; Rerkasem, K.; Phrommintikul, A. Effects of short-term bisoprolol on perioperative myocardial injury in patients undergoing non-cardiac surgery: A randomized control study. *Sci. Rep.* **2021**, *11*, 22006. [CrossRef] [PubMed]
163. Oprea, A.D.; Wang, X.; Sickeler, R.; Kertai, M.D. Contemporary personalized beta-blocker management in the perioperative setting. *J. Anesth.* **2020**, *34*, 115–133. [CrossRef] [PubMed]
164. Lewis, S.R.; Pritchard, M.W.; Schofield-Robinson, O.J.; Alderson, P.; Smith, A.F. Continuation versus discontinuation of antiplatelet therapy for bleeding and ischaemic events in adults undergoing non-cardiac surgery. *Cochrane Database Syst. Rev.* **2018**, *7*, CD012584. [CrossRef] [PubMed]
165. Rodriguez, A.; Guilera, N.; Mases, A.; Sierra, P.; Oliva, J.C.; Colilles, C.; REGISTRESTENTS Group. Management of antiplatelet therapy in patients with coronary stents undergoing noncardiac surgery: Association with adverse events. *Br. J. Anaesth.* **2018**, *120*, 67–76. [CrossRef]
166. Howell, S.J.; Hoeks, S.E.; West, R.M.; Wheatcroft, S.B.; Hoeft, A.; Network, O.I.o.E.S.o.A.C.T. Prospective observational cohort study of the association between antiplatelet therapy, bleeding and thrombosis in patients with coronary stents undergoing noncardiac surgery. *Br. J. Anaesth.* **2019**, *122*, 170–179. [CrossRef]
167. Tarrant, S.M.; Kim, R.G.; McGregor, K.L.; Palazzi, K.; Attia, J.; Balogh, Z.J. Dual Antiplatelet Therapy and Surgical Timing in Geriatric Hip Fracture. *J. Orthop. Trauma.* **2020**, *34*, 559–565. [CrossRef]
168. Yang, M.H.; Li, B.; Yao, D.C.; Zhou, Y.; Zhang, W.C.; Wang, G.; Zhang, P.; Zhu, S.W.; Wu, X.B. Safety of early surgery for geriatric hip fracture patients taking clopidogrel: A retrospective case-control study of 120 patients in China. *Chin. Med. J.* **2021**, *134*, 1720–1725. [CrossRef]
169. Kim, C.; Kim, J.S.; Kim, H.; Ahn, S.G.; Cho, S.; Lee, O.H.; Park, J.K.; Shin, S.; Moon, J.Y.; Won, H.; et al. Consensus Decision-Making for the Management of Antiplatelet Therapy before Non-Cardiac Surgery in Patients Who Underwent Percutaneous Coronary Intervention With Second-Generation Drug-Eluting Stents: A Cohort Study. *J. Am. Heart Assoc.* **2021**, *10*, e020079. [CrossRef]
170. Lee, S.H.; Kim, J.A.; Heo, B.; Kim, Y.R.; Ahn, H.J.; Yang, M.; Jang, J.; Ahn, S. Association between intraoperative hypotension and postoperative myocardial injury in patients with prior coronary stents undergoing high-risk surgery: A retrospective study. *J. Anesth.* **2020**, *34*, 257–267. [CrossRef]
171. Jantzen, C.; Madsen, C.M.; Abrahamsen, B.; Van Der Mark, S.; Duus, B.R.; Howland, J.; Lauritzen, J.B.; Jorgensen, H.L. Pre-fracture medication use as a predictor of 30-day mortality in hip fracture patients: An analysis of 141,201 patients. *Hip. Int.* **2020**, *30*, 101–106. [CrossRef]
172. Langerhuizen, D.W.G.; Verweij, L.P.E.; van der Wouden, J.C.; Kerkhoffs, G.; Janssen, S.J. Antihypertensive drugs demonstrate varying levels of hip fracture risk: A systematic review and meta-analysis. *Injury* **2022**, *53*, 1098–1107. [CrossRef] [PubMed]
173. Zhao, N.; Xu, J.; Singh, B.; Yu, X.; Wu, T.; Huang, Y. Nitrates for the prevention of cardiac morbidity and mortality in patients undergoing non-cardiac surgery. *Cochrane Database Syst. Rev.* **2016**, CD010726. [CrossRef] [PubMed]
174. Duncan, D.; Sankar, A.; Beattie, W.S.; Wijeysundera, D.N. Alpha-2 adrenergic agonists for the prevention of cardiac complications among adults undergoing surgery. *Cochrane Database Syst. Rev.* **2018**, *3*, CD004126. [CrossRef]
175. Park, J.; Lee, J.H. Myocardial injury in noncardiac surgery. *Korean. J. Anesthesiol.* **2022**, *75*, 4–11. [CrossRef] [PubMed]
176. Khan, J.; Alonso-Coello, P.; Devereaux, P.J. Myocardial injury after noncardiac surgery. *Curr. Opin. Cardiol.* **2014**, *29*, 307–311. [CrossRef] [PubMed]
177. Sakuma, M.; Endo, N.; Oinuma, T. Serum 25-OHD insufficiency as a risk factor for hip fracture. *J. Bone Miner. Metab.* **2007**, *25*, 147–150. [CrossRef] [PubMed]
178. Feng, Y.; Cheng, G.; Wang, H.; Chen, B. The associations between serum 25-hydroxyvitamin D level and the risk of total fracture and hip fracture. *Osteoporos. Int.* **2017**, *28*, 1641–1652. [CrossRef]
179. Wang, N.; Chen, Y.; Ji, J.; Chang, J.; Yu, S.; Yu, B. The relationship between serum vitamin D and fracture risk in the elderly: A meta-analysis. *J. Orthop. Surg. Res.* **2020**, *15*, 81. [CrossRef]
180. Dretakis, K.; Igoumenou, V.G. The role of parathyroid hormone (PTH) and vitamin D in falls and hip fracture type. *Aging Clin. Exp. Res.* **2019**, *31*, 1501–1507. [CrossRef]
181. Lo, I.L.; Siu, C.W.; Tse, H.F.; Lau, T.W.; Leung, F.; Wong, M. Pre-operative pulmonary assessment for patients with hip fracture. *Osteoporos. Int.* **2010**, *21*, S579–S586. [CrossRef]
182. Laulund, A.S.; Lauritzen, J.B.; Duus, B.R.; Mosfeldt, M.; Jorgensen, H.L. Routine blood tests as predictors of mortality in hip fracture patients. *Injury* **2012**, *43*, 1014–1020. [CrossRef] [PubMed]
183. Mosfeldt, M.; Pedersen, O.B.; Riis, T.; Worm, H.O.; Mark, S.; Jorgensen, H.L.; Duus, B.R.; Lauritzen, J.B. Value of routine blood tests for prediction of mortality risk in hip fracture patients. *Acta Orthop.* **2012**, *83*, 31–35. [CrossRef] [PubMed]

184. Cabrerizo, S.; Cuadras, D.; Gomez-Busto, F.; Artaza-Artabe, I.; Marin-Ciancas, F.; Malafarina, V. Serum albumin and health in older people: Review and meta analysis. *Maturitas* **2015**, *81*, 17–27. [CrossRef]
185. Bohl, D.D.; Shen, M.R.; Hannon, C.P.; Fillingham, Y.A.; Darrith, B.; Della Valle, C.J. Serum Albumin Predicts Survival and Postoperative Course Following Surgery for Geriatric Hip Fracture. *J. Bone Jt. Surg. Am.* **2017**, *99*, 2110–2118. [CrossRef] [PubMed]
186. Ryan, S.; Politzer, C.; Fletcher, A.; Bolognesi, M.; Seyler, T. Preoperative Hypoalbuminemia Predicts Poor Short-term Outcomes for Hip Fracture Surgery. *Orthopedics* **2018**, *41*, e789–e796. [CrossRef]
187. Higashikawa, T.; Shigemoto, K.; Goshima, K.; Horii, T.; Usuda, D.; Morita, T.; Moriyama, M.; Inujima, H.; Hangyou, M.; Usuda, K.; et al. Mortality and the Risk Factors in Elderly Female Patients with Femoral Neck and Trochanteric Fractures. *J. Clin. Med. Res.* **2020**, *12*, 668–673. [CrossRef]
188. Shin, K.H.; Kim, J.J.; Son, S.W.; Hwang, K.S.; Han, S.B. Early Postoperative Hypoalbuminaemia as a Risk Factor for Postoperative Pneumonia Following Hip Fracture Surgery. *Clin. Interv. Aging* **2020**, *15*, 1907–1915. [CrossRef]
189. Tian, Y.; Zhu, Y.; Zhang, K.; Tian, M.; Qin, S.; Li, X. Relationship Between Preoperative Hypoalbuminemia and Postoperative Pneumonia Following Geriatric Hip Fracture Surgery: A Propensity-Score Matched and Conditional Logistic Regression Analysis. *Clin. Interv. Aging* **2022**, *17*, 495–503. [CrossRef]
190. Gringauz, I.; Weismann, J.; Justo, D.; Adunsky, A.; Segal, G. Alanine aminotransferase blood levels and rehabilitation outcome in older adults following hip fracture surgery. *Int. J. Rehabil. Res.* **2018**, *41*, 41–46. [CrossRef]
191. Kim, K.J.; Hong, N.; Yu, M.H.; Lee, S.; Shin, S.; Kim, S.G.; Rhee, Y. Elevated gamma-glutamyl transpeptidase level is associated with an increased risk of hip fracture in postmenopausal women. *Sci. Rep.* **2022**, *12*, 13947. [CrossRef]
192. Powell, J.; Michael, A. Peri-operative derangement in liver function tests in older patients with neck of femur fracture. *Osteoporos. Int.* **2021**, *32*, 1027–1030. [CrossRef] [PubMed]
193. Cannada, L.K. CORR Insights(R): Hip Fractures in Patients with Liver Cirrhosis: Worsening Liver Function is Associated with Increased Mortality. *Clin. Orthop. Relat. Res.* **2022**, *480*, 1089–1090. [CrossRef] [PubMed]
194. Tseng, F.J.; Gou, G.H.; Wang, S.H.; Shyu, J.F.; Pan, R.Y. Chronic liver disease and cirrhosis increase morbidity in geriatric patients treated surgically for hip fractures: Analysis of the US Nationwide Inpatient Sample. *BMC Geriatr.* **2022**, *22*, 150. [CrossRef] [PubMed]
195. Hundersmarck, D.; Groot, O.Q.; Schuijt, H.J.; Hietbrink, F.; Leenen, L.P.H.; Heng, M. Hip Fractures in Patients With Liver Cirrhosis: Worsening Liver Function Is Associated with Increased Mortality. *Clin. Orthop. Relat. Res.* **2022**, *480*, 1077–1088. [CrossRef] [PubMed]
196. Onochie, E.; Kayani, B.; Dawson-Bowling, S.; Millington, S.; Achan, P.; Hanna, S. Total hip arthroplasty in patients with chronic liver disease: A systematic review. *SICOT J.* **2019**, *5*, 40. [CrossRef]
197. Ryan, G.; Nowak, L.; Melo, L.; Ward, S.; Atrey, A.; Schemitsch, E.H.; Nauth, A.; Khoshbin, A. Anemia at Presentation Predicts Acute Mortality and Need for Readmission Following Geriatric Hip Fracture. *JB JS Open Access* **2020**, *5*, e20.00048. [CrossRef]
198. Hagino, T.; Ochiai, S.; Sato, E.; Maekawa, S.; Wako, M.; Haro, H. The relationship between anemia at admission and outcome in patients older than 60 years with hip fracture. *J. Orthop. Traumatol.* **2009**, *10*, 119–122. [CrossRef]
199. Vochteloo, A.J.; Borger van der Burg, B.L.; Mertens, B.; Niggebrugge, A.H.; de Vries, M.R.; Tuinebreijer, W.E.; Bloem, R.M.; Nelissen, R.G.; Pilot, P. Outcome in hip fracture patients related to anemia at admission and allogeneic blood transfusion: An analysis of 1262 surgically treated patients. *BMC Musculoskelet. Disord.* **2011**, *12*, 262. [CrossRef]
200. Fisher, A.; Srikusalanukul, W.; Fisher, L.; Smith, P. The Neutrophil to Lymphocyte Ratio on Admission and Short-Term Outcomes in Orthogeriatric Patients. *Int. J. Med. Sci.* **2016**, *13*, 588–602. [CrossRef]
201. Forget, P.; Dillien, P.; Engel, H.; Cornu, O.; De Kock, M.; Yombi, J.C. Use of the neutrophil-to-lymphocyte ratio as a component of a score to predict postoperative mortality after surgery for hip fracture in elderly subjects. *BMC Res. Notes.* **2016**, *9*, 284. [CrossRef]
202. Aali-Rezaie, A.; Alijanipour, P.; Shohat, N.; Vahedi, H.; Foltz, C.; Parvizi, J. Red Cell Distribution Width: An Unacknowledged Predictor of Mortality and Adverse Outcomes Following Revision Arthroplasty. *J. Arthroplasty* **2018**, *33*, 3514–3519. [CrossRef] [PubMed]
203. Yin, P.; Lv, H.; Li, Y.; Meng, Y.; Zhang, L.; Zhang, L.; Tang, P. Hip fracture patients who experience a greater fluctuation in RDW during hospital course are at heightened risk for all-cause mortality: A prospective study with 2-year follow-up. *Osteoporos. Int.* **2018**, *29*, 1559–1567. [CrossRef] [PubMed]

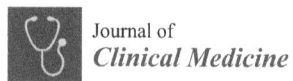

Article

Long Term Effectiveness of ESWT in Plantar Fasciitis in Amateur Runners

Joanna Kapusta [1,*] and Marcin Domżalski [2]

[1] Department of Internal Diseases, Rehabilitation and Physical Medicine, Medical University of Łódź, 70-445 Lodz, Poland
[2] Department of Orthopaedics and Trauma, Veteran's Memorial Hospital, Medical University of Lodz, Zeromskiego 113, 90-549 Lodz, Poland
* Correspondence: joanna.kapusta@umed.lodz.pl

Abstract: Background: Shock wave therapy is one of the modern methods of treatment used to treat diseases of muscles, tendons, and entheses in orthopedics, as well as in sports medicine. The therapy is increasingly used in the treatment of plantar fasciitis—a disease that is very difficult and burdensome to treat. Where basic conservative treatment for heel spurs fails, the only alternative consists of excision of the bone outgrowth, and shock wave therapy: a modern, minimally invasive, and relatively safe method. The aim of the study was to determine the long-term effectiveness of extracorporeal shock wave therapy in the treatment of painful ailments occurring in the course of plantar fasciitis in amateur runners. Materials and methods: The study includes a group of 39 men and women, aged 34–64 (mean age 54.05 ± 8.16), suffering from chronic pain in one or both feet, occurring in the course of plantar fasciitis. The patients had to meet five criteria to qualify for the study. The group was divided into two subgroups: those who had not undergone other physiotherapeutic procedures prior to the extracorporeal shock wave therapy (ESWT-alone; 23 people), and those who had received other procedures (ESWT-plus; 16 people). The therapy was performed using extracorporeal shock wave (ESWT). No local anesthesia was used. The effectiveness of the extracorporeal shock wave therapy was evaluated using the visual analogue scale of pain (VAS), Modified Laitinen Pain Index Questionnaire, the AOFAS scale (American Orthopedic Foot and Ankle Society), and a survey questionnaire consisting of 10 questions concerning metrics and subjective assessment of the effects of therapy. The interview was conducted before ESWT, and again five years later. Results: The use of extracorporeal shock wave therapy reduced the intensity and frequency of pain, and improved daily and recreational activity. Moreover, a reduction in the level of pain sensation on the VAS scale and pain symptoms during walking was demonstrated. More favorable results were obtained in the ESWT-plus group; however, the first effects were observed later than in the ESWT-alone group. Conclusions: Extracorporeal shock wave therapy is an effective form of therapy for amateur runners. It reduces pain associated with plantar fasciitis that amateur runners may experience at rest, while walking, and during daily and recreational activity.

Keywords: extracorporeal shock wave; heel spur; plantar fascia; rehabilitation; sports medicine

Citation: Kapusta, J.; Domżalski, M. Long Term Effectiveness of ESWT in Plantar Fasciitis in Amateur Runners. *J. Clin. Med.* **2022**, *11*, 6926. https://doi.org/10.3390/jcm11236926

Academic Editor: Umile Giuseppe Longo

Received: 12 November 2022
Accepted: 21 November 2022
Published: 24 November 2022

Publisher's Note: MDPI stays neutral with regard to jurisdictional claims in published maps and institutional affiliations.

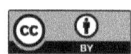

Copyright: © 2022 by the authors. Licensee MDPI, Basel, Switzerland. This article is an open access article distributed under the terms and conditions of the Creative Commons Attribution (CC BY) license (https://creativecommons.org/licenses/by/4.0/).

1. Introduction

Plantar fasciitis with an accompanying heel spur is very burdensome and difficult to treat disease [1–5]. It most often arises as a result of degenerative changes of the proximal plantar fascia and the tissues surrounding the aponeurosis, occurring due to continuous irritation of the area and resulting micro-injuries [6,7].

The main symptom of plantar fasciitis is pain in the heel area; this worsens over time, increasingly occurring upon loading and eventually, even at rest. Redness and swelling are also observed in the heel. The risk of the disease is increased by being overweight, working a job that requires long periods of standing, lifting heavy objects, intensive running, and practicing jumping sports [6–8].

Conservative treatment consists of strengthening the long muscles of the foot, relieving the painful area with special orthopedic insoles that have an opening for the heel in the place corresponding to the presence of bone growth. Appropriate body weight should be maintained and prolonged overloading of the foot should be avoided. While pharmacotherapy, radiation with X-rays [9,10] and physical therapy can be used, this conservative treatment is very frequently insufficient, and the only alternative is surgery consisting of excision of bone spurs. As such, shockwave therapy is becoming increasingly popular among doctors [4,6–9].

Shock wave therapy is a modern method based on the application of mechanical pressure waves directly to the affected tissues. Although it was initially used for crushing inoperable kidney stones, it is increasingly used in the treatment of lesions located within the musculoskeletal apparatus [1–3].

The mechanical waves can be generated by extracorporeal shock wave therapy (ESWT) or radial shock wave therapy (RSWT) [1,2,4]. An extracorporeal shock wave is characterized by deep penetration, a short pulse rise time with the steepness of the wave formed in the tissue, a frequency within the range of 1–22 Hz, as well as a very high energy of generated pulses, reaching even 120 MPa within the treated location [11–14]. The extracorporeal shock wave treatment has a very intense impact, and therefore local anesthesia is very often necessary during the procedure [12–14]. Radial shock wave therapy (RSWT), in contrast, is characterized by lower parameters, lower impact force, and a smaller range of penetration. Despite this, the two wave types have very similar therapeutic effects [1,2,4,15,16].

The mechanism of shockwave functioning is not fully understood. Initially, it was believed that the therapy induced positive therapeutic effects due to a structural breakdown of cells at the microstructural level, resulting in the activation of tissue regeneration processes [3,12,17]. It is now known that, at energy levels below the tissue destruction level, the shock wave also causes a range of other tissue responses and metabolic effects. These changes can increase joint mobility, and result in long-term pain relief and the restoration of normal muscle tone. The principal effects observed during shock wave therapy include reduction of pain, elimination of the source of pain, reduction of muscle tension, and improvement of the function of tissue structures, as well as induction of congestion and activation of regenerative processes [1,4]. However, the shock wave can also cause adverse effects, such as reddening of the skin, hematomas, or local swelling [1,12,17].

The Aim of the Study

The aim of the study was to determine the long-term effectiveness of extracorporeal shock wave therapy in the treatment of painful ailments occurring in the course of plantar fasciitis in amateur runners.

2. Materials and Methods
2.1. Characteristics of the Study Participants

A group of 48 consecutive patients with the diagnosis of plantar fasciitis were identified and examined. Of these, 39 met inclusion criteria and were enrolled in the study.

Inclusion criteria comprised the following: plantar fasciitis (with/without heel spur) confirmed by sonographic examination, prescribed shock wave therapy treatments, no participation in other physical therapy procedures during ESWT therapy, consent given by the subject. The exclusion criteria comprised any lesion or rupture of the plantar fascia found during sonographic examination, systemic inflammatory or autoimmune disorders, previous surgeries of the lower limbs, hereditary deformations of the skeleton, any other contraindications to participating in the study. Patients included in the study did not receive any physical therapy prior to inclusion.

Patient age, sex, involvement side, height, weight, and type of work performed were collected from medical records. The effectiveness of extracorporeal shock wave therapy (ESWT) was determined using the visual analogue scale of pain (VAS), Modified Laitinen

Pain Index Questionnaire, AOFAS score (American Orthopedic Foot and Ankle Society) and a questionnaire about the subjective assessment of the effects of therapy.

Prior to participation, the patients were informed of the study objectives and how the study would be conducted, after which they provided their informed consent to participate in the study. The study was conducted according to the guidelines of the Declaration of Helsinki and approved by the Bioethics Committee of the Medical University of Lodz, Poland (approval number RNN/879/11/KB).

2.2. Study Program

After the initial qualification of patients for the study, in order to avoid bias, patients were randomly assigned to groups by a person from the research team who had no previous contact with qualified patients. The subjects were divided into two groups: the first group, ESWT-alone (23 people), comprised those who had not participated in other physiotherapeutic procedures before the commencement of ESWT therapy. The second group, ESWT-plus (16 people) comprised those who had participated in ultrasound and laser treatments before ESWT therapy.

All patients in the ESWT-plus group received ultrasound and laser treatments for two weeks before the shockwave therapy was started. The ultrasound was performed daily, for 5 min, using the following parameters: continuous mode, base frequency of 1 MHz to produce a deeper penetration, power of 2 W/cm^2 into the areas of the painful heel and the myofascial junction at the dorsum of the heel. Laser therapy was also performed daily, after the ultrasound treatment, for 5 min. All patients were treated with laser at a power of 50 mW. The laser probe was applied to the areas of the painful heel, on the medial calcaneal area, and at the dorsum of the heel, for a total dose of 8 J/cm^2 for 200 s. The selection of parameters during the study was based on previous studies and available literature [18].

The shock wave therapy was performed using extracorporeal shock wave (ESWT). The patients underwent four treatments separated by weekly breaks. Treatment parameters: applied 1000 beats/min at a power density of 0.25 mJ/mm^2. Local anesthesia was not used during the therapy. When selecting the parameters during the study, previous studies and available literature were taken into account [19].

The extracorporeal shock wave penetrates much deeper than the radial shock wave, and is therefore more suitable for this treatment [20,21].

Laser therapy, ultrasound therapy, and ESWT were performed by using the BTL-5000 SWT Power extended version of device.

The patients were interviewed to determine pain symptoms resulting from the presence of plantar fasciitis and the impact of the disease on the activity of everyday life and motor activity using the VAS scale, Laitinen questionnaire, AOFAS score, and a questionnaire for evaluating the effects of therapy. The interviews took place only at two time points: the first was before the extracorporeal shock wave therapy was performed (December 2015 to March 2016), and the second was five years after the procedure to check whether the pain had reappeared (December 2020 to March 2021). For the second interview, the patients were contacted by telephone. The therapeutic effects of the therapy were analyzed in terms of the parameters studied and the level of satisfaction throughout the period under study.

2.3. Statistical Analysis

The statistical analysis was performed using STATISTICA PL 13.3 software (StatSoft Polska, Krakow, Poland) and the R environment. Variables measured are described based on mean and standard deviation (SD), while those involving positional measurements are given as median (Me), inter-quartile range (IQR), and minimum and maximum (Min–Max). For variables measured, only positional measures are provided. For non-measurable variables, the number of observations with a given feature variant (N) and the corresponding percentage (%) are given.

The normality of the variables was verified using the Shapiro–Wilk test. As their distribution was not normal, the non-parametric Mann–Whitney U test was used to compare the two independent groups. Two-way order ANOVA with repeated measurements was used to compare the groups with repeated measures (i.e., before and after treatment).

For the qualitative variables, the groups were compared with the chi-square test of independence. Additionally (where it was justified), the effect size was calculated using the form effect size measurement: $r = z/\sqrt{N}$ (where z is the value of the z statistic in the Wilcoxon pairwise test and N is the sample size). The effect is considered weak when $r \in (0.10–0.40)$, average when $r \in (0.40–0.60)$, and too strong when $r \in 0.60$ [22]. Statistically significant results were obtained with $p < 0.05$.

3. Results

Evaluation of Basic Characteristics

Of the 39 patients included in the initial study, all 39 were included in the final follow-up. The group comprised 22 women (56.41%) and 17 men (43.59%), aged 34–64 (mean age 54.05 ± 8.16). Among the patients who underwent shock wave therapy, 23 (58.97%) had not previously undergone any rehabilitation procedures (ESWT-alone), while 16 (41.03%) had previously participated in other rehabilitation procedures (ESWT-plus).

The mean BMI (body mass index) value was 28.46 ± 3.92 kg/m² (range 20.05 kg/m² to 37.13 kg/m²). In half of the patients, BMI did not exceed 28.41 kg/m² (IQR: 25.89–31.14 kg/m²). No statistically significant difference in BMI was found between the groups ($p = 0.2925$); however, almost 61% of the study group (ESWT-alone) were overweight, while 37.5% of the comparative group (ESWT-plus) were overweight. The characteristics of both groups in terms of sex, age, and BMI are presented in Tables 1–3.

Table 1. The structure of the treatment groups according to sex.

Group	N (%)	Sex		p-Level
		Male	Female	
ESWT-alone	N	8	15	
	%	34.78	65.22	0.1831
ESWT-plus	N	9	7	
	%	56.25	43.75	

No statistically significant difference was found between the groups in terms of sex ($p = 0.1831$).

Table 2. Characteristics of patients from the two treatment groups by age and BMI.

Variable	Measure	ESWT-Alone	ESWT-Plus	p-Level
Age	Mean ± SD	52.17 ± 9.49	56.75 ± 4.84	
	Me (IQR)	56 (48–60)	55.5 (52.5–61.5)	0.2628
	Min–Max	34–64	51–64	
BMI	Mean ± SD	28.51 ± 3.61	28.40 ± 4.46	
	Me (IQR)	28.41 (25.86–31.14)	28.06 (24.46–30.80)	0.6414
	Min–Max	20.05–36.26	23.44–37.13	

There were no statistically significant differences between the groups in terms of age and body mass index (respectively: $p = 0.2628$ and $p = 0.6414$).

Table 3. Structure of patients by BMI.

Group	N (%)	BMI				p-Level
		Normal	Overweight	Obesity I	Obesity II	
ESWT-Alone	N	3	14	4	2	
	%	13.04	60.87	17.39	8.70	0.2925
ESWT-plus	N	6	6	2	2	
	%	37.50	37.50	12.50	12.50	

Table 4 presents the assessment of pain intensity by the two treatment groups according to the VAS scale, before and after therapy. No significant intergroup difference was observed before or after therapy (ESWT-alone vs. ESWT-plus: $p = 0.9809$ before therapy and $p = 0.9200$ after therapy); however, a significant intragroup reduction in pain over time was observed in both groups ($p < 0.0001$). In both groups, the obtained effect should be considered strong; however, it was slightly greater in the ESWT-plus group.

Table 4. Assessment of pain intensity according to the VAS scale before and after therapy in the compared groups.

Group	Measure	Before Therapy	After Therapy	Effect Size	p-Level (before vs. after)
ESWT-alone	Me (IQR)	8 (7–10)	2 (1–3)	0.8384	<0.0001
	Min–Max	6–10	0–6		
ESWT-plus	Me (IQR)	8 (7.5–9.5)	1.5 (1–2)	0.8797	<0.0001
	Min–Max	5–10	1–4		

p-level (group comparison): before therapy: 0.9809; after therapy: 0.9200.

Table 5 presents the characteristics of the two treatment groups before and after therapy, with regard to pain intensity assessed according to the modified Laitinen scale. No significant intergroup differences were noted before or after therapy (ESWT-alone vs. ESWT-plus: $p = 0.8840$ before therapy and $p = 0.9687$ after therapy). Significant intragroup reductions in pain, measured on the Laitinen scale, were found in both groups over time ($p < 0.0001$). In both groups, the obtained effect should be considered strong, while it was slightly higher in the ESWT-plus group.

Table 5. Assessment of pain intensity according to the Laitinen scale before and after therapy in the compared groups.

Group	Measure	Before Therapy	After Therapy	Effect Size	p-Level (before vs. after)
ESWT-alone	Me (IQR)	10 (7–12)	2 (0–3)	0.8402	<0.0001
	Min–Max	6–13	0–6		
ESWT-plus	Me (IQR)	9 (7.5–10)	1 (0–2)	0.8860	<0.0001
	Min–Max	7–11	0–3		

p-level (group comparison): before therapy: 0.8840; after therapy: 0.9687.

The following results were obtained from the questionnaire: the intensity of pain decreased in 91.31% of the respondents in ESWT-alone, and in 100% in ESWT-plus. A significant improvement in the frequency of occurrence of pain was achieved after therapy in ESWT-alone; only two respondents experienced frequent pains. In ESTW-plus, none of the subjects experienced frequent or continuous pain after the therapy. Both groups reported not needing to take painkillers after therapy. Finally, in both groups, 100% reported improvement in physical activity; however, partial limitation of physical activity was half as common in the ESWT-plus group after shock wave therapy.

Table 6 presents the AOFAS (total score) results before and after therapy. No significant intergroup differences were found before or after therapy (ESWT-alone vs. ESWT-plus: $p = 0.9645$ before therapy and $p = 0.8380$ after therapy), while a statistically significant ($p < 0.0001$) intragroup increase was observed in each group over time. In both groups, the obtained effect should be considered strong, while it was slightly higher in ESWT-plus.

Table 6. Assessment of the AOFAS index (total score) before and after therapy in the compared groups.

Group	Measure	Before Therapy	After Therapy	Effect Size	p-Level (before vs. after)
ESWT-alone	Me (IQR)	63 (48–80)	90 (83–100)	0.8351	<0.0001
	Min–Max	22–90	61–100		
ESWT-plus	Me (IQR)	66 (44.5–90)	90 (86.5–100)	0.8484	<0.0001
	Min–Max	30–90	76–100		

p-level (group comparison): before therapy: 0.9645; after therapy: 0.8380.

Table 7 presents the pain assessment (AOFAS—Pain) results before and after treatment. No significant intergroup differences were found before or after therapy (ESWT-alone vs. ESWT-plus: $p = 0.9535$ before therapy and $p = 0.7676$ after therapy). Significant intragroup increases in AOFAS score were found in both groups over time ($p < 0.0001$). In both groups, the obtained effect should be considered strong, while it was slightly higher in the comparative group (with previous rehabilitation treatments).

Table 7. Assessment of the AOFAS index (pain points) before and after therapy in the compared groups.

Group	Measure	Before Therapy	After Therapy	Effect Size	p-Level (before vs. after)
ESWT-alone	Me (IQR)	20 (20–20)	40 (30–40)	0.8473	<0.0001
	Min–Max	0–30	20–40		
ESWT-plus	Me (IQR)	20 (10–30)	40 (40–40)	0.8551	0.0001
	Min–Max	0–30	30–40		

p-level (group comparison): before therapy: 0.9535; after therapy: 0.7676.

Table 8 presents the function point scores (AOFAS—Function) before and after therapy. No significant intergroup differences were found before or after therapy (ESWT-alone vs. ESWT-plus: $p = 0.9396$ before therapy and $p = 0.9574$ after therapy); however, statistically significant intragroup increases in the AOFAS-function score were found in both groups over time ($p = 0.0001$ and $p = 0.0013$). In both groups, the obtained effect should be considered strong, while it was slightly higher in ESWT-alone.

Table 8. Assessment of the AOFAS index (function points) before and after therapy in the compared groups.

Group	Measure	Before Therapy	After Therapy	Effect Size	p-Level (before vs. after)
ESWT-alone	Me (IQR)	38 (33–50)	50 (41–50)	0.7054	0.0001
	Min–Max	19–50	35–50		
ESWT-plus	Me (IQR)	41 (31.5–50)	50 (42.5–50)	0.6903	0.0013
	Min–Max	23–50	39–50		

p-level (group comparison): before therapy: 0.9396; after therapy: 0.9574.

Table S1 (Supplementary Materials) presents the time at which the first treatment effects were noted in the groups. A statistically significant difference was found between the groups, with the effects of therapy being observed earlier in the ESWT-alone group than in the ESWT-plus group (almost 70% of patients after the first treatment) ($p = 0.0190$).

In addition, in the ESWT-alone group, 91.30% of patients reported feeling more physically fit after the treatments; in contrast, in the ESWT-plus group, 100% reported an improvement in physical fitness. Tables S2 and S3 (Supplementary Materials) show the structure of the patients of both groups according to the assessment of the efficiency and effectiveness of the therapy. Although no statistically significant difference was found between the groups (ESWT-alone vs. ESWT-plus: $p = 0.6362$; $p = 0.3049$, respectively), the vast majority of patients assessed the therapy as very effective.

4. Discussion

Based on the results of our research, it can be seen that ESWT works better in conjunction with other treatment modalities. Although there were no significant differences between ESWT-alone and ESWT-plus therapy, ESWT-plus therapy resulted in clinically significant results as reported by 100% recovery in terms of pain and limitation to physical activity compared to 91% of ESWT-alone.

Extracorporeal shock wave therapy (ESWT) is increasingly used in orthopedics and sports medicine in the treatment of the lesions located within the musculoskeletal apparatus. Although the mechanism of action is not fully known, its positive effects in conditions resulting from overload are probably related to microdestruction [3,12,17]. Low level shock waves are known to cause various tissue responses and metabolic effects. It is presumed that the application of focused strokes causes microcracking of avascular tissues and of tissues poor in blood vessels, thus stimulating the revascularization process by releasing local growth factors and recruiting appropriate stem cells. The resulting changes increase joint mobility, prolong pain relief, and restore normal muscle tone [1,4,23,24].

In our study, after therapy, a significant reduction was noted in the intensity of pain experienced by patients during physical activity, assessed using the VAS scale and the Laitinen scale.

Krishnan et al. [25] showed positive reports that substantiate the effectiveness of ESWT on the treatment of plantar fasciitis by reporting the mean VAS scores to be decreased from an average of 9.2 to 3.4, at four weeks after treatment. In a study conducted on 60 patients, aged 45–68 years (mean age 55.6 years), Cosentino et al. [26] observed a reduction in pain intensity when awake, at rest, while walking, and during daily activities, measured using VAS, one month and three months after shock wave application. In addition, they also noted a reduction in the largest diameter of calcification in X-ray (>1 mm). Similar results were not obtained in their control group. Similar results were obtained in Metzner's study [27], which used ESWT on 63 patients with plantar aponeurosis inflammation. Each patient got 1000 impulses of ESWT; the stream density of the emitted energy was 0.35 mJ/mm^2. The pain on VAS was examined 6 weeks, 18 months, and 72 months after the end of ESWT. The level of pain decreased, and an initial 30% of patients without pain increased to 81% of the patients after 6 weeks, 88% of the patients after 18 months, and 96% of the patients in the last examination 72 months after the end of ESWT. On the basis of the results, the authors concluded that the used ESWT doses successfully decreased the pain, and the treatment effects gave satisfying long-term results. In the study by Koch et al. [28], after the completion of therapy, a significant reduction in pain was also achieved, with the same satisfactory results (VAS and Laitinen scale) in the morning, during the day, and in the evening. The effects were achieved after the 5th ESWT treatment and remained one week after the end of treatment. Similar results were obtained in a study of the effectiveness of shock wave treatments in 22 patients with heel spur [29]. The patients underwent five treatment sessions, with four to six day breaks between sessions. The procedure was performed on the three most painful locations, which were detected manually. Significant reductions in pain were noted after therapy in the morning and at night, and the symptoms were significantly reduced after therapy, during the standing test, and during manual examination of the pain points in the foot. Moretti et al. [30] evaluated the analgesic efficacy of low doses of ESWT for foot plantar fasciitis in 54 runners-athletes. The subjects received a weekly shockwave of 1000 impulses with 0.06 mJ/mm^2 energy density. The pain was assessed on VAS. ESWT treatment continued for four weeks, then the patients were examined after 45 days, and 6 and 24 months after the last session. The clinical results were excellent in 59% of cases, good in 12% of cases, satisfactory in 21%, and clearly unsatisfactory in 8%. The low-energy ESWT seems to be a good means to treat inflammation of foot plantar fascia in runners, because the resulting improvement persisted for 24 months from the end of ESWT. Additionally, Hammer et al. [31] assessed the analgesic efficacy of ESWT in 57 patients with painful chronic inflammation of the plantar fascia. Patients treated with ESWT were given 3000 impulses of shocks with energy density of 0.2 mJ/mm^2 at weekly intervals. Two years after the end of treatment, the level of pain on a VAS scale in patients treated with ESWT decreased 94%.

In addition, in our study, therapy was found to have a positive effect on the symptoms experienced during walking and recreational activity, as indicated by the AOFAS score.

A previous study on ESWT on the level of pain and reduction of functional disorders in patients with plantar fasciitis and the accompanying heel spur yielded similar results [31]. The study compared the effects of ESWT alone with those of ESWT preceded by non-steroidal anti-inflammatory drugs and diclofenac iontophoresis. Pain complaints experienced by patients during rest, daily activities, and standing on one leg were assessed. The results indicate that the pain was significantly reduced after 12 weeks of ESWT; however, no significant differences were found between the two groups. Additionally, Samar G

Soliman [32] assessed the efficacy of extracorporeal shock-wave therapy compared with local platelet-rich plasma injection for treatment of plantar fasciitis. This study included 60 patients, comprising 48 female and 12 male patients with plantar fasciitis diagnosed clinically and by ultrasound. Thirty patients received single local PRP injection and thirty patients received three sessions of ESWT weekly. VAS and AOFAS ankle-hind foot scale score in patients with calcaneal spur show more improvement in the ESWT group at 1 month after treatment ($p = 0.019$ and $p = 0.009$, respectively). Another study on patients undergoing ESWT also noted a significant reduction in pain at night, at rest, and under pressure, and an increase in the distance that the participants could walk without the need to rest [33]. Additionally, multiple meta-analyses of randomized controlled trial (RCTs) showed that ESWT decreases pain and improves function [21,31,34–37]. ESWT was found to yield significant improvements in all 20 tested patients suffering from pain in the joints of the feet in one study [4]. In addition, another study found ESWT to yield improvements in heel spurs in about 90% of cases: the patients experienced a great deal of relief when starting to walk, and then less problems when putting weight on the foot. Treatment also resulted in a strong analgesic effect immediately after the first application; however, a transient crisis may occur after the second or third treatment [5].

Chronic pain is a common problem in primary care that not only limits functions, but also adversely affects the quality of life of patients [38]. Therefore, the reduction of pain is a very important therapeutic target in the treatment of many diseases, including plantar fasciitis. In our study, the effect of extracorporeal shock wave therapy was confirmed as an effective and safe method of treating pain associated with plantar fasciitis.

Additionally, in the present study, the subjects from the ESWT-alone group demonstrated earlier effects than those who had received other procedures before therapy. It is possible that this difference may derive from assigning even a minimal improvement in the perception of pain to shock wave therapy, suppressing the effects of therapy by previously performed treatments. It may also be influenced by the habits of patients and their resulting higher expectations. This is our assumption, based on the available literature on the effectiveness of ultrasound and laser therapy. According to the literature [18], both ultrasound and laser therapy have an analgesic effect [39,40], so perhaps it was more difficult for these patients to isolate the analgesic effect of the shock wave. In addition, the study is based on the subjective feelings of patients, so we suspect that a possible reason for the later observation of improvement was the greater expectations of patients. Nevertheless, the effects were observed after each treatment.

Further clinical evidence confirming the positive effects of therapy in the treatment of orthopedic diseases continues to accumulate. In addition, the procedure is non-invasive and significantly reduces the need for orthopedic surgeries. In the literature, ESWT is also comparable to surgical plantar fasciotomy without surgical risk and gives good long-term results [41].

Strengths and limitations of the study. A key strength of our study is its relatively long five-year observation period which confirms that improvement lasted more than a few months. Moreover, all patients received the same type and dose of shock wave, and the power, frequency, and time between treatments did not differ from trial to trial, allowing us to assess the specific type of shockwave and the effect of a specific dose. Finally, the lack of local anesthesia during ESWT therapy increased the homogeneity between the compared trials. However, the presented study had some limitations. Firstly, the subgroups were quite small. The sample size should have been calculated, but this was not done, due to the small number of subjects who met all the eligibility criteria for the study. We selected 39 subjects; this was a necessary selection, as only these patients met the criterion "that patients did not receive any physical therapy prior to inclusion." Secondly, although the patients were randomly assigned to the groups by a person from the research team who had no previous contact with the eligible patients, there is always a risk of bias, because this person had access to the data of all patients. In addition, the study did not analyze the potential mechanisms of the observed improvement, for example, by assessing blood supply improvement or structural changes using Doppler ultrasound. Ultrasound imaging was performed in the study to confirm the presence of plantar fasciitis, but the findings are based on the subjective assessment of patients and not objective tests, such as ultrasonography or blood flow. There were only two time points in the study at which patient information was collected: the first was before the extracorporeal shock wave therapy was performed (December 2015 to March 2016), and the second was five years after the procedure to check whether the pain had reappeared (December 2020 to March 2021). Therefore, important methodological limitation is the lack of other time points and diagnostic tests, within that 5-year follow-up period. Patient responses are mainly based on delayed recall, therefore the data obtained is subjective and may be inaccurate. As such, care should be taken when interpreting our findings.

5. Conclusions

Extracorporeal shock wave therapy is an effective form of therapy for plantar fasciitis experienced by amateur runners. Our observations also show that ESWT works better when combined with other treatments. These observations may be the starting point for further research on the effectiveness of the shock wave in combination with other treatments.

Supplementary Materials: The following supporting information can be downloaded at: https://www.mdpi.com/article/10.3390/jcm11236926/s1, Table S1. The time that the first treatment effects were noted according to treatment group; Table S2. Patient fitness assessment according to treatment group; Table S3. Patient assessment of the effectiveness of therapy according to treatment group.

Author Contributions: J.K., creator of the idea and action plan, development of research assumptions and methods, collection of source materials and research, data collection, interpretation of the obtained results, preparation of the text, review and editing, M.D., substantive evaluation, review and editing. All authors have read and agreed to the published version of the manuscript.

Funding: The authors have not received financial support for the research, authorship, and/or publication of this article.

Institutional Review Board Statement: Approval from the Bioethics Committee of the Medical University of Lodz to conduct the study was obtained.

Informed Consent Statement: Informed consent was obtained from all subjects involved in the study.

Data Availability Statement: The data underlying this article cannot be shared publicly for the privacy of individuals that participated in the study.

Conflicts of Interest: The authors declare no conflict of interest.

References

1. Król, P.; Franek, A.; Zinka, W.; Kubacki, J.; Polak, A.; Franek, E. Extracorporeal and radial shock waves in orthopedics and physiotherapy. *Physiother. Pol.* **2009**, *9*, 1–20.
2. Szczuc, M. Shock waves in competitive sport. *Rehabil. Pract.* **2008**, *4*, 32–34.
3. Thiel, M. Application of shock waves in medicine. *Clin. Orthop. Relat. Res.* **2001**, *387*, 18–21. [CrossRef]
4. Gomulec, G. Extracorporeal shock wave therapy. *Rehabil. Pract.* **2011**, *1*, 42–45.
5. Agatowski, K. Experience of everyday work with a shock wave. *Rehabil. Pract.* **2011**, *5*, 46–49.
6. Dziak, A. *Closed Damage to Soft Tissues of the Musculoskeletal System*; PZWL: Warsaw, Poland, 1985.
7. Strzyżewski, H. Distortions and diseases of tendons, ligaments and connective tissue. In *Orthopedics and Rehabilitation*; Dega, W., Ed.; PZWL: Warsaw, Poland, 1984; Volume 2, p. 656.
8. Kozłowski, P.; Olejniczak, A.; Synder, M. Diseases from overload. In *Outline of Orthopedics, Traumatology and Rehabilitation of Motor Organs*; Zwierzchowski, H., Ed.; Medical Academy: Łódź, Poland, 1995; pp. 118–126.
9. Marciniak, W.; Szulc, A. (Eds.) *Wiktora Dega, Orthopedics and Rehabilitation*; PZWL: Warsaw, Poland, 2004; Volume 2, pp. 294–296.
10. Miszczyk, L.; Woźniak, G.; Jochymek, B.; Trela, K.; Urban, A. Evaluation of the effectiveness of radiotherapy of painful heel spurs. *Musculoskelet. Surg. Orthop. Pol.* **2003**, *68*, 191–195.
11. Melegati, G.; Tornese, D.; Bandi, M.; Rubini, M. Comparison of two ultrasonographic localization techniques for the treatment of lateral epicondylitis with extracorporeal shock wave therapy: A randomised study. *Clin. Rehabil.* **2004**, *18*, 366–370. [CrossRef] [PubMed]

12. Rompe, J.D.; Meurer, A.; Nafe, B.; Hofmann, A.; Gerdesmeyer, L. Repetitive low-energy shock wave application without local anesthesia is more efficient than repetitive low-energy shock wave application with local anesthesia in the treatment of chronic plantar fasciitis. *J. Orthop. Res.* **2005**, *23*, 931–941. [CrossRef]
13. Speed, C.A.; Nichols, D.; Richards, C.; Humphreys, H.; Wies, J.T.; Burnet, S.; Hazleman, B.L. Extracorporeal shock wave therapy for lateral epicondylitis—A double blind randomised controlled study. *J. Orthop. Res.* **2002**, *20*, 895–898. [CrossRef]
14. Schmitt, J.; Haake, M.; Tosch, A.; Hildebrand, R.; Deike, B.; Griss, P. Low-energy extracorporeal shock-wave treatment (ESWT) for tendinitis of the supraspinatus: A prospective, randomised study. *J. Bone Jt. Surg. Br.* **2001**, *83-B*, 873–876. [CrossRef]
15. Gerdesmeyer, L.; Weil, L.W. *Extracorporeal Shock Wave Therapy, Technologies, Basics, Clinical Results*; Data Trace Publishing: Towson, MD, USA, 2007; ISBN 978-1-57400-115-0.
16. Heller, K.D.; Niethard, F. Der Einsatz der extrakorporalen Stoßwellentherapie in der Orthopädie-eine Metaanalyse. *Zeitschrift für Orthopädie und ihre Grenzgebiete* **1998**, *136*, 390–401. [CrossRef]
17. Ogden, J.A.; Toth-Kischkat, A.; Schultheiss, R. Principles of shock wave therapy. *Clin. Orthop. Relat. Res.* **2001**, *387*, 8–17. [CrossRef] [PubMed]
18. Ulusoy, A.; Cerrahoglu, L.; Orguc, S. Magnetic Resonance Imaging and Clinical Outcomes of Laser Therapy, Ultrasound Therapy, and Extracorporeal Shock Wave Therapy for Treatment of Plantar Fasciitis: A Randomized Controlled Trial. *J. Foot Ankle Surg.* **2017**, *56*, 762–767. [CrossRef]
19. Ali, G.Ü.R.; İrfan, K.O.C.A.; Karagüllü, H.; Altindağ, Ö.; Madenci, E.; Tutoğlu, A.; Boyaci, A.; Işik, M. Comparison of the effectiveness of two different extracorporeal shock wave therapy regimens in the treatment of patients with myofascial pain syndrome. *Arch. Rheumatol.* **2014**, *29*, 186–193.
20. Fiani, B.; Davati, C.; Griepp, D.W.; Lee, J.; Pennington, E.; Moawad, C.M. Enhanced Spinal Therapy: Extracorporeal Shock Wave Therapy for the Spine. *Cureus* **2020**, *12*, e11200. [CrossRef] [PubMed]
21. Wang, C.J.; Wang, F.S.; Yang, K.D.; Weng, L.H.; Ko, J.Y. Long-term results of extracorporeal shockwave treatment for plantar fasciitis. *Am. J. Sports Med.* **2006**, *34*, 592–596. [CrossRef] [PubMed]
22. Salvatore, S. Mangiafico, 2016, Summary and Analysis of Extension Program Evaluation in R. Available online: https://rcompanion.org/handbook/F_06.html (accessed on 12 August 2022).
23. Razali, H.; Raj, N.B.; Wan-Arfah, N.; Yusoff, Z.; Ramalingam, V. Effectiveness of Physiotherapy Interventions on Symptom Severity and Hand Function in Patients with Idiopathic CTS. *IJMAES* **2022**, *8*, 1287–1301.
24. Simplicio, C.L.; Purita, J.; Murrell, W.; Santos, G.S.; Dos Santos, R.G.; Lana, J.F.S.D. Extracorporeal shock wave therapy mechanisms in musculoskeletal regenerative medicine. *J. Clin. Orthop. Trauma* **2020**, *11* (Suppl. S3), S309–S318. [CrossRef] [PubMed]
25. Krishnan, A.; Sharma, Y.; Singh, S. Evaluation of therapeutic effects of extracorporeal shock wave therapy in resistant plantar fasciitis patients in a tertiary care setting. *Med. J. Armed Forces India* **2012**, *68*, 236–239. [CrossRef] [PubMed]
26. Cosentino, R.; Falsetti, P.; Manca, S.; De Stefano, R.; Frati, E.; Frediani, B.; Baldi, F.; Selvi, E.; Marcolongo, R. Efficacy of Extracorporeal shock wave treatment in calcaneal enthesophytosis. *Ann. Rheum. Dis.* **2001**, *60*, 1064–1067. [CrossRef]
27. Metzner, G.; Dohnalek, C.; Aigner, E. High-energy Extracorporeal Shock-Wave Therapy (ESWT) for the treatment of chronic plantar fasciitis. *Foot Ankle Int.* **2010**, *31*, 790–796. [CrossRef] [PubMed]
28. Koch, M.; Chochowska, M.; Marcinkowski, J.T. Efficacy of extracorporeal shock wave therapy in treatment of heel spurs. *Hygeia Public Health* **2014**, *49*, 838–844.
29. Wasilewski, L. (Ed.) *Report on the Treatment of Patients Suffering from Degenerative Changes in the Area of the Heel Bone Tumor—"Heel Spur" with a Shock Wave*; Department of Rehabilitation and Physical Therapy, Prague Hospital in Warsaw: Warsaw, Poland, 2011.
30. Moretti, B.; Garofalo, R.; Patella, V.; Sisti, G.L.; Corrado, M.; Mouhsine, E. Extracorporeal shock wave therapy in runners with a symptomatic heel spur. *Knee Surg. Sports Traumatol. Arthrosc.* **2006**, *14*, 1029–1032. [CrossRef]
31. Hammer, D.S.; Adam, F.; Kreutz, A.; Kohn, D.; Seil, R. Extracorporeal Shock Wave Therapy (ESWT) in Patients with Chronic Proximal Plantar Fasciitis: A 2-Year Follow-up. *Foot Ankle Int.* **2003**, *24*, 823–828. [CrossRef]
32. Soliman, S.G.; Labeeb, A.A.; Abd Allah, E.A.; Abd-Ella, T.F.; Abd-El Hady Hammad, E.A. Platelet rich plasma injection versus extracorporeal shock-wave therapy in treatment of plantar fasciitis. *Menoufia Med. J.* **2020**, *33*, 186–190.
33. Rompe, J.D.; Hopf, C.; Nafe, B.; Bürger, R. Low-energy extracorporeal shock wave therapy for painful heel: A prospective controlled single-blind study. *Arch. Orthop. Trauma Surg.* **1996**, *115*, 75–79. [CrossRef]
34. Buchbinder, R.; Ptasznik, R.; Gordon, J.; Buchanan, J.; Prabaharan, V.; Forbes, A. Ultrasound-guided extracorporeal shock wave therapy for plantar fasciitis: A randomized controlled trial. *JAMA* **2002**, *288*, 1364–1372. [CrossRef]
35. Wang, C.J. Extracorporeal shockwave therapy in musculoskeletal disorders. *J. Orthop. Surg. Res.* **2012**, *7*, 11. [CrossRef]
36. Rompe, J.D.; Furia, J.; Weil, L.; Maffulli, N. Shock wave therapy for chronic plantar fasciopathy. *Br. Med. Bull.* **2007**, *81–82*, 183–208. [CrossRef]
37. Dizon, J.N.; Gonzalez-Suarez, C.; Zamora, M.T.; Gambito, E.D. Effectiveness of extracorporeal shock wave therapy in chronic plantar fasciitis: A meta-analysis. *Am. J. Phys. Med. Rehabil.* **2013**, *92*, 606–620. [CrossRef]
38. Hadi, M.A.; McHugh, G.A.; Closs, S.J. Impact of Chronic Pain on Patients' Quality of Life: A Comparative Mixed-Methods Study. *J. Patient Exp.* **2019**, *6*, 133–141. [CrossRef]
39. Chen, F.R.; Manzi, J.E.; Mehta, N.; Gulati, A.; Jones, M. A Review of Laser Therapy and Low-Intensity Ultrasound for Chronic Pain States. *Curr. Pain Headache Rep.* **2022**, *26*, 57–63. [CrossRef]

40. Jorge, A.E.S.; Simão, M.L.S.; Fernades, A.C.; Chiari, A.; de Aquino Junior, A.E. Can combined ultrasound and laser therapy enhance the treatment of symptomatic osteoarthritis? Case report. *J. Nov. Physiother.* **2017**, *7*, 372. [CrossRef]
41. Assad, S.; Ahmad, A.; Kiani, I.; Ghani, U.; Wadhera, V.; Tom, T.N. A novel and conservative approach to the effective treatment of plantar fasciitis. *Kureusz* **2016**, *8*, e913. [CrossRef]

Fibula Nail versus Locking Plate Fixation—A Biomechanical Study

Felix Christian Kohler [1,*], Philipp Schenk [2], Theresa Nies [1], Jakob Hallbauer [1], Gunther Olaf Hofmann [1,3], Uta Biedermann [4], Heike Kielstein [5], Britt Wildemann [1], Roland Ramm [6] and Bernhard Wilhelm Ullrich [1,3]

[1] Department of Trauma, Hand and Reconstructive Surgery, Jena University Hospital, Friedrich Schiller University Jena, 07747 Jena, Germany
[2] Department of Science, Research and Education, BG Klinikum Bergmannstrost Halle gGmbH, 06112 Halle, Germany
[3] Department of Trauma and Reconstructive Surgery, BG Klinikum Bergmannstrost Halle gGmbH, 06112 Halle, Germany
[4] Institute of Anatomy I, Jena University Hospital, Friedrich Schiller University Jena, 07743 Jena, Germany
[5] Institute of Anatomy and Cell-Biology, Halle University-Hospital, Martin Luther University, 06108 Halle, Germany
[6] Fraunhofer Institute for Applied Optics and Precision Engineering (IOF), Albert-Einstein-Str. 7, 07745 Jena, Germany
* Correspondence: felix.kohler@med.uni-jena.de; Tel.: +49-3641-9322855

Abstract: In the treatment of ankle fractures, complications such as wound healing problems following open reduction and internal fixation are a major problem. An innovative alternative to this procedure offers a more minimally invasive nail stabilization. The purpose of this biomechanical study was to clarify whether this method was biomechanically comparable to the established method. First, the stability (range of motion, diastasis) and rotational stiffness of the native upper ankle were evaluated in eight pairs of native geriatric specimens. Subsequently, an unstable ankle fracture was created and fixed with a locking plate or a nail in a pairwise manner. The ankles showed significantly less stability and rotational stiffness properties after nail and plate fixations than the corresponding native ankles ($p < 0.001$ for all parameters). When comparing the two methods, both showed no differences in their range of motion ($p = 0.694$) and diastasis ($p = 0.166$). The nail also presented significantly greater rotational stiffness compared to the plate ($p = 0.001$). However, both fixations remained behind the native stability and rotational stiffness. Due to the comparable biomechanical properties of the nail and plate fixations, an early weight-bearing following nail fixation should be assessed on a case-by-case basis considering the severity of fractures.

Keywords: trauma surgery; open reduction and internal fixation; syndesmosis; upper ankle joint; syndesmotic screw; biomechanical; osteosynthesis; geriatric fracture; geriatric trauma; fibular nail

1. Introduction

Ankle fractures are among the most common fractures experienced by individuals [1–3]. Dislocated ankle fractures and injuries involving the syndesmotic complex are usually treated surgically to restore the integrity of the ankle joint [4]. Open reduction and internal fixation (ORIF) using plate and screws is an established standard practiced in the field [5–7].

Older age and comorbidities lead to higher rates of complications ranging from 7 to 13% as a result of ORIF [8–12].

Closed reduction and nail fixation (CRNF) is an alternative minimally invasive treatment option for ankle fractures [13–17]. Less frequent complication rates [18–21] and the immediate possibility of full weightbearing postoperatively [18,22] seem to be the advantages of CRNF.

To the authors' knowledge, to date, there are only three relevant biomechanical studies on human specimens on the fibula nail [10,11,23].

Smith et al. compared intramedullary fibular nail fixation using one fibulotibial syndesmotic screw with non-locking plate fixation without a fibulotibial syndesmotic screw in an OTA/AO B-Typ fracture model. They observed greater torque to failure and a better preservation of the fibular construct in the nail group [10]. The main limitation of this study seems to be that only in the nail group was a fibulotibial syndesmotic screw used. However, a fibulotibial syndesmotic screw was not necessary for the fracture simulated in this study with plate osteosynthesis.

Switaj et al. compared the nail with a locking plate using only one syndesmotic screw in each group. They observed the nail to present less external rotational stiffness in highly unstable ankle fractures, while syndesmotic diastasis exhibited failure characteristics comparable to a locking plate [11]. One limitation of this study is that only one fibulotibial syndesmotic screw was used, providing the nail with less potential for rotational stabilization.

Carter et al. created an OTA/AO B-Type fracture and tested fibula nail fixation with one fibulotibial syndesmotic screw against a locking plate fixation without a fibulotibial syndesmotic screw. They observed no significant differences when testing to failure [23]. The biomechanical results remained inconsistent regarding the achieved biomechanical stability.

The present research investigated the biomechanics of fibula nail fixation using both fibulotibial syndesmotic screws and compared it with a locking plate fixation using two fibulotibial syndesmotic screws. A fracture model corresponding to a highly unstable injury was attempted to simulate a worst-case scenario. We aimed to address the above-mentioned limitations of the pre-studies.

We hypothesize that the fixation of rotationally unstable ankle fractures with a fibula nail is biomechanically comparable to fixation using a locking plate regarding the stabilization of the syndesmotic complex and rotational stiffness. Furthermore, the stability of both fixation methods was compared to the native, non-fractured condition.

2. Materials and Methods

2.1. Specimen

For the present study, eight fresh, deep-frozen ($\leq -20\ °C$) lower-leg specimens following disarticulation in the knee joint were used (six males and two females, age: 86 ± 6 years). The donors' history did not include musculoskeletal diseases or known injuries of the upper ankle joint. To analyze the bone quality and exclude relevant differences between the specimens, each frozen specimen underwent diagnostic computed tomography (CT) and bone mineral density (BMD) measurements by quantitative computed tomography (qCT) in the cancellous metaphyseal regions of the tibia, the distal fibula, and the talus body (Device GE Revolution EVO, 128 lines, Solingen, Germany).

For further biomechanical testing, the specimens were thawed over 18 h. Initially, the muscles and soft tissue up to 10 cm above the joint level of the upper ankle were removed. In order to be able to detect only the movements of the upper ankle joint at the syndesmotic level, arthrodesis of the lower ankle joint and Lisfranc joint was performed using talocalcaneal screws (Fa. Synthes, Johnson & Johnson Medical GmbH, Norderstedt, Germany, diameter: 4 mm, length: 60 mm, Figure 1). In addition, the hindfoot was fixed with a spongiosa screw (Fa. Stryker, diameter: 6 mm, length: 85 mm, Figure 1). The foot was submerged in methylmethacrylate (PMMA, TECHNOVIT®, Kulzer GmbH, Hanau, Germany) and the tibial plateau was fixed into portable frames using Schanz screws.

2.2. Standardized Instability and Fixation

A standardized lesion simulating a Weber C fracture with rotationally unstable pronation external rotation (PER) injury according to Lauge–Hansen (stage 4) was set (Figures 1C and 2B). For this purpose, an osteotomy of the fibula was performed at a 45° angle to the axis using an oscillating saw 1.5 cm above the syndesmotic level. To generate the relevant instability within the fracture zone, a 0.5–1 cm wide bone segment was removed at this height to simulate a zone of fragmentation. The entire syndesmotic complex (anterior, intermedius, and posterior talofibular ligaments) and the deltoid ligament were cut. The interosseous membrane was distally incised up to the fracture level. All other ligaments or bones remained intact.

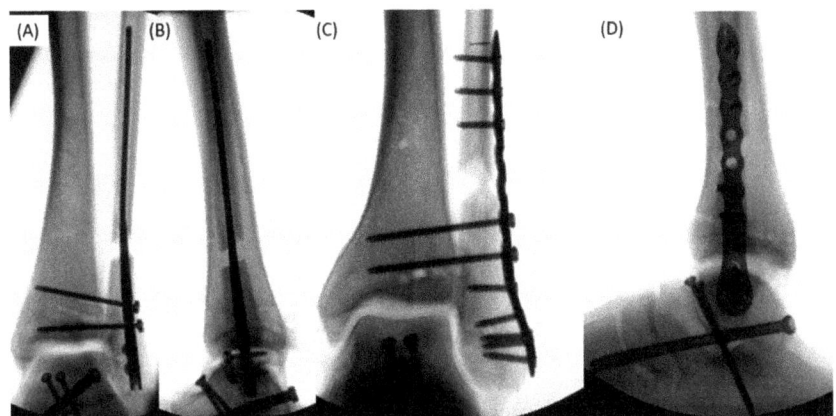

Figure 1. X-ray (**A,B**) fixations with the Vitus-Fi Fibula Nail System (nail group) with two locking and two syndesmotic screws in anterior–posterior and lateral radiographs; X-ray (**C,D**) fixations with locking plate (plate group) with two syndesmotic screws in the anterior–posterior and lateral radiographs.

For the fixation, the donors' left and right specimens were randomized in plate or nail groups to avoid side-specific bias.

The following fixation methods were used:

Nail group: The Vitus-Fi Fibula Nailing System (Fa. Dieter Marquardt Medizintechnik GmbH, Spaichingen, Germany) was used following the surgical instructions. Distally, the nail was locked twice with screws and two tricortical syndesmotic screws were placed over the target system (Figure 1A,B)

Plate group: A locking plate fixation (Variax, Fa. Stryker, Duisburg, Germany, 12-hole plate) was performed. Two fibulotibial tricortical syndesmotic screws were inserted in addition to the locking screws (Figure 1C,D).

Fixation was performed by two of the authors (FK and BU) who were surgically experienced to avoid creating differences in the quality of the fixations performed.

2.3. Experimental Setup

The biomechanical tests were performed with a constant axial preload of 750 N by a pneumatic device (to simulate body weight). A material testing machine (zwickiLine Z1.0 from Zwick/Roell, Ulm, Germany) was used to expose standardized rotational torque to the specimens (Figure 2A). The actuator of the testing machine was connected by a lever arm to the portable frame in which the specimen was proximally fixed. Therefore, the external and internal rotations of the tibial plateau could be applied against the fixed foot, simulating the external or internal rotations of the foot (Figures 2A and 3). Rotational loads were applied starting at 2 nm and were subsequently increased in 2 nm steps up to 12 nm. A total of 10 cycles in each direction (external and internal rotations) were performed. First, the loading cycles were performed on the native, followed by the testing of the destabilized and osteosynthesized specimens.

2.3.1. Movement Measuring

During the biomechanical tests, the movements of the distal fibula and tibia were recorded using an optical 3D measurement system that tracks two marker plates (kolibri CORDLESS, Fraunhofer IOF, Jena, Germany; measurement uncertainty of 20–100 µm) [24].

Each marker plate consisted of three passive, spherical markers 6.5 mm in diameter attached to a jet-black plate with a 2.5 cm diameter. The marker plates (hereafter referred to as M1 and M2) positioned tibially (M1) and fibularly (M2) were applied in the same manner to the syndesmotic plane on each specimen, as shown in Figures 2C and 3.

2.3.2. Biomechanical Parameters

In order to compare the stability of the native and stabilized specimens, and both fixation methods, the following parameters were used: the angle of rotation between the fibula and tibia (ROM), rotational stiffness (RS), and the diastasis between the fibula and tibia. These parameters were measured and calculated as follows.

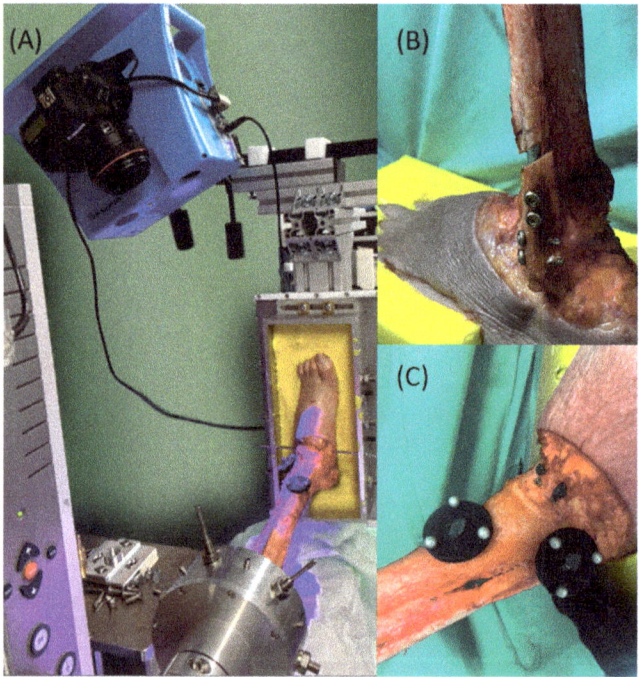

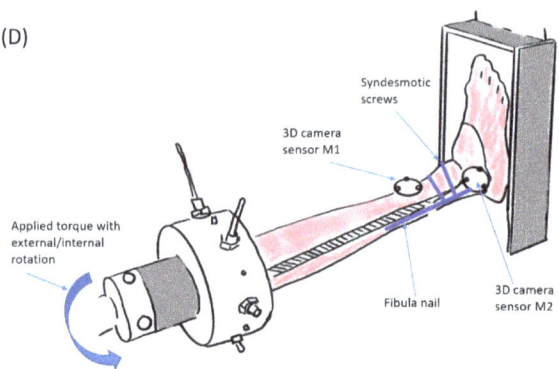

Figure 2. (**A**) The test setup with the material testing machine and optical 3D measuring system, (**B**) a prepared specimen with implanted vitus fibula nail, (**C**) the arrangement of the marker plates M1 (distal tibia) and M2 (distal fibula), (**D**) test setup with the placement of the marker plates M1 and M2. Torque was applied by repeated external/internal rotations of the tibia plateau against the fixed foot.

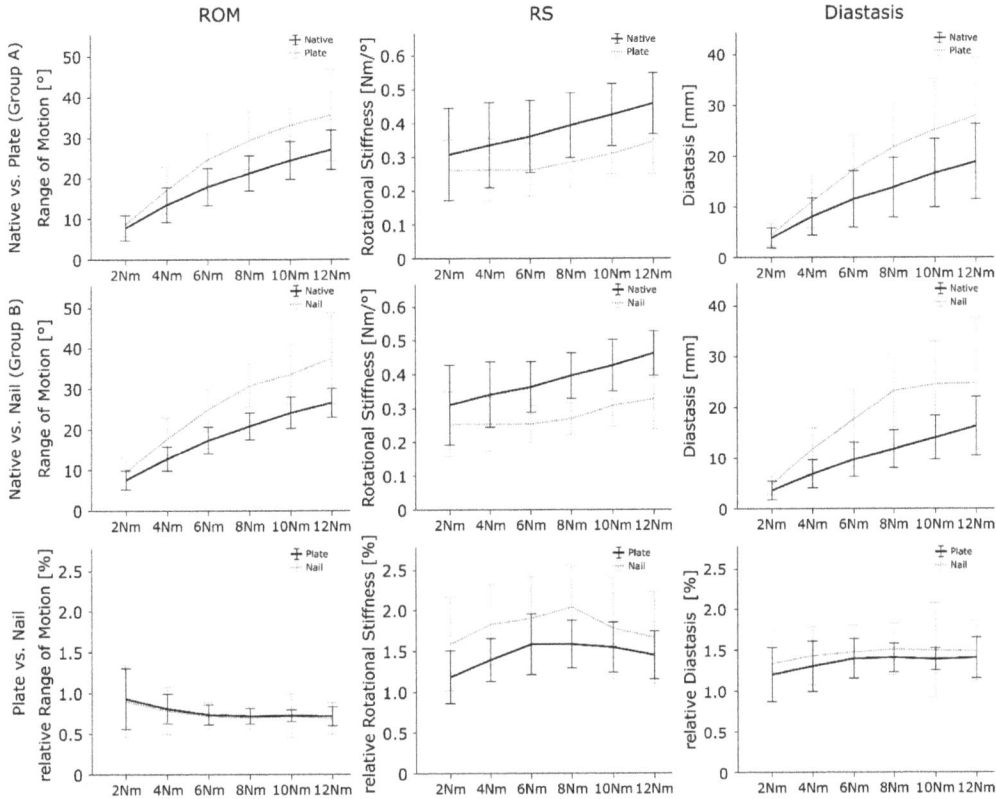

Figure 3. Results for the ROM, RS, and diastasis for native condition versus plate fixation (row 1), native condition versus nail fixation (row 2), and plate versus nail fixation (row 3). The data are presented with 95% confidence intervals. Non-overlapping intervals indicate significant differences.

2.3.3. Range of Motion (ROM)

The ROM in degree was measured as the transversal angle of rotation in the tibial plateau against the fixed embedded foot. The ROM was recorded for each load level as the sum of the maximal degree of the internal and external rotational angles. The greater the ROM, the greater the movement in the ankle joint and thus the instability.

2.3.4. Rotational Stiffness (RS)

For each load level, the RS in Nm/° was calculated based on the applied force in Nm and the angle of rotation of the tibia against the foot in the transversal plane. The data were calculated separately for external and internal rotations. The higher the value of RS, the greater the rotational stiffness, and consequently the stability of the upper ankle joint.

2.3.5. Diastasis

To evaluate the diastasis in mm, the maximum change in distance between M1 (tibia) and M2 (fibula) at each load level was measured.

2.3.6. Normalized ROM, RS, and Diastasis

To compare the stability between both fixation methods, avoiding side-related bias, ROM, RS, and diastasis were normalized by the results in the native condition for each load level, respectively.

2.4. Statistics

The differences in the mean BMD between the plate and nail groups were analyzed using Welch tests. A statistical analysis of the differences between native and stabilized specimens (fixed factor) was performed using separate general linear mixed models (GLMs) using ROM, RS, and diastasis as dependent variables. Bonferroni post hoc tests were used to perform pairwise comparisons. To compare both stabilization methods, the normalized values of ROM, RS, and diastasis were used in separate GLMs with the group as the fixed factor, respectively.

Due to the small sample size, effect sizes (ESs) such as Cohen's d (0.2 = small, 0.5 = medium, 0.8 = large effects) were presented for the comparison of fixation versus native condition and the comparison of both methods for the main effects, in addition to p-values. If a significant interaction effect between the load level and fixed factor could be observed, the p-values were presented. Otherwise, no statement was exhibited. Descriptive statistics are presented as the mean and standard deviation. For a visual comparison and statistical interpretation of the pairwise comparisons, the results were presented graphically as the means and 95% confidence intervals as error bars. This means that the true mean is within these limits 95% of the time and non-overlapping error bars indicate significant differences.

SPSS version 26 (IBM SPSS Statistics for Windows, IBM Corp., Armonk, NY, USA) was used for statistical analyses. The significance level was set to $p = 0.05$.

3. Results

3.1. Bone Mineral Density

The BMD did not differ between both groups ($p = 0.943$), with 226 ± 62 g/cm^3 in the plate group and 229 ± 59 g/cm^3 in the nail group ($p = 0.943$). Thus, the BMD was assumed to not be different between the two sides, and the effect of the BMD on the stability of the fixation was assumed to produce an effect in a comparable manner.

3.2. Native versus Plate and Nail

3.2.1. Range of Motion

When comparing the ROM of the specimens in the plate group with the corresponding native specimen, the fixed specimens showed significantly greater ROM values ($p < 0.001$; native: $18.7 \pm 8.0°$; plate: $24.8 \pm 11.0°$; ES: 0.51, Figure 3). Furthermore, the ROM was significantly affected by the torque level; as the torque level increased, the ROM also increased ($p < 0.001$).

The ROM of the specimens following fibula nail fixation significantly differed from the native specimens ($p < 0.001$; native: $18.2 \pm 7.5°$; nail: $25.7 \pm 11.0°$; ES: 0.65, Figure 3). The ROM was again significantly affected by the level of torque ($p < 0.001$).

3.2.2. Rotational Stiffness

The stiffness significantly decreased after plate fixation compared to the native situation ($p < 0.001$; native: 0.38 ± 0.12 Nm/°; plate: 0.29 ± 0.08 Nm/°; ES: 1.39, Figure 3). The upper ankle joints of the specimen with the fibula nail fixation showed significantly less RS compared to the native specimens ($p < 0.001$; native: 0.38 ± 0.11 Nm/°; nail: 0.28 ± 0.08 Nm/°; ES: 1.15, Figure 3). For both techniques, the load level showed no significance in the post hoc pairwise comparisons ($p < 0.085$).

3.2.3. Diastasis

The diastases were significantly greater after plate fixation compared to the native condition ($p < 0.001$; native: 12.1 ± 7.6 mm; plate: 18.0 ± 10.7 mm; ES: 0.83, Figure 3). Diastasis increased with greater loads ($p < 0.001$).

A significant greater diastasis value was observed for the nail fixed specimen also comparted to native tissue ($p < 0.001$; native: 10.4 ± 5.9 mm; nail: 17.7 ± 9.7 mm; ES: 0.83) (Figure 3). With an increase in the load level, the diastasis also increased ($p < 0.001$).

A significant interaction effect between nail fixation and load level was observed with $p = 0.010$.

3.3. Plate vs. Nail

3.3.1. Range of Motion

Comparing the two methods, no significant difference and low ES in the normalized ROM was observed for the mean of all force levels ($p = 0.694$; plate: 0.77 ± 0.22; nail: 0.75 ± 0.31; ES: 0.08, Table 1, Figure 3). In general, the load level showed no significant effect on the ROM ($p = 0.541$).

Table 1. Results of the biomechanical tests of the nail and plate fixations for each load level, normalized to the native condition. Values greater than 1 indicate greater movement (range of motion (ROM) and diastasis) or stiffness; lower values vice versa. To compare both stabilization methods, the normalized values of ROM, RS, and diastasis were used in separate GLMs with the group as the fixed factor, respectively. The p-values and effect size (ES, Cohen's d) are presented for each pairwise comparison and for the mean values of all force levels. The significance level was set at ≤ 0.05. The ES values as Cohen's d mean: 0.2 = small effect, 0.5 = medium effect, 0.8 = large effect.

	Load Level, [Nm]	Nail	Plate	p-Value	ES
Normalized ROM [%]	2	0.90 ± 0.53	0.93 ± 0.40	0.896	0.07
	4	0.78 ± 0.35	0.81 ± 0.20	0.862	0.09
	6	0.72 ± 0.20	0.74 ± 0.13	0.854	0.10
	8	0.70 ± 0.17	0.72 ± 0.09	0.768	0.15
	10	0.72 ± 0.22	0.72 ± 0.07	0.974	0.02
	12	0.69 ± 0.12	0.72 ± 0.07	0.686	0.30
Mean values		0.75 ± 0.31	0.77 ± 0.22	0.694	0.08
Normalized RS [%]	2	1.59 ± 0.69	1.18 ± 0.35	0.172	0.73
	4	1.83 ± 0.59	1.40 ± 0.28	0.095	0.91
	6	1.91 ± 0.61	1.59 ± 0.40	0.253	0.60
	8	2.04 ± 0.62	1.59 ± 0.28	0.094	0.90
	10	1.78 ± 0.59	1.55 ± 0.29	0.416	0.50
	12	1.67 ± 0.23	1.45 ± 0.24	0.270	0.91
Mean values		1.80 ± 0.59	1.46 ± 0.33	<0.001	0.76
Normalized diastasis [%]	2	1.33 ± 0.47	1.20 ± 0.36	0.547	0.31
	4	1.43 ± 0.43	1.30 ± 0.33	0.527	0.33
	6	1.48 ± 0.39	1.40 ± 0.26	0.650	0.24
	8	1.51 ± 0.38	1.41 ± 0.17	0.512	0.33
	10	1.50 ± 0.47	1.39 ± 0.13	0.648	0.32
	12	1.49 ± 0.23	1.41 ± 0.16	0.582	0.41
Mean values	12	1.46 ± 0.39	1.35 ± 0.26	0.166	0.32

3.3.2. Rotational Stiffness

The nail fixation showed significantly higher normalized RS values than the plate fixation for the mean of all force levels ($p < 0.001$; plate: 1.46 ± 0.33; nail: 1.80 ± 0.59; ES: 0.76, Table 1, Figure 3). The ES underlines this significance and presents a strong effect. The load level showed no significant impact on RS ($p = 0.246$).

3.3.3. Diastasis

No significant difference was observed between the two methods and their influence on upper ankle diastasis for the mean of all force levels ($p = 0.166$; plate: 1.35 ± 0.26; nail: 1.46 ± 0.39; ES: 0.32, Table 1, Figure 3). ES showed a minor effect. The load level had no significant influence on the diastasis ($p = 0.722$).

4. Discussion

The purpose of this biomechanical cadaver study was to investigate whether the stabilization of unstable ankle fractures (PER injury stage 4 according to Lauge-Hansen [25]) using a Vitus-Fi Fibula Nail System is biomechanically comparable to locking plate fixation.

In our biomechanical study, both OS, ORIF using a locking plate, and CRNF using a fibula nail were observed to remain behind native stability in a highly unstable PER injury. A biomechanical comparison of the two OS showed comparable results. A significantly greater rotational stiffness was observed in the nail OS.

There is evidence in the clinical trials that the fibula nail may present advantages due to fewer wound complications [26–28]. A systematic review and meta-analysis conducted in 2022 that included randomized clinical trials concluded that there is good evidence for comparable clinical outcomes between the fibula nail and ORIF [29]. With moderate safety, to date, fewer postoperative complications can be expected [29]. A technique-related disadvantage is that closed reduction makes the anatomical restoration of the ankle difficult. These results suggest that nail fixation is a good alternative to open reduction and locking plate fixation for a geriatric patient population [13,18]. In addition, full weight-bearing should be possible postoperatively [18,22], which would offer clear advantages, especially for elderly people, because the absence of weight-bearing is often not possible at all.

In our biomechanical study, the comparison of the two techniques (nail and locking plate) with the corresponding native specimens showed significant differences in all three parameters (ROM, RS, and diastasis) toward reduced stability and rotational stiffness after fixation. It seems to be very clear that both fixation techniques failed to restore the native stability. With a PER (Stage 4) injury and a fracture segment at the Weber C level, a highly unstable situation was created in our study, which may be one explanation for the lower stability even after fixation. What this means for clinical recommendations is that it cannot be concluded from the biomechanical results alone. For functional stability under real-life conditions, the additional stabilizing effect of muscle forces and ankle joint passing tendons has to be considered. However, the question is how our results are reasonably put into practice, since we only tested specimens without muscles and soft tissues in the artificial injured area. We share an opinion similar to Switaj et al. on the question of weight-bearing following surgery. Due to the significant increase in diastasis following OS, weight-bearing should also be decided as a case decision depending on the severity of the injury [11]. When comparing the two fixation methods, there were no significant differences for the ROM and diastasis of the ankle. The effect sizes showed weak effects for ROM (ES = 0.08) and diastasis (ES = 0.32), indicating very comparable stability conditions with regard to these two parameters. However, there was a significant difference in RS to greater RS in nail fixation. The high ES value of 0.76 underlines the difference in the overall mean of the measured values. In contrast, the pairwise comparison showed no significant differences between specimens (Table 1). Overall, this result was unexpected regarding the existing literature. In contrast to Switaj et al., who observed a lower RS value for the nail than for the plate fixation across the syndesmosis, we could not demonstrate similar results. With regard to diastasis, Switaj et al. also observed no differences between nail and plate OS values. However, the nail probably remained below its potential in the study by Switaj et al. because only one syndesmotic screw was used [11]. This could be an explanation for the lower rotational stiffness observed by Switaj et al. [11]. This study also highlighted that diastasis showed even lower values for the locking plate compared to the native condition. The diastasis occurring following nail OS increased by only 0.7 mm. In our study, both OS values remained significantly lower than the native sample for all measurement parameters. Here, similar to Switaj et al.'s study, a dislocation model with a highly unstable situation was selected [11]. In addition to the complete transection of the syndesmotic ligaments and simulation of a fibular fragmentation zone, the deltoid ligament at the medial malleolus was also transected. This created a worst-case scenario, which has never before been biomechanically investigated for the fibula nail in this form and could be an explanation for the lower stability to the native condition. The study conducted by Smith et al. compared the fixation following a simulated supination-eversion injury (AO 44 B2, stage 3 according to Lauge-Hansen). Stability under an 800 N axial preload and external rotation loading was investigated [10]. The failure angle, the applied torque at failure, and the failure pattern were compared. In this case, the nail was only simply locked proximally and distally, and therefore most likely did not present the optimal results. In elderly patients, who frequently also present osteoporotic bone quality, the comparison of the lag screw and non-locking plate fixation did not seem optimal either. This was also illustrated by the nature of the failure observed in this study. In the non-locking one-third tubular plate construct, the screws failed, whereas in the nail, the lateral ligament structures ruptured. Thus, the nail seemed to be clearly superior to the non-locking plate construct. With a PER stage 4 injury, we created a more unstable situation than Smith et al. [10]. In addition, the comparison with a locking plate and dual syndesmotic screw provided a more clinically realistic comparison overall.

Carter et al. compared the fibula nail with a locking plate in a supination external rotation injury in geriatric specimens. However, the fibula nail was again used with only one syndesmotic screw [23]. The fixations were tested again to failure; therefore, a different biomechanical approach was employed than that used in our study. The comparison of OS using a nail with a syndesmotic screw versus a locking plate without stabilization of the syndesmosis does not seem to be a fair comparison. Despite the mean torque to failure result favoring the intramedullary nail by 1.9 Nm, the statistical significance was demonstrated only in the angle of failure, which favored the intramedullary nail by a mean of 13.2 degrees.

In our study, the fibula nail was tested for the first time, biomechanically fixed with two syndesmotic screws in addition to double distal locking, as required by the system. However, unlike the plate, these two screws were an integral part of the fibula nail system and inserted regardless of the stage of syndesmosis injury. To compare the fixation process, a standardized fracture model was fixed with two syndesmotic screws each for both the plate and nail. We observed an advantage here compared to the previous biomechanical studies, as the fibula nail obviously received an increase in stiffness and stability due to additional bony fixation points. From a biomechanical perspective, the fibula nail is shown to be an alternative to the locking plate.

Limitations

A limitation of this biomechanical study was the low number of specimens, but this has similarly been reported in other comparable studies [22–25]. One explanation for the low number of specimens is certainly the availability of body donors, which is limited. The transfer of the biomechanical results to the clinic is not immediately possible due to the lack of muscular stabilization compared to living humans. Further clinical studies are needed to compare the two OS values in clinical practice. The instability model of PER injury reflects only a part of the possible injuries and instabilities at the ankle joint. An attempt was made to produce the worst-case scenario in order to maximally challenge the implants. Despite this, the results cannot simply be transferred to other injuries. Comparability to studies with failure testing is limited, as these were not performed. The biomechanical model chosen here with internal and external rotations did not correspond to the normal cyclic loading of an ankle joint in a walking cycle, but was an abstraction in the laboratory model.

5. Conclusions

The results show that both fixation techniques achieved comparable biomechanical stability values in the case of highly unstable ankle fractures. The nail offers an advantage over the plate for rotational stability. However, both fixations fell short of native stability and rotational stiffness. Therefore, full weight-bearing following osteosynthesis in a highly unstable situation such as pronation external rotation injury should not be considered in general terms, but rather on a case-by-case basis.

Author Contributions: Conceptualization, F.C.K., P.S., T.N. and B.W.U.; Methodology, F.C.K., P.S., T.N. and B.W.U.; Software, F.C.K., P.S. and B.W.U.; Validation, F.C.K., P.S. and B.W.U.; Formal analysis, F.C.K., P.S., T.N., J.H., G.O.H., U.B., B.W., H.K., R.R. and B.W.U.; Investigation, F.C.K., T.N., J.H. and B.W.U.; Resources, F.C.K., P.S., T.N. and B.W.U.; Data curation, F.C.K., P.S., T.N. and B.W.U.; Writing—original draft preparation, F.C.K., P.S., T.N. and B.W.U.; Writing—review and editing, F.C.K., P.S., T.N., J.H., G.O.H., U.B., B.W., H.K., R.R. and B.W.U.; Visualization, F.C.K., P.S. and T.N.; Supervision, J.H., G.O.H. and B.W.U.; Project administration, F.C.K. and B.W.U.; Funding acquisition, F.C.K. and B.W.U. All authors have read and agreed to the published version of the manuscript.

Funding: This research was funded by Dieter Marquardt Medizintechnik GmbH (Spaichingen, Germany) with EUR 5000.

Institutional Review Board Statement: The study was conducted in accordance with the Declaration of Helsinki and approved by the Ethics Committee of Jena University Hospital (approval number: 2020-1949-Material).

Informed Consent Statement: Informed consent was obtained from all subjects involved in the study before death.

Data Availability Statement: The data presented in the study are stored on secure servers at University Hospital Jena. Donor consent forms are stored at the Anatomical Institute of the University Hospital in Jena. The data are available on request from the corresponding author.

Acknowledgments: We would like to thank AO Trauma Germany for the support in the context of the promotion of young scientists.

Conflicts of Interest: The study was partially funded by Dieter Marquardt Medizintechnik GmbH (Spaichingen, Germany) with EUR 5000. No employee of the company was involved in either the experimental procedure, evaluation, interpretation, or writing of the present manuscript. BU received honoraria for lectures from the company BB Aesculap (Tuttlingen, Germany). The lectures are not related to the present study.

References

1. Court-Brown, C.M.; McBirnie, J.; Wilson, G. Adult ankle fractures—an increasing problem? *Acta Orthop. Scand.* **1998**, *69*, 43–47. [CrossRef]
2. Rupp, M.; Walter, N.; Pfeifer, C.; Lang, S.; Kerschbaum, M.; Krutsch, W.; Baumann, F.; Alt, V. The incidence of fractures among the adult population of Germany: An analysis from 2009 through 2019. *Dtsch. Ärzteblatt Int.* **2021**, *118*, 665.
3. Elsoe, R.; Ostgaard, S.E.; Larsen, P. Population-based epidemiology of 9767 ankle fractures. *Foot Ankle Surg.* **2018**, *24*, 34–39. [CrossRef] [PubMed]
4. Weber, B. Lengthening osteotomy of the fibula to correct a widened mortice of the ankle after fracture. *Int. Orthop.* **1981**, *4*, 289–293. [CrossRef] [PubMed]
5. Pettrone, F.A.; Gail, M.; Pee, D.; Fitzpatrick, T.; Van Herpe, L.B. Quantitative criteria for prediction of the results after displaced fracture of the ankle. *J. Bone Jt. Surg. Am. Vol.* **1983**, *65*, 667–677. [CrossRef]
6. Phillips, W.; Schwartz, H.; Keller, C.; Woodward, H.R.; Rudd, W.S.; Spiegel, P.; Laros, G. A prospective, randomized study of the management of severe ankle fractures. *J. Bone Jt. Surg. Am. Vol.* **1985**, *67*, 67–78. [CrossRef]
7. Ali, M.; McLaren, C.; Rouholamin, E.; O'Connor, B. Ankle fractures in the elderly: Nonoperative or operative treatment. *J. Orthop. Trauma* **1987**, *1*, 275–280. [CrossRef]
8. Varenne, Y.; Curado, J.; Asloum, Y.; de Chou, E.S.; Colin, F.; Gouin, F. Analysis of risk factors of the postoperative complications of surgical treatment of ankle fractures in the elderly: A series of 477 patients. *Orthop. Traumatol. Surg. Res.* **2016**, *102*, S245–S248. [CrossRef]
9. Zaghloul, A.; Haddad, B.; Barksfield, R.; Davis, B. Early complications of surgery in operative treatment of ankle fractures in those over 60: A review of 186 cases. *Injury* **2014**, *45*, 780–783. [CrossRef]
10. Smith, G.; Mackenzie, S.P.; Wallace, R.J.; Carter, T.; White, T.O. Biomechanical comparison of intramedullary fibular nail versus plate and screw fixation. *Foot Ankle Int.* **2017**, *38*, 1394–1399. [CrossRef]
11. Switaj, P.J.; Fuchs, D.; Alshouli, M.; Patwardhan, A.G.; Voronov, L.I.; Muriuki, M.; Havey, R.M.; Kadakia, A.R. A biomechanical comparison study of a modern fibular nail and distal fibular locking plate in AO/OTA 44C2 ankle fractures. *J. Orthop. Surg. Res.* **2016**, *11*, 100. [CrossRef] [PubMed]
12. Lynde, M.J.; Sautter, T.; Hamilton, G.A.; Schuberth, J.M. Complications after open reduction and internal fixation of ankle fractures in the elderly. *Foot Ankle Surg.* **2012**, *18*, 103–107. [CrossRef]

13. Bugler, K.; Watson, C.; Hardie, A.; Appleton, P.; McQueen, M.; Court-Brown, C.; White, T. The treatment of unstable fractures of the ankle using the Acumed fibular nail: Development of a technique. *J. Bone Jt. Surg. Br. Vol.* **2012**, *94*, 1107–1112. [CrossRef] [PubMed]
14. Giordano, V.; Boni, G.; Godoy-Santos, A.L.; Pires, R.E.; Fukuyama, J.M.; Koch, H.A.; Giannoudis, P.V. Nailing the fibula: Alternative or standard treatment for lateral malleolar fracture fixation? A broken paradigm. *Eur. J. Trauma Emerg. Surg.* **2021**, *47*, 1911–1920. [CrossRef] [PubMed]
15. Sain, A.; Garg, S.; Sharma, V.; Meena, U.K.; Bansal, H. Osteoporotic Distal Fibula Fractures in the Elderly: How to Fix Them. *Cureus* **2020**, *12*, e6552. [CrossRef]
16. Carter, T.H.; Mackenzie, S.P.; Bell, K.R.; Bugler, K.E.; MacDonald, D.; Duckworth, A.D.; White, T.O. Optimizing long-term outcomes and avoiding failure with the fibula intramedullary nail. *J. Orthop. Trauma* **2019**, *33*, 189–195. [CrossRef]
17. Dabash, S.; Eisenstein, E.D.; Potter, E.; Kusnezov, N.; Thabet, A.M.; Abdelgawad, A.A. Unstable ankle fracture fixation using locked fibular intramedullary nail in high-risk patients. *J. Foot Ankle Surg.* **2019**, *58*, 357–362. [CrossRef]
18. White, T.O.; Bugler, K.; Appleton, P.; Will, E.; McQueen, M.; Court-Brown, C. A prospective randomised controlled trial of the fibular nail versus standard open reduction and internal fixation for fixation of ankle fractures in elderly patients. *Bone Jt. J.* **2016**, *98*, 1248–1252. [CrossRef]
19. Jain, S.; Haughton, B.A.; Brew, C. Intramedullary fixation of distal fibular fractures: A systematic review of clinical and functional outcomes. *J. Orthop. Traumatol.* **2014**, *15*, 245. [CrossRef]
20. Jordan, R.; Chapman, A.; Buchanan, D.; Makrides, P. The role of intramedullary fixation in ankle fractures—A systematic review. *Foot Ankle Surg.* **2018**, *24*, 1–10. [CrossRef]
21. Asloum, Y.; Bedin, B.; Roger, T.; Charissoux, J.-L.; Arnaud, J.-P.; Mabit, C. Internal fixation of the fibula in ankle fractures. A prospective, randomized and comparative study: Plating versus nailing. *Orthop. Traumatol. Surg. Res.* **2014**, *100*, S255–S259. [CrossRef] [PubMed]
22. Challagundla, S.R.; Shewale, S.; Cree, C.; Hawkins, A. Intramedullary fixation of lateral malleolus using Fibula Rod System in ankle fractures in the elderly. *Foot Ankle Surg.* **2018**, *24*, 423–426. [CrossRef] [PubMed]
23. Carter, T.H.; Wallace, R.; Mackenzie, S.A.; Oliver, W.M.; Duckworth, A.D.; White, T.O. The fibular intramedullary nail versus locking plate and lag screw fixation in the management of unstable elderly ankle fractures: A cadaveric biomechanical comparison. *J. Orthop. Trauma* **2020**, *34*, e401–e406. [CrossRef]
24. Ramm, R.; Heinze, M.; Kühmstedt, P.; Christoph, A.; Heist, S.; Notni, G. Portable solution for high-resolution 3D and color texture on-site digitization of cultural heritage objects. *J. Cult. Herit.* **2022**, *53*, 165–175. [CrossRef]
25. Lauge-Hansen, N. Fractures of the ankle. II. Combined experimental-surgical and experimental-roentgenologic investigations. *Arch. Surg.* **1950**, *60*, 957–985. [CrossRef]
26. Appleton, P.; McQueen, M. The fibula nail for treatment of ankle fractures in elderly and high risk patients. *Tech. Foot Ankle Surg.* **2006**, *5*, 204–208. [CrossRef]
27. Dingemans, S.; Rammelt, S.; White, T.; Goslings, J.; Schepers, T. Should syndesmotic screws be removed after surgical fixation of unstable ankle fractures? A systematic review. *Bone Jt. J.* **2016**, *98*, 1497–1504. [CrossRef]
28. Rajeev, A.; Senevirathna, S.; Radha, S.; Kashayap, N. Functional outcomes after fibula locking nail for fragility fractures of the ankle. *J. Foot Ankle Surg.* **2011**, *50*, 547–550. [CrossRef]
29. Walsh, J.P.; Hsiao, M.S.; LeCavalier, D.; McDermott, R.; Gupta, S.; Watson, T.S. Clinical outcomes in the surgical management of ankle fractures: A systematic review and meta-analysis of fibular intramedullary nail fixation vs. open reduction and internal fixation in randomized controlled trials. *Foot Ankle Surg.* **2022**, *28*, 836–844. [CrossRef] [PubMed]

Disclaimer/Publisher's Note: The statements, opinions and data contained in all publications are solely those of the individual author(s) and contributor(s) and not of MDPI and/or the editor(s). MDPI and/or the editor(s) disclaim responsibility for any injury to people or property resulting from any ideas, methods, instructions or products referred to in the content.

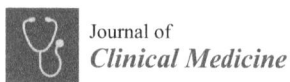

Article

Blade Augmentation in Nailing Proximal Femur Fractures—An Advantage despite Higher Costs?

Alexander Böhringer *, Raffael Cintean, Alexander Eickhoff, Florian Gebhard and Konrad Schütze

Department of Trauma, Hand and Reconstructive Surgery Ulm University, Albert-Einstein-Allee 23, 89081 Ulm, Germany
* Correspondence: alexander.boehringer@uniklinik-ulm.de; Tel.: +49-73150054561

Abstract: Background: Proximal femoral fractures occur with increasing incidence, especially in the elderly. Commonly used implants for surgical treatment are cephalomedullary nails. To increase stability, a perforated femoral neck blade can be augmented with cement. The study investigated whether this results in a relevant clinical advantage and justifies the higher cost. Materials and methods: This is a single-center retrospective study of 620 patients with proximal femur fractures treated with cephalomedullary nailing. Between January 2016 and December 2020, 207 male and 413 female patients were surgically treated with a proximal femur nail (DePuy Synthes) using a perforated blade and cement augmentation in cases with severe osteoporosis. Primary outcome measures were the rate of cut-out, tip apex distance and the positioning of the blade in the femoral head. Secondary outcome measures were the implant costs and operating times. Results: Of the 620 femoral neck blades, 299 were augmented with cement. A total of six cut-outs were seen in the first 3 months after the operation. There were three in the cement-augmented group (CAB = cement-augmented blade) and three in the conventional group (NCAB = non-cement-augmented blade). There was a significant positive correlation between age and augmentation, with a mean difference of 11 years between the two groups (CAB 85.7 ± 7.9 vs. NCAB 75.3 ± 15.1; $p < 0.05$). There was no difference in the tip-apex distance (CAB 15.97 vs. 15.69; $p = 0.64$) or rate of optimal blade positions between the groups (CAB 81.6% vs. NCAB 83.2%; $p = 0.341$). Operation times were significantly longer in the cemented group (CAB 62.6 21.2 min vs. NCAB 54.1 7.7 min; $p < 0.05$), and the implant cost nearly doubled due to augmentation. Conclusion: When the principles of anatomic fracture reduction, optimal tip-apex distance and optimal blade position are combined with cement augmentation in cases of severe osteoporosis, a cut-out rate of less than 1% can be achieved. Nevertheless, it should be noted that augmentation remains expensive and prolongs surgery time without definite proof of mechanical superiority.

Keywords: proximal femur and hip fracture; tip-apex distance; helical blade position; cut-out rate; cement augmentation; osteoporosis

1. Introduction

Proximal femur fractures occur with increasing incidence, especially in the elderly population due to demographic change, osteoporosis and increased activity level with unsteady walking [1]. Prompt surgical care within 24 h is recommended to avoid serious complications and achieve better patient outcomes [2,3]. Various surgical procedures and implants have been developed, including wires, screws, plates, and intramedullary nails. Despite several treatment options, the risk of mechanical failures, such as the femoral neck blade cutting through the femoral head, has been reported in the literature to be as high as 17% [4–8]. In comparison, a recent study by Bojan et al. [9] showed an osteosynthesis failure rate of only 2% using the "gamma nail" and state-of-the-art implantation techniques. Although the risk of mechanical osteosynthesis failure has been reduced, there is still a need for improvement, as the mortality rate in the first year is as high as 56% when revision surgery is required [10,11].

One of the most commonly used implants today for treating proximal femoral fractures is the PFNA ("proximal femur nail anti-rotation"; DePuy Synthes). To increase stability in the femoral head, the perforated helical femoral neck blade can be augmented with cement [12]. Biomechanical experiments have shown higher osteosynthesis stability by cement augmentation of the femoral neck blade. More test cycles to mechanical osteosynthesis failure, higher rotational stability, and higher pullout strength were achieved on the cadaveric model [13–15]. The first promising clinical results of cement-augmented blades (CAB) in the femoral head were shown by Kammerlander et al. [16].

In this study, no mechanical failure was observed in 105 patients with CAB. In contrast, 6 of the 118 patients in the non-cement-augmented blade (NCAB) group showed osteosynthesis failure. In a study with only 67 patients [17], there was no significant difference in complications but also fewer mechanical failures in the CAB group (CAB cut-out 2% vs. NCAB 14%). Schuetze et al. [18] demonstrated in 152 cases that PFNA blade augmentation is a safe and good procedure with no increase in complications and mortality. There was no cement leakage into the joint, while blood pressure changes occurred during augmentation. The aim of the study was to evaluate if there is an advantage and at what cost with the use of CAB compared to NCAB in a large cohort of patients.

2. Materials and Methods

Approval was obtained from our ethics committee for the use of patient data prior to the evaluation. All patients between January 2016 and December 2020 who had undergone PFNA surgery for proximal femur fracture were retrospectively analyzed for this study. We included all patients with radiographic follow-ups after at least 3 months. We excluded patients with pathologic fractures or additional surgeries for other injuries in the same hospital stay. For all cases, a perforated helical femoral neck blade was used (Fa. DePuy Synthes). The decision for or against cement augmentation (TRAUMACEM V+ Injectable Bone Cement system; Fa. DePuy Synthes) was made by the surgeon, taking into account patient age, fracture pattern, and intraoperative assessment of bone quality. Specific criteria included previously diagnosed and treated osteoporosis in the patient record, unstable fracture patterns, such as multiple fragments, severe dislocation, and varus tilt, as well as intraoperatively tested bone quality during guide-wire insertion and femoral neck blade reaming. Before blade augmentation with cement, a contrast agent was injected to avoid possible leakage into the hip joint. The treating surgeon decided intraoperatively on the final amount of cement (about 4–7 mL).

To investigate the post-operative outcome, radiographs were evaluated before discharge, after six weeks and after 3 months. A total of nine different blade positions were defined across two radiographic planes (anterior/posterior = a.p. and Lauenstein = axial). In a.p. view, the inferior, center or superior blade positions were evaluated. The axial view was used to determine the center, anterior or posterior. The blade position was determined, and the distance of the blade tip to the apex of the femoral head was measured as described by Baumgaertner et al. [19]. The measurement method for determining the tip-apex distance (TAD) and the blade position is illustrated by two examples in Figure 1. Radiographs at 6 weeks and 3 months were analyzed by two independent investigators for signs of mechanical failure. Patient charts, patient records, and anesthesia protocols were evaluated regarding surgical and non-surgical complications during hospital stays. Costs for cement augmentation were measured by the price of the augmentation kit (Traumacem V+ cement, Fa. DePuy Synthes) and the additional operating time. Data collection was performed with SAP using ICD-10 and OPS codes. Data analysis was performed with Microsoft Excel (2019 MSO) and IBM SPSS Statistics (V27.0). Demographic characteristics were described as means and as standard deviations. Due to the low number of mechanical failures, logistic regression was not possible. Therefore, group comparisons were performed using the chi-square test for frequencies, Fischer's exact test for small sample sizes, and the Student's *t*-test or Welch's test for the comparisons of means.

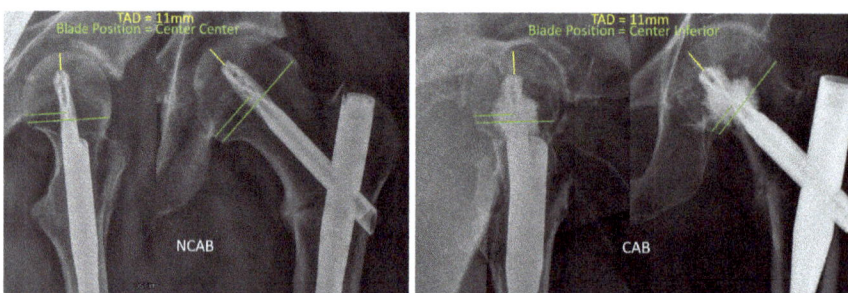

Figure 1. Measurement of the TAD (tip apex distance = yellow lines) and the blade position (position of the blade in the area of the femoral head = green lines). Left side: NCAB; right side: CAB.

3. Results

3.1. Patient Population

The medical records of the 620 patients were retrospectively reviewed. In 299 (48.2%) cases, cement augmentation of the blade was performed and was not performed in 321. The mean age was 80 ± 13 years and showed a significant difference between the groups (CAB 86 ± 7; NCAB 75 ± 15; $p < 0.05$). Out of the 620 patients, 207 were male, and 413 were female. Significantly more women were treated with cement augmentation of the blade ($p < 0.05$). In the CAB group, 78.3% of the patients were female, and 21.7% were male; in the NCAB group, 55.8% of the patients were female and 44.2% male. There was no significant difference between the two groups in terms of fracture classification according to AO (Arbeitsgemeinschaft für Osteosynthesefragen). Type 31-A2 was the most common, with 150 cases in the CAB group and 143 cases in the NCAB group. The ASA score (American Society of Anesthesiologists Classification) also showed no significant differences in the distribution of grades 1–4 in the two groups. As expected, there was no difference in time to surgery. The increased time required for cement augmentation of the femoral neck blade was significant at 8 min ($p < 0.001$). The hospital stay of both groups of patients did not differ significantly. The optimal blade position was achieved with center-center or center-inferior in both groups with >80%. Likewise, the tip-apex distance showed no significant difference in both groups, with 16 ± 7.3 mm in CAB and 15.7 ± 7.6 mm in NCAB. In each of the two groups, three cases with a blade cut-out occurred. Regarding the risks of post-operative hematoma and wound infection, there was no significant difference between the two groups (although close at $p = 0.101$ for hematoma). Finally, in hospital, death and one-year mortality rates were significantly higher in the CAB group. Follow-up was possible for 3 months in all patients and up to 1 year postoperatively in 313 patients. The main results are shown in Table 1 and Figure 2.

Table 1. Patient demographics.

Variable		CAB	NCAB	p-Value (s/ns)
Patients		299	321	
Age (years)		86 ± 8	75 ± 15	$p < 0.001$ (Welch)
Sex		m: 21.7% vs. f: 78.3%	m: 44.2% vs. f: 55.8%	$p < 0.001$ (Chi-Qua)
AO classification				
	31-A1	88	97	
	31-A2	150	143	
	31-A3	61	81	
ASA score				$p = 0.13$ (t-test)
	1	2	9	
	2	28	39	
	3	199	205	
	4	70	68	
Time to surgery [h]		10.6 ± 4.2	11.9 ± 14.8	$p = 0.44$ (Chi-Qua)
OP time [min]		62.6 ± 21.2	54.01 ± 7.1	$p < 0.001$ (Chi-Qua)
Hospital stay [days]		10.6 ± 4.2	11.9 ± 2.8	$p = 0.66$ (Chi-Qua)
Optimal blade position		81.6%	83.2%	$p = 0.46$ (Chi-Qua)
Tip-apex [mm]		16 ± 7.3	15,7 ± 7.6	$p = 0.640$ (T-Test)
Cut-out		3	3	$p = 0.832$ (Chi-Qua)
Hematoma		13	6	$p = 0.101$ (Fischer)
Surgical site infection		3	3	$p = 1$ (Fischer)
Hospital death		8.7%	4%	$p < 0.017$ (Chi-Qua)
One-year mortality		26.3%	15.3%	$p < 0.016$ (Chi-Qua)

The significant values have been highlighted in bold.

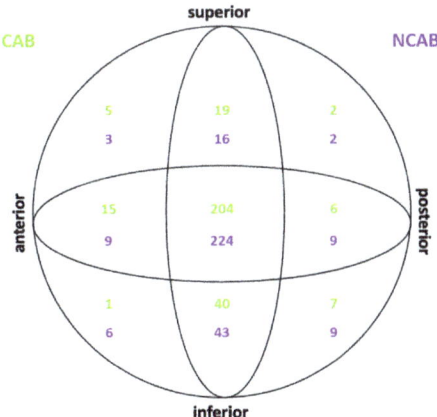

Figure 2. Blade positions of patients without mechanical failure.

3.2. Mechanical Failure, Blade Position and Cement Augmentation

At the follow-up at 3 months, only six patients showed signs of mechanical failure. Of these, three were in the CAB group and three in the NCAB group. The respective cases are shown in Table 2 and Figure 3. The overall cut-out rate was 0.97%. The blade position between the CAB and NCAB groups did not differ significantly. An optimal blade position was achieved in 511 (82.4%) of the 620 cases. The implant positions are shown in Figure 2. No significant differences were found in the tip-apex distance between the two groups (CAB 16 ± 7.3 vs. NCAB 15.7 ± 7.6, $p = 0.640$) with an overall mean of 15.8 ± 7.5 mm.

Table 2. All patients with mechanical failure.

Case	Age	Sex	AO-Classification	Tip Apex	First Signs	Augmentation
(A)	77	female	31-A3	16 mm	39 days	no
(B)	84	female	31-A2	19 mm	56 days	no
(C)	88	female	31-A2	16 mm	10 days	yes
(D)	98	female	31-A2	13 mm	14 days	yes
(E)	93	female	31-A3	2 mm	6 days	yes
(F)	65	female	31-A2	11 mm	41 days	no

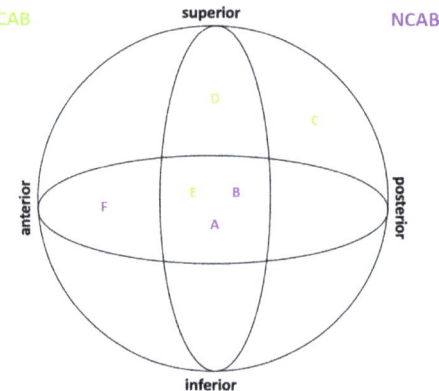

Figure 3. Blade positions of patients with mechanical failure.

3.3. Costs

The mean hospital reimbursement per case was USD 7154 ± 834. Implant costs for the nail system without augmentation (nail, blade, and locking screw) were USD 484 US dollars. For augmentation, the TRAUMACEM V+ Injectable Bone Cement system (Fa. DePuy Synthes) was used with an overall cost of USD 432. The price of the augmentation system included the TRAUMACEM™ V+ Injectable bone cement, TRAUMACEM™ V+ syringe kit and TRAUMACEM™ V+ Injection cannula (Fa. DePuy Synthes). The mean operating time was about 8 min longer in the CAB group (CAB 62.6 ± 21.2 min vs. NCAB 54.01 ± 7.1; $p < 0.05$).

3.4. Complications and Mortality

Surgical site infections occurred in only 0.97% of the cases without a significant difference between the groups. The post-operative hematoma was detected in 3.1% of patients, showing no significant difference between the groups. Hospital mortality (CAB 8.7% vs. NCAB 4.0%; $p < 0.05$; $n = 620$) and 1 year mortality (CAB 26.3% vs. NCAB 15.3%; $p < 0.05$; $n = 313$) were significantly higher in the cement augmentation group.

4. Discussion

Mechanical failure of osteosynthesis in the proximal femur is a feared complication when treating elderly patients with osteoporotic bone. In the literature, the cut-out of the femoral neck blade through the femoral head was reported in between 1.8% and 16.5% of cases [3,7,8,20]. In the study by Bojan et al. [9], a failure rate of 1.8% was observed in 3066 hip fractures treated with the gamma nail between 1990 and 2002. Davis et al. [5] investigated the causes of mechanical osteosynthesis failure in a prospective study of 230 hip screws and Y-nails. The study found 12.4% cut-out and 16.5% further implant failures.

The aim of this study was to evaluate the mechanical failure rate of a large number of patients using a cement-augmented helical femoral neck blade if patient characteristics suggested severe osteoporosis. Using cement augmentation of the blade in about 50% of the cases, the overall mechanical failure rate was lower than in the mentioned studies and evaluated under 1%. Notwithstanding, cement augmentation of the blade extended the operating time by 8 min and nearly doubled the implant costs. Overall, six patients showed signs of mechanical failure, resulting in revision surgery with arthroplasty. If revision surgery was required due to mechanical osteosynthesis failure, a high rate of complications, reoperation, significant loss of function, and pain can be expected [21].

After revision surgery, mortality increases up to 56% in the first year. In addition, according to Palmer et al. [10], a considerable increase in treatment costs with a simultaneous poor prognosis can also be expected. If cement augmentation proves to prevent costly revision surgery, the increased implant costs might be justified. To prevent mechanical failure, Erhart et al. [15] tested the anchorage of PFNA blades augmented with bone cement in eight fresh frozen femoral heads, showing increased rotational stability and higher pullout strength. There is limited clinical evidence evaluating cement augmentation of the femoral neck blade.

Yee and Kammerlander et al. [16,17] addressed the cut-out rate of PFNA blades. Yee et al. [17] studied 76 patients (47 in the CAB group and 29 in the NCAB group) in their retrospective study. The cut-out rate was 2.1% in the CAB group and 13.8% in the NCAB group. Thirty-one patients (29%) could not be followed-up until 6 months postoperatively. In a prospective, multicenter, randomized, and patient-blinded study in 2018, Kammerlander et al. [16] investigated 223 patients (105 in the CAB group and 118 in the NCAB group). There was no cut-out in the CAB group compared to the six cases (5%) in the NCAB not reaching statistical significance due to the low number of cases. One conclusion of the study was that although blade augmentation does not improve patients' ability to walk, it may have the potential to prevent revision surgery by strengthening the osteosynthesis construct. Compared with these studies, augmentation was performed in 48% of patients (299 of 620) in the present study. The average OR time with augmentation was 8 min longer, apart from the additional implant costs. The patients in the CAB group were, on average, 11 years older, and the proportion of women was significantly higher. Both values, age and female gender, are known risk factors for osteoporosis. Nevertheless, the cut-out rate between these two groups in our study showed no significant difference (CAB 1% vs. NCAB 0.9%). Therefore, despite the higher costs and not reaching statistical significance, this might confirm the higher stability of augmented femoral neck blades in patients with severe osteoporosis. In line with the literature [12–15], there was no significant difference in the cut-out rate between the groups. Due to the low overall cut-out rate of less than 1%, the study cohort needs to be even larger than the 620 evaluated patients.

With regard to the low cut-out rate in our NCAB group, the authors would like to emphasize the value of the anatomical reduction, tip-apex distance (TAD) of less than 25 mm, and a center-center or inferior-center blade position. In 2008, Lobo-Escolar et al. [3] showed in their case-control study that an unfavorable tip-apex distance and blade position are significant risk factors for cut-out. The study evaluated 916 proximal femur fractures treated with a gamma nail resulting in a mechanical failure rate of 3.3%. This is in line with several studies [22–24]. Ibrahim et al. [25] analyzed 313 patients for fracture pattern, TAD, Parker's ratio and reduction quality and demonstrated that insufficient fracture reduction also was a significant predictor of implant failure.

The study has certain limitations. This is a retrospective study with a short follow-up of only 3 months in all patients and up to 1 year in only 313 patients. However, mechanical implant failure may occur even later. There is a huge selection bias due to the significant age and gender differences in both groups as well as the unrandomized design of the study. Furthermore, no functional or emotional data were collected. To show a significant difference between the groups, a large RCT with a long follow-up period must be performed because the cut-out rate of modern implants is very low with correct indications and surgical techniques. Clinical parameters, such as ROM (range of motion), HHS (Harris hip score), and VAS (visual analogue scale), etc., could then be included.

5. Conclusions

In conclusion, this study evaluated, by far, the largest cohort of patients with proximal femoral fractures treated with augmented blades compared to non-augmented blades. A significant difference between the groups could not be established despite increased implant costs and longer operating times. However, treating proximal femoral fractures with cephalomedullary nails can achieve a mechanical failure rate of less than 1% of anatomical reduction, a tip-apex distance of less than 25 mm, an optimal blade position is achieved, and cement augmentation is used in cases with severe osteoporosis. Therefore, the authors recommend the augmentation of the blade in osteoporotic patients. However, it should be noted that augmentation is expensive and prolongs surgery time without definite proof of its mechanical superiority.

Author Contributions: All authors contributed equally to the study. All authors have read and agreed to the published version of the manuscript.

Funding: This research received no external funding.

Institutional Review Board Statement: This retrospective chart review study involving human participants was in accordance with the ethical standards of the institutional and national research committee and with the 1964 Helsinki Declaration and its later amendments or comparable ethical standards. The local Human Investigation Committee (IRB) approved this study.

Informed Consent Statement: Consent to participate: In accordance with the local ethics committee, due to the retrospective design, obtaining consent to participate was not necessary. Consent for publication: In accordance with the local ethics committee, due to the retrospective design, consent to publication was not necessary.

Data Availability Statement: All authors decided that the data and material would not be deposited in a public repository.

Conflicts of Interest: The authors declare no conflict of interest. No company had influence in the collection of data or contributed to or had influence on the conception, design, analysis and writing of the study. No further funding was received.

References

1. Court-Brown, C.M.; Caesar, B. Epidemiology of adult fractures: A review. *Injury* **2006**, *37*, 691–697. [CrossRef] [PubMed]
2. Müller-Mai, C.; Raestrup, U.S.; Kostuj, T.; Dahlhoff, G.; Günster, C.; Smektala, R. One-year outcomes for proximal femoral fractures: Posthospital analysis of mortality and care levels based on health insurance data. *Unfallchirurg* **2015**, *118*, 780–794. [CrossRef] [PubMed]
3. Lobo-Escolar, A.; Joven, E.; Iglesias, D.; Herrera, A. Predictive factors for cutting-out in femoral intramedullary nailing. *Injury* **2010**, *41*, 1312–1316. [CrossRef]
4. von Rüden, C.; Augat, P. Failure of fracture fixation in osteoporotic bone. *Injury* **2016**, *47* (Suppl. S2), S3–S10. [CrossRef]
5. Davis, T.; Sher, J.; Horsman, A.; Simpson, M.; Porter, B.; Checketts, R. Intertrochanteric femoral fractures. Mechanical failure after internal fixation. *J. Bone Jt. Surg. Br.* **1990**, *72*, 26–31. [CrossRef]
6. Bonnaire, F.; Weber, A.; Bösl, O.; Eckhardt, C.; Schwieger, K.; Linke, B. "Cutting out" in pertrochanteric fractures–problem of osteoporosis? *Der Unf.* **2007**, *110*, 425–432. [CrossRef] [PubMed]
7. Bojan, A.J.; Beimel, C.; Taglang, G.; Collin, D.; Ekholm, C.; Jönsson, A. Critical factors in cut-out complication after gamma nail treatment of proximal femoral fractures. *BMC Musculoskelet. Disord.* **2013**, *14*, 1. [CrossRef] [PubMed]
8. Lizaur-Utrilla, A.; Reig, J.S.; Miralles-Muñoz, F.A.; Tufanisco, C.B. Trochanteric gamma nail and compression hip screw for trochanteric fractures: A randomized, prospective, comparative study in 210 elderly patients with a new design of the gamma nail. *J. Orthop. Trauma* **2005**, *19*, 229–233. [CrossRef] [PubMed]
9. Bojan, A.J.; Beimel, C.; Speitling, A.; Taglang, G.; Ekholm, C.; Jonsson, A. 3066 consecutive Gamma Nails. 12 years experience at a single centre. *BMC Musculoskelet. Disord.* **2010**, *11*, 133. [CrossRef] [PubMed]
10. Palmer, S.J.; Parker, M.J.; Hollingworth, W. The cost and implications of reoperation after surgery for fracture of the hip. *J. Bone Jt. Surg. Br.* **2000**, *82*, 864–866. [CrossRef]
11. Tucker, A.; Warnock, M.; McDonald, S.; Cusick, L.; Foster, A.P. Fatigue failure of the cephalomedullary nail: Revision options, outcomes and review of the literature. *Eur. J. Orthop. Surg. Traumatol.* **2017**, *28*, 511–520. [CrossRef] [PubMed]
12. Neuerburg, C.; Gosch, M.; Blauth, M.; Bocker, W.; Kammerlander, C. Augmentation techniques on the proximal femur. *Der Unf.* **2015**, *118*, 755–764. [CrossRef] [PubMed]

13. Von Der Linden, P.; Gisep, A.; Boner, V.; Windolf, M.; Appelt, A.; Suhm, N. Biomechanical evaluation of a new augmentation method for enhanced screw fixation in osteoporotic proximal femoral fractures. *J. Orthop. Res.* **2006**, *24*, 2230–2237. [CrossRef]
14. Fensky, F.; Nüchtern, J.; Kolb, J.; Huber, S.; Rupprecht, M.; Jauch, S.; Sellenschloh, K.; Püschel, K.; Morlock, M.; Rueger, J.; et al. Cement augmentation of the proximal femoral nail antirotation for the treatment of osteoporotic pertrochanteric fractures—A biomechanical cadaver study. *Injury* **2013**, *44*, 802–807. [CrossRef]
15. Erhart, S.; Schmoelz, W.; Blauth, M.; Lenich, A. Biomechanical effect of bone cement augmentation on rotational stability and pull-out strength of the Proximal Femur Nail Antirotation™. *Injury* **2011**, *42*, 1322–1327. [CrossRef] [PubMed]
16. Kammerlander, C.; Hem, E.S.; Klopfer, T.; Gebhard, F.; Sermon, A.; Dietrich, M.; Bach, O.; Weil, Y.; Babst, R.; Blauth, M. Cement augmentation of the Proximal Femoral Nail Antirotation (PFNA)—A multicentre randomized controlled trial. *Injury* **2018**, *49*, 1436–1444. [CrossRef]
17. Yee, D.K.H.; Lau, W.; Tiu, K.L.; Leung, F.; Fang, E.; Pineda, J.P.S.; Fang, C. Cementation: For better or worse? Interim results of a multi-centre cohort study using a fenestrated spiral blade cephalomedullary device for pertrochanteric fractures in the elderly. *Arch. Orthop. Trauma Surg.* **2020**, *140*, 1957–1964. [CrossRef]
18. Schuetze, K.; Ehinger, S.; Eickhoff, A.; Dehner, C.; Gebhard, F.; Richter, P.H. Cement augmentation of the proximal femur nail antirotation: Is it safe? *Arch. Orthop. Trauma Surg.* **2021**, *141*, 803–811. [CrossRef] [PubMed]
19. Baumgaertner, M.R.; Curtin, S.L.; Lindskog, D.M.; Keggi, J.M. The value of the tip-apex distance in predicting failure of fixation of peritrochanteric fractures of the hip. *J. Bone Jt. Surg. Am.* **1995**, *77*, 1058–1064. [CrossRef] [PubMed]
20. Kukla, C.; Heinz, T.; Gaebler, C.; Heinze, G.; Vécsei, V. The Standard Gamma Nail: A Critical Analysis of 1000 Cases. *J. Trauma Inj. Infect. Crit. Care* **2001**, *51*, 77–83. [CrossRef]
21. Liu, P.; Jin, D.; Zhang, C.; Gao, Y. Revision surgery due to failed internal fixation of intertrochanteric femoral fracture: Current state-of-the-art. *BMC Musculoskelet. Disord.* **2020**, *21*, 573. [CrossRef] [PubMed]
22. Buyukdogan, K.; Caglar, O.; Isik, S.; Tokgozoglu, M.; Atilla, B. Risk factors for cut-out of double lag screw fixation in proximal femoral fractures. *Injury* **2016**, *48*, 414–418. [CrossRef] [PubMed]
23. Geller, J.A.; Saifi, C.; Morrison, T.A.; Macaulay, W. Tip-apex distance of intramedullary devices as a predictor of cut-out failure in the treatment of peritrochanteric elderly hip fractures. *Int. Orthop.* **2010**, *34*, 719–722. [CrossRef] [PubMed]
24. De Bruijn, K.; den Hartog, D.; Tuinebreijer, W.; Roukema, G. Reliability of Predictors for Screw Cutout in Intertrochanteric Hip Fractures. *J. Bone Jt. Sur. Am. Vol.* **2012**, *94*, 1266–1272. [CrossRef] [PubMed]
25. Ibrahim, I.; Appleton, P.T.; Wixted, J.J.; DeAngelis, J.P.; Rodriguez, E.K. Implant cut-out following cephalomedullary nailing of intertrochanteric femur fractures: Are helical blades to blame? *Injury* **2019**, *50*, 926–930. [CrossRef] [PubMed]

Disclaimer/Publisher's Note: The statements, opinions and data contained in all publications are solely those of the individual author(s) and contributor(s) and not of MDPI and/or the editor(s). MDPI and/or the editor(s) disclaim responsibility for any injury to people or property resulting from any ideas, methods, instructions or products referred to in the content.

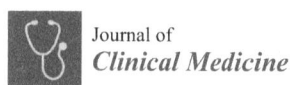

Article

Value of Diagnostic Tools in the Diagnosis of Osteomyelitis: Pilot Study to Establish an Osteomyelitis Score

Roslind K. Hackenberg [1,2,*], Fabio Schmitt-Sánchez [1], Christoph Endler [3], Verena Tischler [4], Jayagopi Surendar [1], Kristian Welle [1], Koroush Kabir [1] and Frank A. Schildberg [1,*]

[1] Department of Orthopedics and Trauma Surgery, University Hospital Bonn, 53127 Bonn, Germany
[2] Department of Hand, Plastic and Reconstructive Surgery, Burn Center, BG Trauma Center Ludwigshafen, University of Heidelberg, 67071 Ludwigshafen, Germany
[3] Department of Diagnostic and Interventional Radiology, University Hospital Bonn, 53127 Bonn, Germany
[4] Institute of Pathology, University Hospital Bonn, 53127 Bonn, Germany
* Correspondence: roslind.hackenberg@bgu-ludwigshafen.de (R.K.H.); frank.schildberg@ukbonn.de (F.A.S.)

Abstract: Osteomyelitis (OM) remains one of the most feared complications in bone surgery and trauma. Its diagnosis remains a major challenge due to lack of guidelines. The aim of this study was to prospectively analyze the value of the most common and available diagnostic tools and to establish an OM score to derive treatment recommendations. All patients with suspected OM were included in a prospective pilot study. All patients underwent blood sampling for C-reactive protein and white blood cell count analysis. Magnetic resonance imaging (MRI), and microbiologic and histopathologic samples, were taken from representative sites of initial debridement. All patients were treated according to their OM test results and followed for at least one year. Subsequently, the value of individual or combined diagnostic tools was analyzed in patients with confirmed OM and in patients in whom OM was ruled out. Based on these findings, an OM score was developed that included MRI, microbiology, and histopathology. The score identified all control patients and all but one OM patient, resulting in a correct diagnosis of 93.3%, which was validated in a second independent larger cohort. This was the first study to analyze the value of the most commonly used tools to diagnose OM. The proposed OM score provides a simple scoring system to safely interpret test results with high accuracy.

Keywords: osteomyelitis; score; diagnostics; histology; MRI

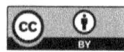

1. Introduction

Osteomyelitis (OM) is an inflammation of the bone caused by infecting microorganisms. The origin can be hematogenous (blood-born spread of bacteria to a predominantly pre-injured bone) or contiguous after open fractures, preceding surgery, adjacent skin ulcer or pressure sore [1,2]. It can be acute with severe localized pain, swelling, erythema, elevated temperature, malaise, exceed to bacteremia, and pyrexia or chronic with only minor clinical symptoms of subtle pain, swelling, redness and temperature elevation. In chronic OM tenderness, soft tissue remodeling, and recurrent sinuses may be present. If not treated adequately, acute OM can become chronic, and chronic OM can stay subclinical for years with a possible acute exacerbation at any time. The discrimination between acute and chronic OM is the presence of dead bone in chronic OM due to destruction and remodeling of the bone [2].

A precise and determined diagnostics is crucial to adequately treat OM, especially in OM of the limbs, where it is localized most frequently with at least 73.8% in the lower and 17.7% in the upper limb [3]. In the treatment of OM, the question of limb salvage versus an inevitable amputation is always raised. Despite medical progress, including more and more elaborate reconstructive procedures and new antibiotics allowing to aim for limb salvage more frequently, the prevalence of OM has been increasing [3]. The diagnostic workup remains a challenge and is the starting point for any treatment.

Besides the assessment of clinical symptoms, which may be subtle and nondescript, plain X-rays of the limb and laboratory workup including white blood count (WBC) and C-reactive protein (CRP) are basic diagnostics. In the early phase, X-rays may be normal, present with unspecific osteopenia or delayed fracture healing, so that differential diagnosis cannot be ruled out. Additionally, an elevated WBC and CRP are not specific for OM and can be present after trauma and surgery and in any inflammatory circumstance of the body [1,4–8]. In addition, a normal WBC and CRP may not rule out an OM, especially in clinically inapparent and chronic cases. Advanced diagnostic workup, including magnetic resonance imaging (MRI) and obtaining histological and microbiological samples, is not performed uniformly, due to a lack of consensus and standardized treatment recommendations [9].

Until now, there has been a vast lack of knowledge about the possibilities of advanced diagnostics, their proper performance, interpretation, and informative value. An adequate diagnostic workup, however, is inevitable and the basis for any treatment and, specifically, limb salvage. Thus, the aim of this study was to prospectively evaluate the value of diagnostic means in the diagnosis of OM and to develop a grading system to facilitate and standardize the diagnosis of OM in the limbs.

2. Materials and Methods

In this prospective monocenter pilot study in a clinic of maximum medical care, all patients with a minimum age of 18 years and a suspected OM of the limbs were included between January 2020 and March 2021. OM was suspected based on medical history and clinical findings such as local swelling, pain, redness, hyperthermia, and wound healing disorders with a persistent wound or recurrence of a wound or fistula, as well as fever and shivering.

Patients with and without a history of trauma and/or surgery at the local site, as well as those with and without local implants, were included. Age, gender, localization of suspected OM, length of hospital stay, treatment, predisposing factors, and complications were recorded. Complications were death, recurrent or persistent soft tissue infection, OM, and wound healing disorders, as well as adverse events necessitating revision surgery or intervention, such as joint dislocation, implant dislocation, postoperative bleeding, pneumonia, urinary tract infection, acute renal failure necessitating dialysis, thromboembolism, and myocardial infarction.

After inclusion into the study, an MRI with contrast medium was performed and a blood sample was taken from each patient to analyze the WBC and CRP. The presence of an implant was no contraindication for an MRI. In case of an implant at the site of suspected OM, the MRI was performed as a metal artifact reduction sequence. A computed tomography (CT) scan instead of an MRI was only considered as sufficient if the CT scan already showed distinct signs of OM. Distinct signs for OM in the CT were destruction of the bone, osteolysis, and the formation of sequestrums. Typical signs for OM in the MRI were as follows: focal decrease in bone marrow signal intensity on T1-weighted images, focal increase in signal intensity in the bone on T2-weighted, fat-suppressed images, focal bone marrow enhancement on gadolinium-enhanced fat suppressed T1-weighted images suggesting bone marrow edema, and in advanced stage, intraosseous abscess with formation of reactive bone surrounding intramedullary pus, subperiosteal abscess, sinus tract, ulceration, and cortical erosion [10–12].

During the first surgical debridement, microbiologic and histopathologic samples, each from soft tissue and bone, were taken and assessed by senior microbiologists and pathologists. Intraoperatively collected tissue specimens were homogenized and plated on Columbia agar with 5% sheep blood, MacConkey agar, chocolate agar, and Sabouraud agar (Becton & Dickinson, Bergen County, NJ, USA). In addition, samples were also cultured in thioglycolate boullion (Becton & Dickinson, Bergen County, NJ, USA). For anaerobic cultures, Schaedler and kanamycin/vancomycin agar plates (Becton & Dickinson, Bergen County, NJ, USA) were used. All cultures were grown at 5% CO_2 and 35 °C for at least 14 days. All histopathologic samples were preserved in formalin, processed as paraffin sections, and stained with hemotoxylin and eosin. All bone samples were decalcified. Inflammation was diagnosed when inflammatory cells, specifically macrophages and granulocytes, were present.

Based on the diagnostic findings, patients were classified as "osteomyelitis" (OM) or "control" (CO) and treated accordingly. Classification was performed blinded and independently by two senior orthopedic and trauma surgeons. In case of disagreement, the case was reviewed by a third orthopedic and trauma surgeon. Patients were classified as "OM" when showing distinct signs of OM in the MRI and either having an active or chronic inflammation in histopathologic bone samples or an isolate of a microbiological pathogen in a bone sample. Patients were also classified as "OM" when only having signs compatible with OM in the MRI, such as minimal or diffuse contrast medium enhancement in the bone marrow, but a proof of active or chronic inflammation in histopathological bone samples combined with an isolate of microbiological pathogens in bone samples. Patients were classified as "CO" when no pathogen was isolated in bone samples, there were no signs of inflammation in histopathological bone samples, and there was an absence of distinct signs of "OM" in the MRI, or only when "OM" could not be completely ruled out. In all other cases, a reevaluation of the pre-analysis was performed, and testing was repeated. All patients were followed-up with for at least one year. Based on further diagnostic findings and the course of treatment, the classification into OM and CO was reevaluated in every patient and, in case of initial misdiagnosis, corrected.

The WBC, CRP, MRI, microbiologic, and histopathologic results were analyzed regarding their diagnostic value to predict the presence of OM between patients with and without a subsequent OM.

Furthermore, an OM score was established concerning the probability of a present OM based on the diagnostic findings. To confirm this score, we retrospectively validated it in a second independent cohort of 55 patients. Patients' diagnostic findings were blindly evaluated according to the OM score and the results were compared with the initial clinician's diagnosis. Descriptive statistical analysis was performed using GraphPad Prism, Version 9 (GraphPad Software, San Diego, CA, USA). Significant differences between the groups were identified using the unpaired t-test in normally distributed variables and the Mann-Whitney U test in non-normally distributed variables. The level of significance was defined at $p < 0.05$.

All patients included were willing to participate in the study and gave their written informed consent. The study was approved by the local ethics committee of the University Hospital Bonn (local review board number 277/19) and performed in accordance with the ethical standards of the institutional and national research committees and the 1964 Helsinki declaration and its later amendments.

3. Results

3.1. Patient Cohort and Clinical Presentation

A total of 15 patients were included in this pilot study. Nine patients had an OM and were assigned to the OM group. In 6 patients an OM was ruled out; thus, these patients were assigned to the CO group. There was no significant difference in the demographic data between the groups as displayed in Table 1.

Table 1. Epidemiologic data.

		OM	CO	p
Number of patients [n]		9	6	-
Age [y] *		55 ± 19 [26; 79]	54 ± 18 [30; 78]	p = 0.910
Gender [n]	Female	3	2	p = 0.490
	Male	6	4	
Number of surgeries [n] *		13 ± 8 [2; 28]	7 ± 4 [3; 15]	p = 0.199
Length of hospital stay [d] *		81 ± 70 [6; 213]	53 ± 34 [5; 94]	p = 0.387
Type of injury [n]	Mono trauma	6	3	p = 0.422
	Polytrauma	3	3	
Complications	Death [n]	1	0	p = 0.465
	Recurrent/persistent infection, OM, wound healing disorder, adverse events [n]	5	2	
Localization [n]	Upper limb	Hand/finger	1	0	-
		Forearm/elbow	0	1	
		Upper arm/shoulder	1	0	
	Lower Limb	Ankle/foot	0	2	
		Lower leg/knee	5	3	
		Thigh/Hip	2	0	

* mean ± standard deviation [minimum; maximum].

In both groups the gender ratio was equivalent with 2:1 in favor of men. Despite, on average, a longer length of hospital stay and higher number of surgeries in patients of the OM group, there was no significant difference between both groups, respectively (length of hospital stay: $p = 0.387$, number of surgeries: $p = 0.199$).

All patients had a history of trauma, of whom 6 had a history of polytrauma (OM group n = 3, control group n = 3). There was no significant difference of the ratio of mono vs. polytrauma between the two groups ($p = 0.422$). There was no idiopathic wound healing disorder or OM. Additionally, in all patients of both groups, at least one risk factor for soft tissue infection and/or OM, such as an open fracture, underlying peripheral artery disease (PAD), underlying immunosuppressive or inflammatory disease or treatment (cancer, chemotherapy, chronic inflammatory autoimmune disease), and perforating injury, could be identified as shown in Table 2.

Of the 9 OM patients, in 6 an acute OM and in 3 a chronic OM was diagnosed. Two patients with chronic OM refused radical bony debridement and bony reconstruction, and so their numbers of surgeries and lengths of hospital stay were comparably low. Excluding both these patients, neither was the length of hospital stay significantly longer (OM group: 101 ± 67 d, CO group: 53 ± 34 d; $p = 0.141$), nor was the number of surgeries significantly higher (OM group: 15 ± 8 surgeries, CO group: 7 ± 4 surgeries; $p = 0.087$). In total, the lower limb (upper limb n = 3, lower limb n = 12) and the lower leg were affected most often in both groups; see Table 1. The rate of complications was not significantly higher in the OM group (n = 6) than the CO group (n = 2), even including 1 death in the OM group ($p = 0.465$). There was found to be no initial misdiagnosis after a follow-up of at least one year, and so no initial diagnosis needed to be corrected.

Table 2. Injury entity and risk factors for soft tissue infection and/or OM.

Injury Entity and Risk Factors		OM	CO
Open fracture	Total	4	2
	With PAD * or immunosuppressive disease/treatment	0	0
Closed fracture	Total	4	3
	With multiple surgeries	1	0
	With PAD or immunosuppressive disease/treatment	1	3
	With multiple surgeries and PAD or immunosuppressive disease/treatment	2	0
Soft tissue/perforating injury without fracture	Total	1	1
	With PAD or immunosuppressive disease/treatment	0	1

* PAD: peripheral artery disease.

3.2. WBC and CRP

On average, both the WBC (OM group: $9.2 \pm 2.8 \times 10^9$/L, CO group: $6.4 \pm 2.0 \times 10^9$/L) and CRP were higher in the OM group (OM group: 46 ± 65 mg/L; CO group: 19 ± 13 mg/L). Despite the average WBC being within the reference range (female: 3.6–10.5×10^9/L; male: 3.9–10.2×10^9/L) in both groups, it was significantly higher in the OM group ($p = 0.046$). In the OM group, 4 patients showed an elevated WBC (>10.5×10^9/L). In the CO group 1 patient had a lowered WBC (<3.6–10.5×10^9/L).

The average CRP was elevated and above the reference range of 0–3 mg/L in both groups, however, not being significantly different between the groups ($p = 0.344$). In the OM group, 1 patient showed a normal value of the CRP while all other patients had an elevated CRP in both groups.

3.3. MRI

In the CO group, 2 patients (33.3%) showed osseous alterations with contrast medium enhancement in the MRI disallowing an exclusion of an OM. The remaining 4 patients had no typical OM-like alterations of the bone. Thus, in the CO group there was no positive MRI for OM; however, in 2 cases, an OM could not be ruled out.

In 8 patients of the OM group an MRI was performed. In 1 patient only a CT was performed and classified as sufficient, since it already showed distinct signs of OM with bone destruction, osteolysis, and sequestrums. In 7 patients (87.5%) of the OM group, OM-typical alterations were found in the MRI and, thus, were classified as positive for OM diagnosis. One OM patient (12.5%) exhibited osseous alterations, however, inconclusive of being in the context of OM or postoperative or stress reaction. This one MRI was not negative for OM, but did not confirm it either. Table 3 presents the essential diagnostic findings of the imaging procedures.

Table 3. Diagnostic findings in MRI, Microbiology and Histopathology.

Patient	Group	MRI	Microbiology	Histopathology
1	OM	**Positive** (Long-segment contrast medium enhancement in the bone as sign of OM)	**Bone**: S. haemolyticus	**Bone**: Chronic granulating inflammation
2	OM	**Positive** (Contrast medium enhancement in the bone adjacent to the fracture zone as signs of OM)	**Bone**: S. epidermidis, Pseudomonas aeruginosa	**Bone**: Active and chronic granulating inflammation in the medullary cavity
3	OM	**Positive** (Contrast medium enhancement in the bone with signs for distinct OM with abscess-forming soft tissue defect)	**Bone**: S. aureus (MSSA *)	**Bone**: Active and chronic granulating inflammation in the medullary cavity
4	OM	**Positive** (Contrast medium enhancement of the bone as a sign of OM)	**Bone**: S. epidermidis	**Bone**: Chronic granulating inflammation
7	OM	**Indistinct** (Slight contrast medium enhancement in the bone marrow of the without affection of the cortical bone, most likely to postoperative reaction; however, an inflammatory process (e.g., OM) cannot be ruled out)	**Bone**: E. faecalis, Klebsiella pneumoniae, S. epidermidis	**Bone**: Chronic active granulating inflammation
5	OM	**Positive** (Contrast medium enhancement in the bone and cortical bone defects with signs for OM and abscess-formation adjacent to a cortical bone defect)	**Bone**: S. aureus (MSSA *)	**Bone**: Chronic granulating inflammation
8	OM	**Positive** (Contrast medium enhancement of the bone with signs for OM)	**Bone**: S. aureus (MSSA *), S. saccrolyticus	**Bone**: Chronic granulating inflammation
6	OM	**CT: Positive** (Bony destruction with osteolysis and formation of bony sequestrums)	**Bone**: S. capitis	**Bone**: Chronic granulating inflammation
9	OM	**Positive** (Erosion of the cortical bone accompanied by signal alterations and contrast medium enhancement compatible with OM)	**Bone**: none **Soft tissue**: Pseudomonas fluorescens	**Soft tissue**: Moderate chronic granulating inflammation
10	CO	**Negative** (No OM-typical alterations with contrast medium enhancement only in the adjacent soft tissue)	**Bone**: none **Soft tissue**: S. haemolyticus, Candida parapsilosis	**Bone**: No signs for inflammation Soft tissue: Periprosthetic membrane, wear particle-induced type
11	CO	**Negative** (No contrast medium enhancement of the bone ruling out an inflammatory process of the bone)	**Bone**: none **Soft tissue**: S. haemolyticus, S. epidermidis, Roseomonas mucosa	**Bone**: No signs for inflammation **Soft tissue**: Chronic soft tissue inflammation
12	CO	**Indistinct** (Diffuse contrast medium enhancement of the bone compatible with stress reaction but also an inflammation, e.g., OM)	**Bone**: none **Soft tissue**: E. cloacae, Acinetobacter bereziniae, Acinetobacter lwoffii	**Bone**: No signs for inflammation and OM
13	CO	**Indistinct** (Diffuse contrast medium enhancement of the dorsal cortical bone compatible with an inflammatory process, such as OM, or stress reacion)	**Bone**: none **Soft tissue**: S. aureus (MSSA *), S. agalactiae	**Bone**: No signs for active inflammation **Soft tissue**: Chronic granulating active ulcerating inflammation with necrosis
14	CO	**Negative** (Minimal contrast medium enhancement of the superficial cortical bone; most likely postoperative reactive)	**Bone**: none **Soft tissue**: S. epidermidis	**Bone**: No signs for active granulating inflammation
15	CO	**Negative** (No contrast medium enhancement of the bone; no sign of OM)	**Bone**: none **Soft tissue**: none	**Bone**: No signs for chronic inflammation or OM **Soft tissue**: Connective tissue with focal purulent inflammation

* MSSA: methicillin-susceptible Staphylococcus aureus.

3.4. Microbiology

During surgical debridement, samples of the bone and soft tissue were taken routinely. In the CO group, no patient had a detection of a microorganism in the bone samples. In 5 of the 6 CO patients, bacteria could be isolated in the soft tissue samples. In 4 of them a polymicrobial infection was present, only 1 patient had an isolation of one pathogen.

In the OM group, 8 patients (88.9%) had an isolation of at least one pathogen in the bone samples. In 1 patient (11.1%) a pathogen could be isolated only in the soft tissue despite the presence of OM. Five patients (55.6%) had a monomicrobial OM. Three patients (33.3%) had a polymicrobial OM, with 2 patients having 2 pathogens and 1 patient having 3 pathogens isolated. Four patients had additional pathogens isolated in the soft tissue and/or the course of treatment. No patient had an infection with a multi-resistant pathogen. Table 3 displays the isolated pathogens in the OM and CO groups.

3.5. Histopathology

Histopathologic samples of the bone and soft tissue were taken in the first debridement in all but 1 OM patient. In 1 OM patient only soft tissue samples were taken, which were positive for inflammation. A repetition was not performed since there was no revision surgery for persistent OM. In 2 CO patients, no additional histopathologic samples of the soft tissue were taken. In all patients of the OM group, the bone samples showed chronic granulating inflammations and, thus, were positive for OM (100%). In all patients of the OM group that had soft tissue samples taken (n = 8), an accompanying chronic granulating inflammation of the soft tissue was also diagnosed.

No patient in the CO group had signs of inflammation in the bone samples. Of the patients with additional soft tissue samples in the CO group, 3 had signs of chronic granulating inflammation in the soft tissue, and in 1 patient a peri-implant membrane formation was present. Based on the histopathologic bone samples, all patients were correctly diagnosed for having OM or ruling out an OM. Table 3 shows the histopathologic results of all patients.

3.6. Osteomyelitis Score

On the sole basis of histopathologic exams, the diagnosis could be made correctly in all cases. Due to the risk of implementation error in taking samples from non-representative areas resulting in false negative results, a combination of diagnostic tools is recommended. Thus, an OM score was established to strengthen the diagnosis.

The OM score includes MRI, microbiology, and histopathology. A CT scan will only be valid instead of an MRI if it already is distinct for OM. Due to a lack of informative value, both laboratory tests—WBC and CRP—were not included in the OM score. For each diagnostic procedure, a point score was assigned, then added up for each patient and interpreted according to Table 4.

By means of the OM score, the presence and absence of OM could be correctly diagnosed in 14 patients (93.3%) and treatment could be derived for all patients according to the score. Based on this OM score, in all patients in the CO group, an OM could be correctly ruled out (n = 6; 100%), as shown in Table 5. All OM patients but 1 could be correctly diagnosed as suffering from an OM. One patient was classified as indistinct. The reevaluation of the diagnostic tools showed that there were no histopathologic samples taken from bone, which could have led to a correct diagnosis of OM. However, despite not having proof of OM, that patient was classified as highly at risk and, OM being probable, was thus treated as having an acute OM.

Table 4. Osteomyelitis Score.

Diagnostics			
Diagnostic Procedure	Points	Findings	
MRI	+1 *	OM-typical alterations making OM very probable	
	0	Unspecific osseous alterations with contrast medium enhancement or edema suggesting postoperative or posttraumatic stress reaction but not ruling out OM	
	−1	No osseous alterations; absence of OM-typical bone reactions	
Microbiology	+1	Isolation of pathogen in bone sample	
	0	Isolation of pathogen only in soft tissue samples, but not in bone samples	
	−1	No isolation of pathogen: neither in bone nor in soft tissue samples	
Histopathology	+1	Granulating inflammation in bone samples	
	0	Granulating inflammation in soft tissue samples, but not in bone samples	
	−1	No granulating inflammation: neither in bone nor in tissue samples	
Interpretation			
Points	Interpretation	Treatment recommendation	
2–3	Presence of OM/OM most likely	Therapy of OM	
1	Presence of OM indistinct	Reevaluate the adequate realization of the diagnostic tool (e.g., MRI performed with contrast medium, samples for microbiology and/or histopathology taken from representative sites?); high risk for developing an OM; thus, treat as OM	
−3–0	Absence of OM/OM very unlikely	Therapy of underlying condition apart from OM, e.g., wound/soft tissue infection	

* A CT with distinct signs for OM (destruction of the bone, osteolysis, and formation of sequestrums) may substitute an MRI and equivalently add +1 point to the score.

To validate the new OM score, we utilized a second independent cohort of 55 patients (female: n = 19, 34.5%; male: n = 36, 65.5%) with a mean age of 59.8 ± 15.7 years. In this cohort, 25 patients (45.5%) were initially clinically diagnosed with OM. Using the OM score, 22 of these patients were also diagnosed with OM. The remaining 3 patients had an OM score of 1 with a recommendation to re-evaluate the test or treat as OM. Upon closer inspection, it was found that 2 patients did not receive complete histopathologic diagnostics, 2 did not have a properly interpreted MRI, and 1 had a false negative microbiologic result after antibiotic treatment. Most importantly, by clinical means alone, 30 patients were diagnosed as not having OM, of which 7 were misdiagnosed. Using the OM score, 23 patients were correctly diagnosed as not having OM and the 7 clinically missed OM were identified by the OM score as highly suspicious for OM (score of 1) with the recommendation to re-evaluate the test or treat as OM. Thus, by clinical means alone, only 87.3% of the patients were correctly diagnosed as having or not having OM and 7 patients with OM (12.7%) were missed (Figure 1). Using the OM score, all patients were correctly identified as having OM, not having OM, or being highly suspicious for OM. There were no false negative diagnoses using the OM score, and the 7 misdiagnosed patients would have been identified.

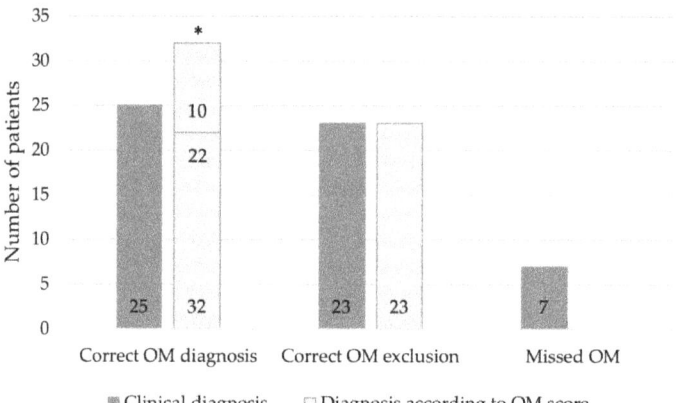

Figure 1. Validation of the OM score. A second independent cohort of 55 patients was used to validate the new OM score. Clinical diagnosis was compared to diagnosis according to OM score and the extent to which both modes correctly diagnosed, excluded, or misdiagnosed OM. * n = 32 patients: 22 patients with the correct diagnosis of OM (OM score of 2–3) and 10 patients with OM score of 1, recommending re-evaluation of diagnostic testing or treatment as OM.

Table 5. Osteomyelitis score.

Group	Patient	MRI	Histo	Mibi	OM-Score
OM	1	1	1	1	3
	2	1	1	1	3
	3	1	1	1	3
	4	1	1	1	3
	5	0	1	1	2
	6	1	0 **	1	2
	7	1	1	1	3
	8	1 *	1	1	3
	9	1	0 **	0	1
CO	1	−1	0	0	−1
	2	−1	0	0	−1
	3	0	0 ***	0	0
	4	0	0	0	0
	5	−1	0 ***	0	−1
	6	−1	0	−1	−2

* Patient was only examined by CT. ** No bone sample was taken. *** No soft tissue sample was taken.

4. Discussion

Overall, OM is a rare disease with a prevalence of 16.7/100,000 inhabitants [3]. However, despite more and more modern treatment options, over a 10-year period from 2008 to 2018, its prevalence has increased by about 10.44% [3]. Its burden on the patient and health care providers, therefore, remains immense. A precise diagnostic is inevitable but crucial. Diagnostic tools such as clinical symptoms and blood tests are unspecific and may only aid as additional criteria. The correct administration and application of further diagnostic tools, specifically MRI, microbiological and histopathological tests, and their precise interpretation, is essential to a proper diagnosis of OM.

As soon as the diagnosis of an OM is set, a treatment consequence is inevitable. The initial diagnosis in early and acute stages may not be difficult to make, and may be correctly made in up to 80% of cases [13]. However, difficulties are specifically encountered in recurrent or persistent OM. Their therapy is crucial and often necessitates vast debridements and resections of bone segments, as well as implant removal in the case of present implants. This often results in the need for segmental bone reconstruction, not infrequently accompanying soft tissue reconstruction. If limb salvage is not possible, the only alternative is an amputation. The encounter with these severe therapeutical consequences may influence the correct interpretation of diagnostic findings and decision making. The honest interpretation of the diagnostic means should not be biased by a clinician's concern regarding the challenging treatment options.

In this context, this is the first prospective study to evaluate the value of the most common diagnostic means for the diagnosis of OM in the limbs. Moreover, the established OM score offers a simple scoring system by which test results can be safely and accurately interpreted. There was no misdiagnosis based on the score. Only one OM patient was diagnosed as indistinct, where OM could not be safely diagnosed; however, treatment was recommended and conducted as having OM. Therefore, there was no missed OM and no overtreatment, and so the predictive value and accuracy of the score were high. The strengths and advantages of the proposed score are that it is easy to assess and that only those diagnostic tools have been included that are ubiquitously available and, thus, feasible for any surgeon.

Clinical symptoms are often subtle so that only 1–3 of the 5 typical signs of infection (pain, swelling, elevated temperature, redness, and loss of function) may be present [14,15]. While WBC is a good marker for sepsis, it has a low value in non-systemic infections and is largely neglected there [7,8,16,17]. CRP levels may be influenced by age, gender, weight, blood pressure [18], liver diseases [19], medications [20], and genetic preconditions [18,21,22]. Besides being elevated in case of infections [23], it may increase in any inflammatory condition such as rheumatoid arthritis, cardiovascular diseases, trauma, and cancer [4–6]. Both WBC and CRP are unspecific, and may be normal despite an OM or elevated without OM, as seen in the presented study population. Clinical symptoms as well as the CRP and WBC may aid in diagnosing OM but are unreliable diagnostic tools and, therefore, were not included in the proposed OM score.

Until today, microbiology has remained the gold standard in diagnosing infections. In bone and joint infections, however, it is known that microbial pathogens may only be isolated in 90% of acute and 51.4% of chronic OM, resulting in a high amount of false negative results [24]. In false negative cases, samples may not have been taken from representative regions of the affected bone, administered antibiotic treatment may have resulted in insufficient diagnostic power, or standardized culture mediums may have failed to isolate small colony variants [25–27]. In the presented study population, microbiologic organisms could also be isolated in only 88.9% of the patients. Hence, the sole diagnosis and consecutive treatment of OM should not be based on microbiology alone but rather on a combination of several diagnostics.

Despite the accuracy of 100% of the histopathology in the current study, a combination of diagnostic tools is still suggested. The risk of samples being taken from non-representative areas of the bone, resulting in false negative results, would have crucial consequences. Histopathological examinations, on the other hand, remain critical when taken from the representative area and can distinguish between acute, chronic, and acute on chronic OM even when microbial pathogens cannot be isolated [24].

In the presented study, performing an MRI belonged to the standard protocol for diagnosing OM. Still, MRI is not uniformly used—specifically, not when implants are present—even though several metal artifact-reducing sequences have well been introduced, and so, contraindications in the presence of orthopedic and trauma implants have become rare [28]. Due to its superiority in visualizing soft tissue contrasts compared to CT scans, it gains an accuracy of 71% to detect OM despite the presence of orthopedic implants and, thus, should always be favored or at least conducted additionally [29].

The advantage of the proposed score is its reduction of the diagnostic tools to the bare minimum and its clear instructions for treatment with strict cut-off levels. In the presented score, two diagnostic procedures may be sufficient if both are positive or negative; a third procedure, however, increases diagnostic safety. In individual cases, even one parameter may be enough to diagnose OM; however, in clinical practice, one parameter seems unsafe, and so a second should always be aimed for. Still, in all diagnostics, the inevitable precondition is that tissue samples are taken from representative areas, suggesting taking no less than 2 samples to reduce false negative results, and that the MRI is performed correctly, e.g., with contrast medium and metal artifact-reducing sequences when implants are present, prior to surgical bony debridement to rule out postoperative stress reactions of the bone, and preferably adjudged by a musculoskeletal radiologist.

As shown in the second retrospectively reviewed independent cohort, the new OM score could be validated without any misdiagnosis, while only 87.3% were correctly diagnosed by clinical means alone. Most importantly, even the 7 clinically missed OM would have been identified by the OM score. Contrary to the clinicians' previous opinion, the score would have had a higher accuracy and the diagnosis of OM would have been more certain if the proposed OM score had been used.

In contrast to the proposed simple OM score, the 2011-introduced Osteomyelitis Diagnosis Score (ODS) to predict an OM contains 104 items and is quite demanding [13]. Furthermore, it contains broad windows with OM being "probable" (8–17 points) and "possible" (2–7 points) [13]. Therefore, until now, the score has not prevailed in everyday clinical practice despite its sensitivity of 82.8% and specificity of 95.8%. In a validation study [30], several items remained negative in all patients and, thus, seem redundant, and the score seems not practicable in everyday clinical practice.

Despite the first description of the score in this study, larger study populations will be needed to validate the score. However, since the score is simple, it may be possible to expand or modify certain parameters to further strengthen the score, e.g., by weighting items or adding subcategories such as the presence of metal implants. So far, however, the benefit of potential modifying factors and subcategories remains unclear, so the score is intended to be as simple and reliable as possible.

Due to the scarce overall incidence of OM and the prospective study design, the number of patients is low. Owing to this, the presented study does not claim to be confirmative but serves as a pilot study. Further studies with larger patient cohorts will be needed to verify the utility of the derived OM score.

Author Contributions: Conceptualization, R.K.H. and F.A.S.; formal analysis, R.K.H., F.S.-S., C.E., V.T., J.S., K.W., K.K. and F.A.S.; investigation, R.K.H., F.S.-S., C.E., V.T., J.S., K.W., K.K. and F.A.S.; writing—original draft preparation, R.K.H. and F.A.S.; writing—review and editing, all authors. All authors have read and agreed to the published version of the manuscript.

Funding: This research received no external funding.

Institutional Review Board Statement: The study was conducted in accordance with the Declaration of Helsinki, and approved by the Institutional Ethics Committee of the University of Bonn (protocol code 277/19 and 8 January 2020).

Informed Consent Statement: Informed consent was obtained from all subjects involved in the study.

Data Availability Statement: Not applicable.

Conflicts of Interest: The authors declare no conflict of interest.

References

1. Lew, D.P.; Waldvogel, F.A. Osteomyelitis. *Lancet* **2004**, *364*, 369–379. [CrossRef]
2. McNally, M.N.K. (iv) Osteomyelitis. *Orthop. Trauma.* **2010**, *24*, 416–429. [CrossRef]
3. Walter, N.; Baertl, S.; Alt, V.; Rupp, M. What is the burden of osteomyelitis in Germany? An analysis of inpatient data from 2008 through 2018. *BMC Infect. Dis.* **2021**, *21*, 550. [CrossRef]
4. Du Clos, T.W.; Mold, C. C-reactive protein: An activator of innate immunity and a modulator of adaptive immunity. *Immunol. Res.* **2004**, *30*, 261–277. [CrossRef] [PubMed]
5. Gabay, C.; Kushner, I. Acute-phase proteins and other systemic responses to inflammation. *N. Engl. J. Med.* **1999**, *340*, 448–454. [CrossRef]
6. Ciubotaru, I.; Potempa, L.A.; Wander, R.C. Production of Modified C-Reactive Protein in U937-Derived Macrophages. *Exp. Biol. Med.* **2005**, *230*, 762–777. [CrossRef]
7. Bottner, F.; Wegner, A.; Winkelmann, W.; Becker, K.; Erren, M.; Gotze, C. Interleukin-6, procalcitonin and TNF-alpha: Markers of peri-prosthetic infection following total joint replacement. *J. Bone Jt. Surg. Br.* **2007**, *89*, 94–99. [CrossRef]
8. Muller, M.; Morawietz, L.; Hasart, O.; Strube, P.; Perka, C.; Tohtz, S. Diagnosis of periprosthetic infection following total hip arthroplasty–evaluation of the diagnostic values of pre- and intraoperative parameters and the associated strategy to preoperatively select patients with a high probability of joint infection. *J. Orthop. Surg. Res.* **2008**, *3*, 31. [CrossRef]
9. AWMF Leitlinie. S2k-Leitlinie "Akute und chronische exogene Osteomyelitis langer Röhrenknochen des Erwachsenen". AWMF-Nr. 012-033. 1 December 2017. Available online: https://register.awmf.org/assets/guidelines/012-033l_S2k_Osteomyelitis_2018-01_1_01.pdf (accessed on 19 February 2023).
10. Massel, D.H.; Jenkins, N.W.; Rush, A.J., III; Trapana, J.E.; Foremny, G.B.; Donnally, C.J., III; Subhawong, T.; Aiyer, A. MRI and Clinical Risk Indicators for Osteomyelitis. *Foot Ankle Spec.* **2021**, *14*, 415–426. [CrossRef] [PubMed]
11. Ledermann, H.P.; Morrison, W.B.; Schweitzer, M.E. MR Image Analysis of Pedal Osteomyelitis: Distribution, Patterns of Spread, and Frequency of Associated Ulceration and Septic Arthritis. *Radiology* **2002**, *223*, 747–755. [CrossRef] [PubMed]
12. Lee, Y.J.; Sadigh, S.; Mankad, K.; Kapse, N.; Rajeswaran, G. The imaging of osteomyelitis. *Quant. Imaging Med. Surg.* **2016**, *6*, 184–198. [CrossRef] [PubMed]
13. Schmidt, H.G.; Tiemann, A.H.; Braunschweig, R.; Diefenbeck, M.; Buhler, M.; Abitzsch, D.; Haustedt, N.; Walter, G.; Schoop, R.; Heppert, V.; et al. Definition of the Diagnosis Osteomyelitis-Osteomyelitis Diagnosis Score (ODS). *Z. Orthop. Unfall.* **2011**, *149*, 449–460. [CrossRef]
14. Baltensperger, M.; Grätz, K.; Bruder, E.; Lebeda, R.; Makek, M.; Eyrich, G. Is primary chronic osteomyelitis a uniform disease? Proposal of a classification based on a retrospective analysis of patients treated in the past 30 years. *J. Cranio-Maxillofac. Surg.* **2004**, *32*, 43–50. [CrossRef]
15. Bühler, M.E.M.; Schmidt, H.G.K. *Septische Postoperative Komplikationen*; Springer: Vienna, Austria; New York, NY, USA, 2003.
16. Canner, G.C.; E Steinberg, M.; Heppenstall, R.B.; Balderston, R. The infected hip after total hip arthroplasty. *J. Bone Jt. Surg.* **1984**, *66*, 1393–1399. [CrossRef]
17. Collins, I.; Wilson-MacDonald, J.; Chami, G.; Burgoyne, W.; Vinayakam, P.; Berendt, T.; Fairbank, J. The diagnosis and management of infection following instrumented spinal fusion. *Eur. Spine J.* **2008**, *17*, 445–450. [CrossRef] [PubMed]
18. Hage, F.G.; Szalai, A.J. C-Reactive Protein Gene Polymorphisms, C-Reactive Protein Blood Levels, and Cardiovascular Disease Risk. *J. Am. Coll. Cardiol.* **2007**, *50*, 1115–1122. [CrossRef]
19. Pankow, J.S.; Folsom, A.R.; Cushman, M.; Borecki, I.B.; Hopkins, P.N.; Eckfeldt, J.H.; Tracy, R.P. Familial and genetic determinants of systemic markers of inflammation: The NHLBI family heart study. *Atherosclerosis* **2001**, *154*, 681–689. [CrossRef]
20. Pepys, M.B.; Hirschfield, G. C-reactive protein: A critical update. *J. Clin. Investig.* **2003**, *111*, 1805–1812. [CrossRef]
21. Eisenhardt, S.U.; Thiele, J.R.; Bannasch, H.; Stark, G.B.; Peter, K. C-reactive protein: How conformational changes influence inflammatory properties. *Cell Cycle* **2009**, *8*, 3885–3892. [CrossRef]
22. Devraj, S.; Venugopal, S.; Jialal, I. Native pentameric C-reactive protein displays more potent pro-atherogenic activities in human aortic endothelial cells than modified C-reactive protein. *Atherosclerosis* **2006**, *184*, 48–52. [CrossRef] [PubMed]
23. Thompson, D.; Pepys, M.B.; Wood, S.P. The physiological structure of human C-reactive protein and its complex with phosphocholine. *Structure* **1999**, *7*, 169–177. [CrossRef] [PubMed]
24. Tiemann, A.; Hofmann, G.O.; Krukemeyer, M.G.; Krenn, V.; Langwald, S. Histopathological Osteomyelitis Evaluation Score (HOES)—An innovative approach to histopathological diagnostics and scoring of osteomyelitis. *GMS Interdiscip. Plast Reconstr. Surg. DGPW* **2014**, *3*, Doc08.
25. Kriegeskorte, A.; König, S.; Sander, G.; Pirkl, A.; Mahabir, E.; Proctor, R.A.; von Eiff, C.; Peters, G.; Becker, K. Small colony variants of *Staphylococcus aureus* reveal distinct protein profiles. *Proteomics* **2011**, *11*, 2476–2490. [CrossRef] [PubMed]
26. Zimmerli, W.; Trampuz, A.; Ochsner, P.E. Prosthetic-joint infections. *N. Engl. J. Med.* **2004**, *351*, 1645–1654. [CrossRef] [PubMed]
27. Spangehl, M.J.; Masri, B.A.; O'connell, J.X.; Duncan, C.P. Prospective Analysis of Preoperative and Intraoperative Investigations for the Diagnosis of Infection at the Sites of Two Hundred and Two Revision Total Hip Arthroplasties*. *J. Bone Jt. Surg. Am.* **1999**, *81*, 672–683. [CrossRef]
28. Buckwalter, K.; Lin, C.; Ford, J. Managing Postoperative Artifacts on Computed Tomography and Magnetic Resonance Imaging. *Semin. Musculoskelet. Radiol.* **2011**, *15*, 309–319. [CrossRef]

29. Na Park, B.; Hong, S.-J.; A Yoon, M.; Oh, J.-K. MRI Diagnosis for Post-Traumatic Osteomyelitis of Extremities Using Conventional Metal-Artifact Reducing Protocols: Revisited. *Acad. Radiol.* **2019**, *26*, e317–e323. [CrossRef]
30. Steinhausen, E.; Lundin, S.; Dahmen, J.; Zulueta La Rosa, G.; Al Malat, T.; Glombitza, M.; Rixen, D. Validation of the Osteomyelitis Diagnosis Score on the Basis of a Retrospective Analysis of 100 Patients with Non-Union of the Tibia. *Z. Orthop Unfall.* **2016**, *154*, 578–582.

Disclaimer/Publisher's Note: The statements, opinions and data contained in all publications are solely those of the individual author(s) and contributor(s) and not of MDPI and/or the editor(s). MDPI and/or the editor(s) disclaim responsibility for any injury to people or property resulting from any ideas, methods, instructions or products referred to in the content.

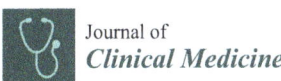

Journal of Clinical Medicine

Article

Using a Traction Table for Fracture Reduction during Minimally Invasive Plate Osteosynthesis (MIPO) of Distal Femoral Fractures Provides Anatomical Alignment

Martin Paulsson [1,2,*], Carl Ekholm [1,2], Roy Tranberg [1,2], Ola Rolfson [1,2] and Mats Geijer [3,4,5]

1 Department of Orthopaedics, Sahlgrenska University Hospital, 41345 Gothenburg, Sweden
2 Department of Orthopaedics, Institute of Clinical Sciences, Sahlgrenska Academy, University of Gothenburg, 41345 Gothenburg, Sweden
3 Department of Radiology, Sahlgrenska University Hospital, 41345 Gothenburg, Sweden
4 Department of Radiology, Institute of Clinical Sciences, Sahlgrenska Academy, University of Gothenburg, 41345 Gothenburg, Sweden
5 Department of Clinical Sciences, Lund University, 22185 Lund, Sweden
* Correspondence: martin.paulsson@vgregion.se

Abstract: Introduction: Fracture reduction and fixation of distal femur fractures are technically demanding. Postoperative malalignment is still commonly reported after minimally invasive plate osteosynthesis (MIPO). We evaluated the postoperative alignment after MIPO using a traction table with a dedicated femoral support. Methods: The study included 32 patients aged 65 years or older with distal femur fractures of all AO/OTA types 32 (c) and 33 (except 33 B3 and C3) and peri-implant fractures with stable implants. Internal fixation was achieved with MIPO using a bridge-plating construct. Bilateral computed tomography (CT) scans of the entire femur were performed postoperatively, and measurements of the uninjured contralateral side defined anatomical alignment. Due to incomplete CT scans or excessively distorted femoral anatomy, seven patients were excluded from analyses. Results: Fracture reduction and fixation on the traction table provided excellent postoperative alignment. Only one of the 25 patients had a rotational malalignment of more than 15° (18°). Conclusions: The surgical setup for MIPO of distal femur fractures on a traction table with a dedicated femoral support facilitated reduction and fixation, resulting in a low rate of postoperative malalignment, despite a high rate of peri-implant fractures, and could be recommended for surgical treatment of distal femur fractures.

Keywords: femur fracture; orthopedic surgical procedure; fracture osteosynthesis; fracture fixation; internal; minimally invasive surgical procedure; operating table; bone misalignment

1. Introduction

Fractures of the distal femur show a bimodal age distribution. One peak comprises high-energy trauma in young males, and the second, more significant, peak comprises elderly females with low-energy trauma [1,2]. Distal femoral fractures are, however, difficult injuries for patients and surgeons alike. It is advantageous to use minimally invasive techniques for obtaining fracture reduction and surgical fixation of distal femoral fractures instead of open surgery. The minimally invasive technique preserves the periosteal blood supply, which is beneficial for fracture healing [3–5]. The minimally invasive plate osteosynthesis (MIPO) technique is typically carried out on a standard operating table, with the patient's leg draped free. However, the lack of clear landmarks in the femur makes per-operative validation of reduction difficult, particularly of rotation, regardless of whether a nail or plate is used, and mal-reduction is not uncommon [4,6–12]. Postoperative malalignment increases the risk of non-union [13,14]. Rotational malalignment has also been shown to have a negative impact on knee function, resulting in articular cartilage shearing, which can, in turn, develop into painful osteoarthritis [15–17].

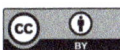

The use of a traction table for fracture reduction and per-operative fracture immobilization is standard for both proximal and femoral shaft fractures. Using a traction table for distal femur fractures has also been described. However, the reports are scarce; they consist of technical notes and a report of one case with a comminuted distal femur fracture [18–20]. The technique of using a traction table equipped with a dedicated femoral support has been employed as the standard surgical setup for operating distal femur fractures in our hospital for more than ten years. However, whether the use of a traction table improves the accuracy of surgical reduction has not previously been reported.

In this prospective cohort study, we aimed to evaluate to what degree anatomic alignment could be achieved if closed reduction of a distal femur fracture on a traction table with a dedicated femoral support was used when performing a minimally invasive plate osteosynthesis (MIPO) plating and to compare results with previously published findings using a conventional operating table setup.

2. Materials and Methods

2.1. Patient Cohort

Patients in this study originate from a randomized controlled trial (RCT) of weight-bearing regimens following fixation of distal femur fracture. All patients were operated with MIPO using a traction table [21]. In the RCT, we included 32 patients aged 65 years or older with a traumatic fracture of the distal part of the femur of 2018 AO/OTA types 33 (A2-3, B1-2, C1-2) and 32(c) (A1-3, B2-3, C2-3) and unified periprosthetic classifications system (UPCS) IV (3B1, 3C-3D) and V (3B1, 3C-3D) [22].

For the current study, 25 out of the original 32 eligible patients were included. Three patients were excluded due to incomplete postoperative computed tomography (CT) scans (the entire length of both femurs was not available), and four due to excessively distorted femoral anatomy from previous fractures or surgery, making measurements unreliable.

The mean age was 81 years (standard deviation, SD, 9.0; range 67–95), mean operation time was 96 min (SD 28.0; range 52–175), and the mean blood loss was 272 mL (SD 147.1; range 75–600). None of the commonly seen complications related to the patient setup on the traction table was observed pre- or postoperatively [23]. The distribution of fracture types according to the 2018 AO/OTA classification [22] is shown in Table 1.

Table 1. AO/OTA Classification.

n	AO/OTA	UM	Q	UCPF
2	32A2.1	(c)		
4	32A2.1	(c)	[12]	
1	32A2.1	(c)		V.3C
1	32A2.1	(c)	[12]	V.3C
2	32B2	(c)	[13]	
2	32B2	(c)	[13]	V.3D
2	32B3	(c)	[13]	
1	32B3	(c)	[13]	IV.3C
1	32B3	(c)	[13]	IV.3C
1	33A2.2			V.3B1
2	33A3.2			V.3B1
1	33A3.2			
1	33A3.2		[7]	V.3B1
1	33A3.2		[7]	IV.3D
1	33B2.1			
1	33C1.1			IV.3C
1	33C2.3			

AO/OTA; Arbeitsgemeinschaft für Osteosynthesefragen/Orthopaedic Trauma Association, UM; Universal Modifiers, Q; Qualifications, UCPF; Unified Classification System for Periprosthetic Fractures.

Sixteen of the 25 patients (64%) had had previous surgery on the injured femur with either a joint replacement (Table 1) or osteosynthesis (four patients with antegrade intramedullary nail and one with hip screws), and one patient had both a total knee replacement and an antegrade intramedullary nail.

2.2. Surgical Intervention

One of seven predetermined consultant orthopedic trauma surgeons performed the surgical procedure according to a written protocol. The patients were supine on an operating table, with the fractured leg in traction. Bi-planar fluoroscopy was used. An adjustable femoral-supporting device (POsterior Reduction Device P.O.R.D. Orthofix™ SRL, Verona, Italy) mounted on the side of the operating table was used for dorsal support of the fracture (Figure 1). Before skin washing and draping, closed reduction was performed. To reduce the fracture's commonly occurring apex posterior angulation, the knee was flexed about 20° by lowering the foot stand, keeping the femur horizontal (Figure 2). To further improve the reduction, the height of the femoral support and the amount of traction on the leg could be adjusted. Only mild traction was allowed. The rotation of the leg was set at neutral, with the foot pointing upwards (Figure 3). For a true lateral view with the image intensifier, the foot rotation could be slightly adjusted to align the dorsal contours of the femoral condyles horizontally. However, as specified by the protocol, no further actions to improve the rotational alignment were undertaken.

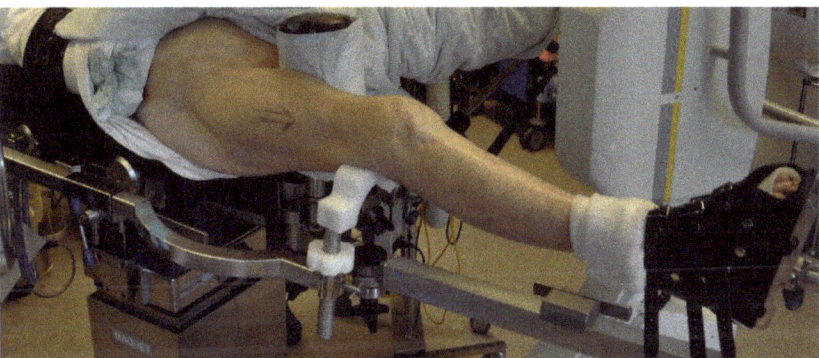

Figure 1. The patient on the traction table with the leg in traction. A femoral support (POsterior Reduction Device P.O.R.D. Orthofix™ SRL, Verona, Italy) [24] is used to reduce the commonly occurring apex posterior angulation of the distal femoral fracture (red arrow).

A small longitudinal incision was made over the lateral epicondyle. The fascia lata was incised longitudinally, and the epicondyle cleared of periosteal tissue. An LCP® Distal Femoral Plate (Synthes™, Oberdorf, Switzerland) was introduced under the fascia lata and fitted to the lateral femoral epicondyle and the femoral diaphysis (Figure 4). A large clamp was used to hold the plate firmly onto the lateral condyle and shaft to achieve best possible contact between the plate and the lateral femoral. When correctly seated, as verified by fluoroscopy, the plate was temporarily fixed with distal and proximal K-wires. The correct plate position is also crucial for optimal distal screw positioning [25,26]. Anatomical reduction of the fracture was prioritized over the approximation of the plate to the femoral proximal shaft (Figures 5 and 6).

A 13-hole plate was used for patients of short stature, while in the other patients, the fractures were fixed with a 15-hole plate. Five bi-cortical locking screws were used in the distal part of the plate, and three bi-cortical locking screws were used in the proximal portion of the plate, the latter through stab incisions. The proximal screws were spaced between 5 holes to distribute the proximal load. The fixation was a bridge-plating construction, and no additional screws or cerclage wires were used across the fracture.

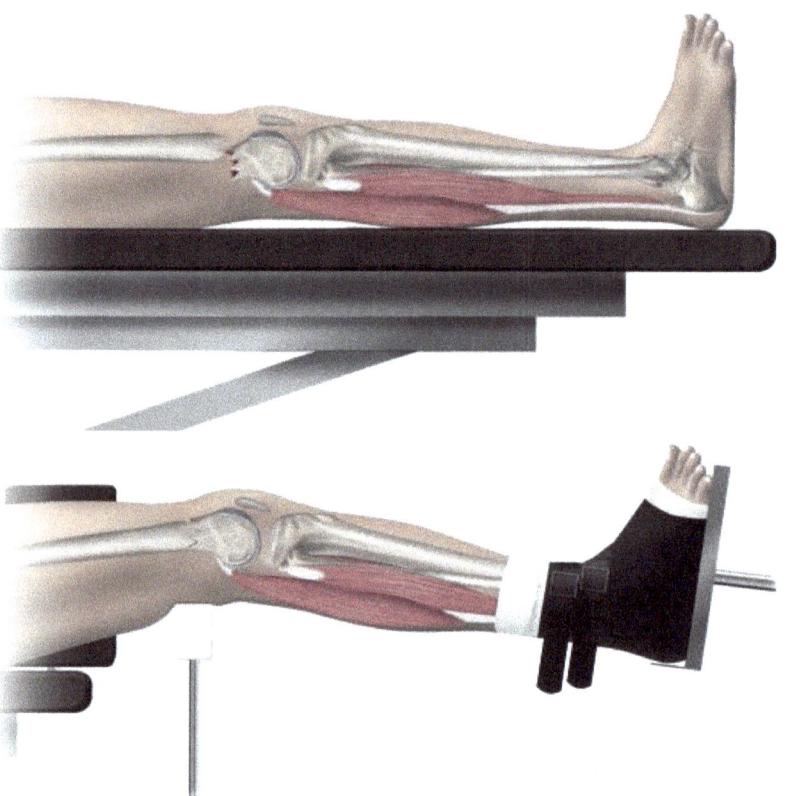

Figure 2. (**Top**) Apex posterior angulation of the distal femoral fracture, which is commonly occurring. The pull of the gastrocnemius muscles attached to the femoral condyles causes the typical displacement pattern. (**Bottom**) With the patient on the traction table, closed reduction was obtained by gentle traction and lowering the foot stand, while the fracture was supported from dorsal by the dorsal femoral support. The reduction could be further improved by adjusting the height of the femoral support, the foot stand, and the amount of traction on the leg.

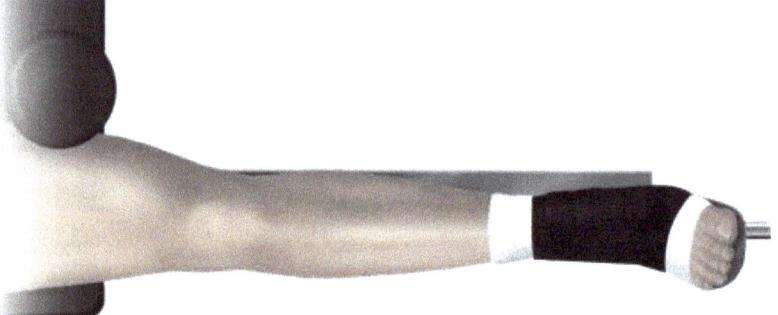

Figure 3. The patient on the traction table with the leg in traction and the foot pointing upwards (seen from above), which reduces preoperative coronal or rotational malalignment. The patient's position on the table is important, as the central post can affect the angulation of the fracture in the frontal plane.

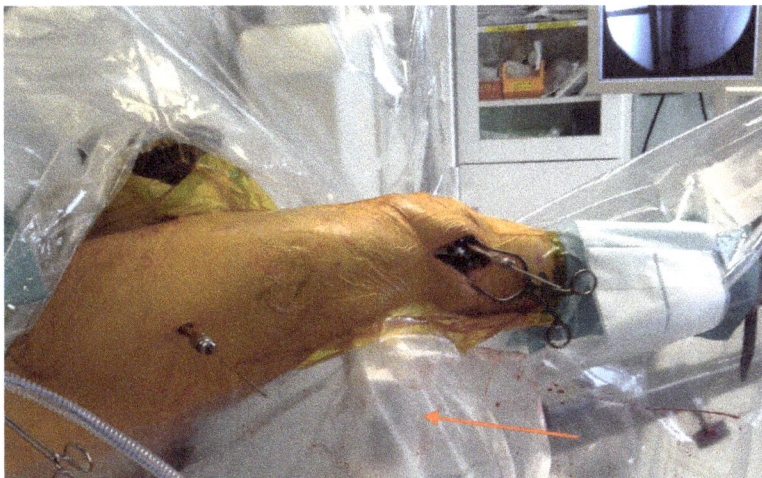

Figure 4. The patient setup on the operating table, with the fractured leg in mild traction and fracture supported by an adjustable femoral-supporting device. The red arrow points towards the femoral support, partly hidden behind the draping. A small incision has been made over the lateral condyle. The fascia lata has been longitudinally incised, and an LCP® Distal Femoral Plate (Synthes™, Oberdorf, Switzerland) has been introduced under the fascia lata and fitted to the lateral femoral epicondyle and the femoral diaphysis. The plate is temporarily fixed with distal and proximal K-wires.

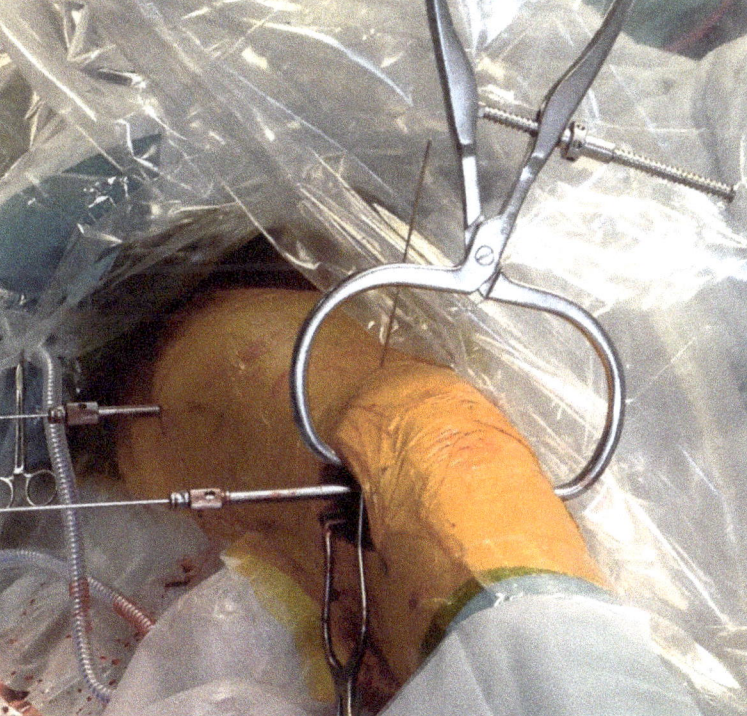

Figure 5. The plate was firmly pressed onto the lateral condyle by a large clamp to achieve as much contact as possible between the plate and the femoral surface.

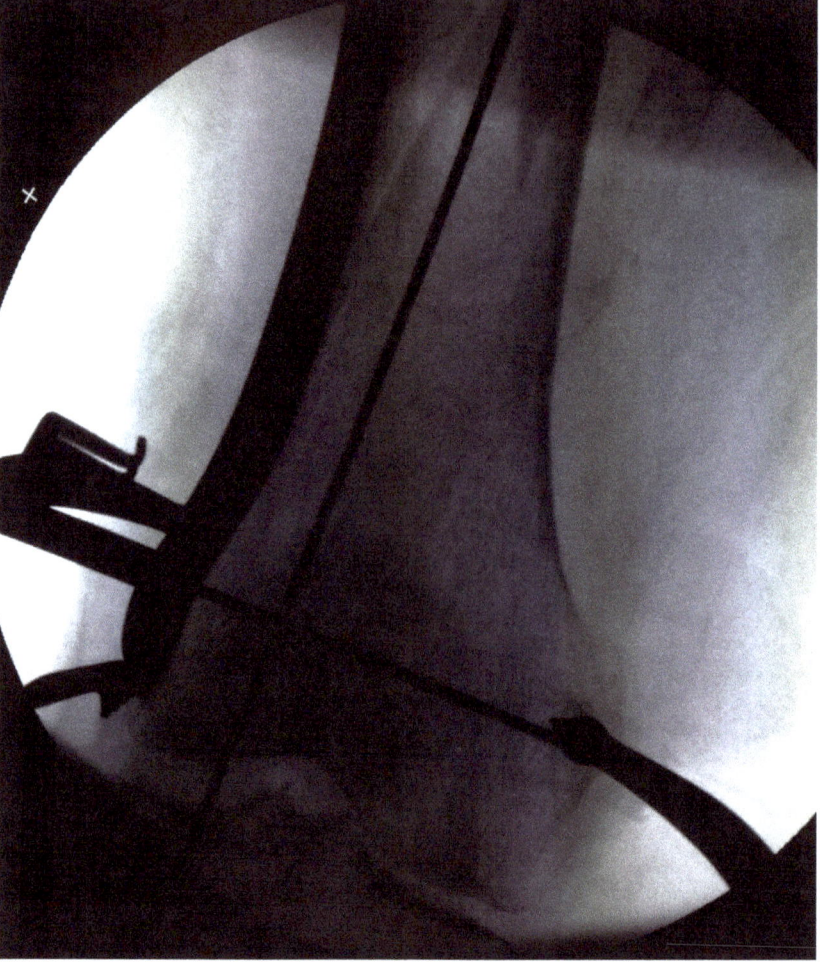

Figure 6. Image from the bi-planar image intensifier. A large clamp firmly pressed the plate onto the lateral condyle and diaphysis. The plate was temporarily fixed with K-wires. The spiral-shaped fracture of the distal shaft was reduced by a combination of traction, a dedicated femoral support, and the application of an LCP® Distal Femoral Plate (Synthes™, Oberdorf, Switzerland), firmly pressed onto the lateral epicondyle.

2.3. Image Evaluation

For the assessment of angular measurements and measurements of femoral length, all patients underwent a CT scan of both complete femurs within one week after surgery using a metal-artifact reduction reconstruction algorithm and archived as 3-mm contiguous slices.

Rotation was measured on axial multiplanar reformations (MPR), oriented perpendicular to the long axis of the femur. The rotational angle was defined as the angle between the dorsal condylar line of the distal femur and a line from the apex of the lesser trochanter through the center of the femoral medullary canal (Figure 7). If the patient had a total knee replacement, the corresponding parts of the prosthesis were used for the distal measurement. The vertical side of the image was used as reference.

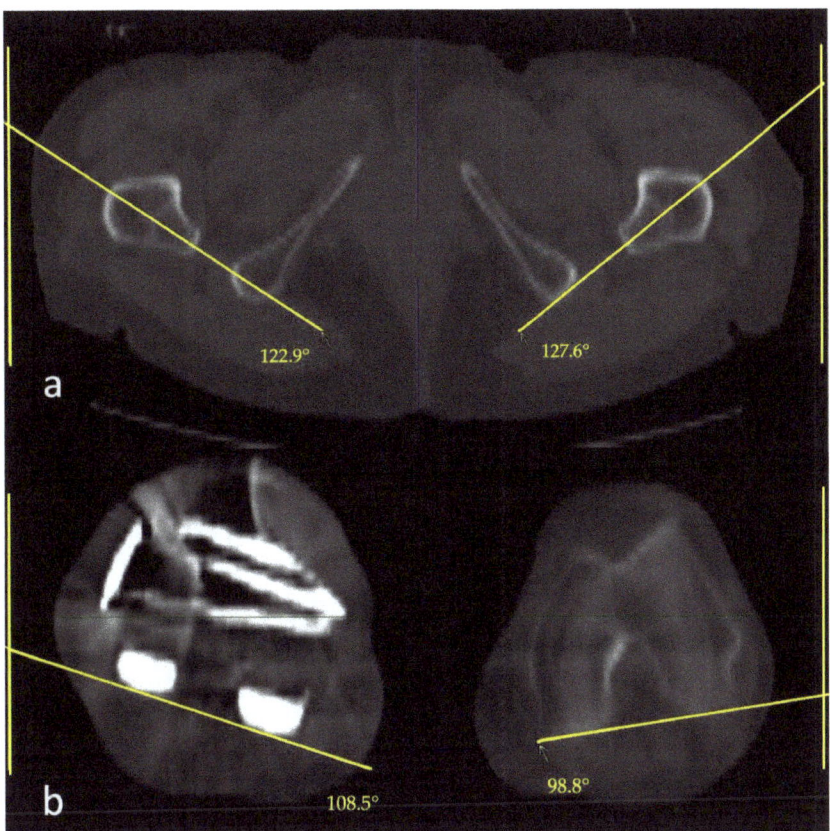

Figure 7. (**a**) Proximal rotational angles were measured by a line passing through the apex of the lesser trochanter and the center of the femoral medullary canal. (**b**) Distal rotational angles were measured using the dorsal condylar line. The vertical side of the image was used for reference.

The length of the femur was measured on a coronal MPR from the most cranial part of the femoral head to the center of the line that connected the most distal contour of the condyles (Figure 8a). CT slice thickness was set to 50 mm to facilitate the determination of the femoral outlines. If the patient had had previous surgery on the proximal part of the femur, the apex of the lesser trochanter was instead used as a measuring reference.

Genu varum/valgum or coronal angulation was measured using the abovementioned plane. CT slice thickness was set to 50 mm to facilitate the determination of the femoral outlines. The angle between the distal joint line and the mechanical axis of the femur was measured (from the center of the femoral head through the center of the knee) (Figure 8b). With a total hip replacement, the center of the femoral head of the prosthesis was used, even though some total hip replacements did not have an anatomical offset.

On a sagittal MPR plane, perpendicular to the dorsal femoral condylar line, genu antecurvatum or recurvatum (sagittal angulation) was measured as the angle between the longitudinal axis of the distal part of the femoral diaphysis and a line cutting the center of the distal metaphysis at the funnel-shaped transition into the flared portion of the distal shaft (Figure 9).

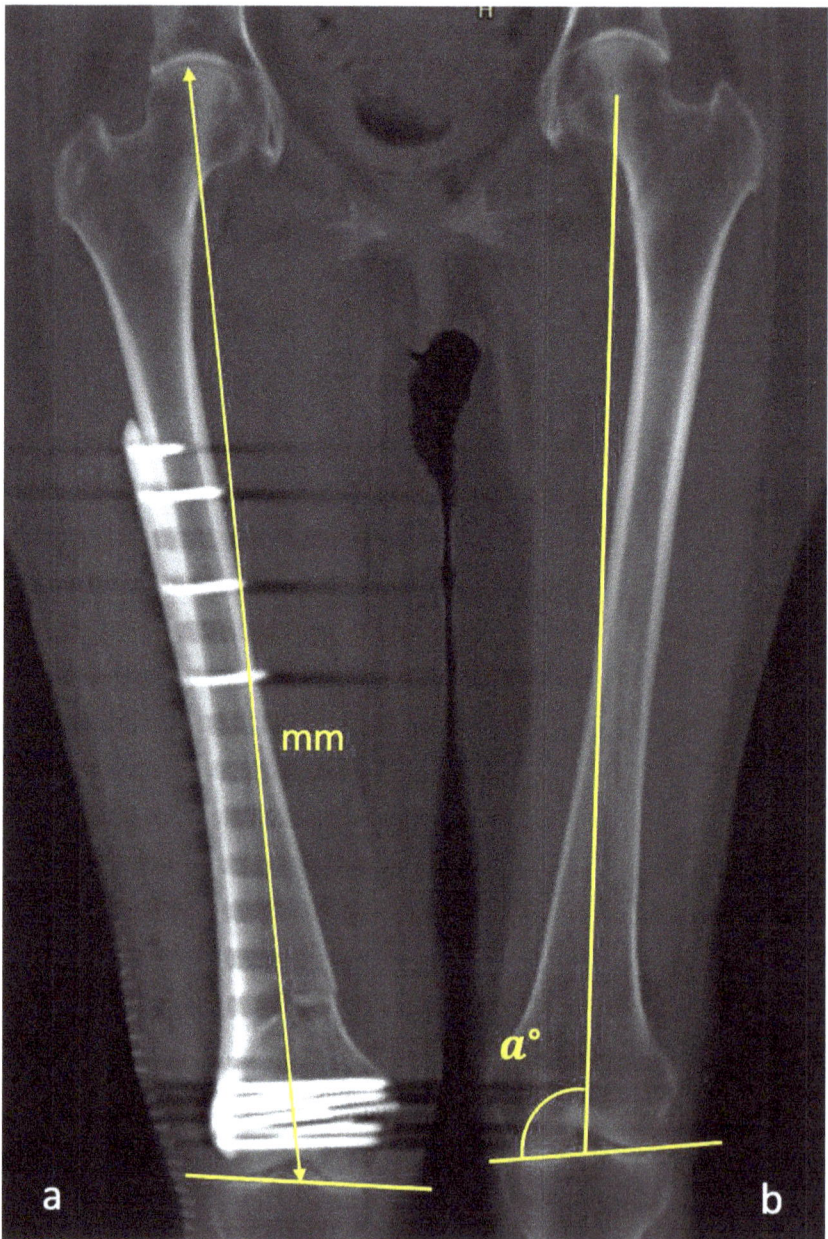

Figure 8. (**a**) The total femoral length was measured from the most cranial part of the femoral head to the center of the line that connected the most distal contour of the medial and lateral condyles. (**b**) The varus/valgus angulation was measured between the joint line using the distal contour of the femoral condyles and the mechanical axis of the femur from the center of the femoral head through the center of the knee.

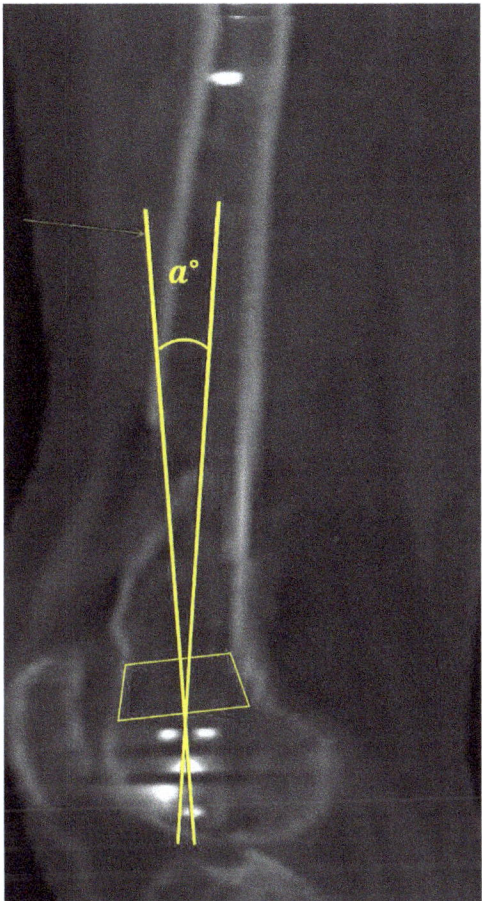

Figure 9. Genu antecurvatum/recurvatum (sagittal angulation) was defined as the angle between a line passing through the center of the distal diaphysis and a line cutting the center of the distal metaphysis at the funnel-shaped transition into the flared shaft on a sagittal multiplanar reformation.

2.4. Statistical Methods

The analysis was performed in SPSS Statistics, Version 28 (IBM, New York, NY, USA). The normality of continuous data was analyzed with Q-Q plots. Data with a normal distribution are presented as mean and standard deviation (SD) and as median and interquartile range (IQR) if the distribution is non-normal. Intraclass correlation (ICC) was used to calculate the accuracy and intra-rater agreement of the CT scan measurements. Single-rater, multiple measurements (CT scans) on the same femur at different time points gave intra-rater reliability ICC with 2-way mixed effects and an absolute agreement of 95% [27].

All measurements were made by the first author (MP) on two occasions, six months apart, using Xero Viewer (web-based software) (AGFA, Mortsel, Belgium). The contralateral femur was used as a reference, and a malalignment score (coronal, sagittal, and length), presented by Handolin et al. [28] was used to evaluate the quality of the postoperative reduction. The mean value of the two independent observations on both femurs is presented.

3. Results

Reduction Measurements

Only the rotational side-to-side difference had a normal distribution. The mean postoperative difference in the rotation was 5.8° (SD 4.3°, range 18.2° internal rotation to 10.6° external rotation). The distribution is presented in Figure 10. The median length difference was 5.0 mm (IQR 3.0–6.8 mm). One patient had a 10 mm-longer fractured femur due to femoral side-to-side variances (Figure 11) [29]. The median coronal angulation difference (varus or valgus) was 1.2° (IQR 0.4–2.0°), and the median sagittal angulation difference (genu antecurvatum or recurvatum angulation) was 0.8° (IQR 0.4–1.2°). Using the threshold values for malalignment suggested by Handolin et al. [28], all patients were categorized as "excellent".

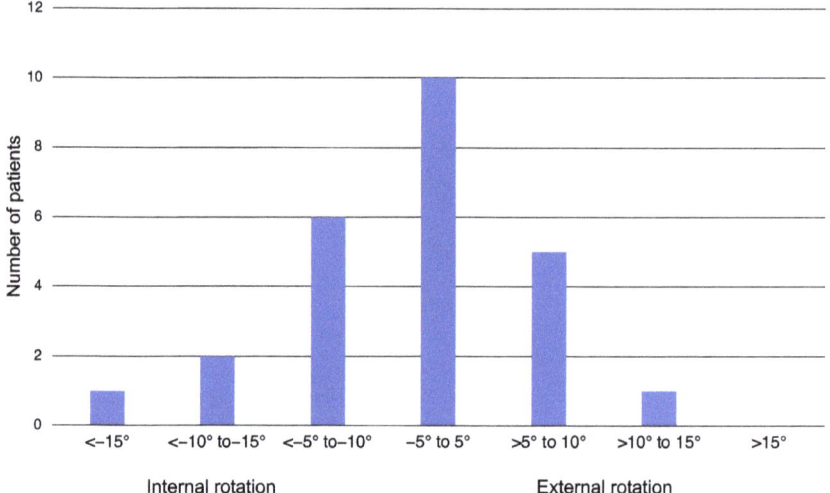

Figure 10. The diagram shows the distribution of postoperative rotational side-to-side differences in the investigated patients. The negative values represent an internal rotation compared with the unfractured femur, and the positive values represent external rotation.

The results of the intra-observer agreement of the reduction measurements assessed by ICC are shown in Table 2.

Table 2. Intraclass correlation, postoperative computed tomography (CT) scans TEST-RETEST.

ROTATION	n	ICC	95% CI
Distal Angle Fracture	25	0.985	(0.964–0.993)
Distal Angle Non-fracture	25	0.951	(0.877–0.975)
Proximal Angle Fracture	25	0.919	(0.823–0.963)
Proximal Angle Non-fracture	25	0.975	(0.823–0.963)
GENU VARUM/VALGUM			
Fracture	25	0.959	(0.909–0.982)
Non-fracture	25	0.968	(0.928–0.986)
LENGTH			
Fracture	25	0.999	(0.998–1.000)
Non-fracture	25	0.999	(0.998–1.000)
GENU ANTE-/RECURVATUM			
Fracture	25	0.596	(0.271–0.800)
Non-fracture	25	0.544	(0.198–0.770)

CI; confidence interval, Fracture; the fractured femur. Non-fracture; the unfractured femur.

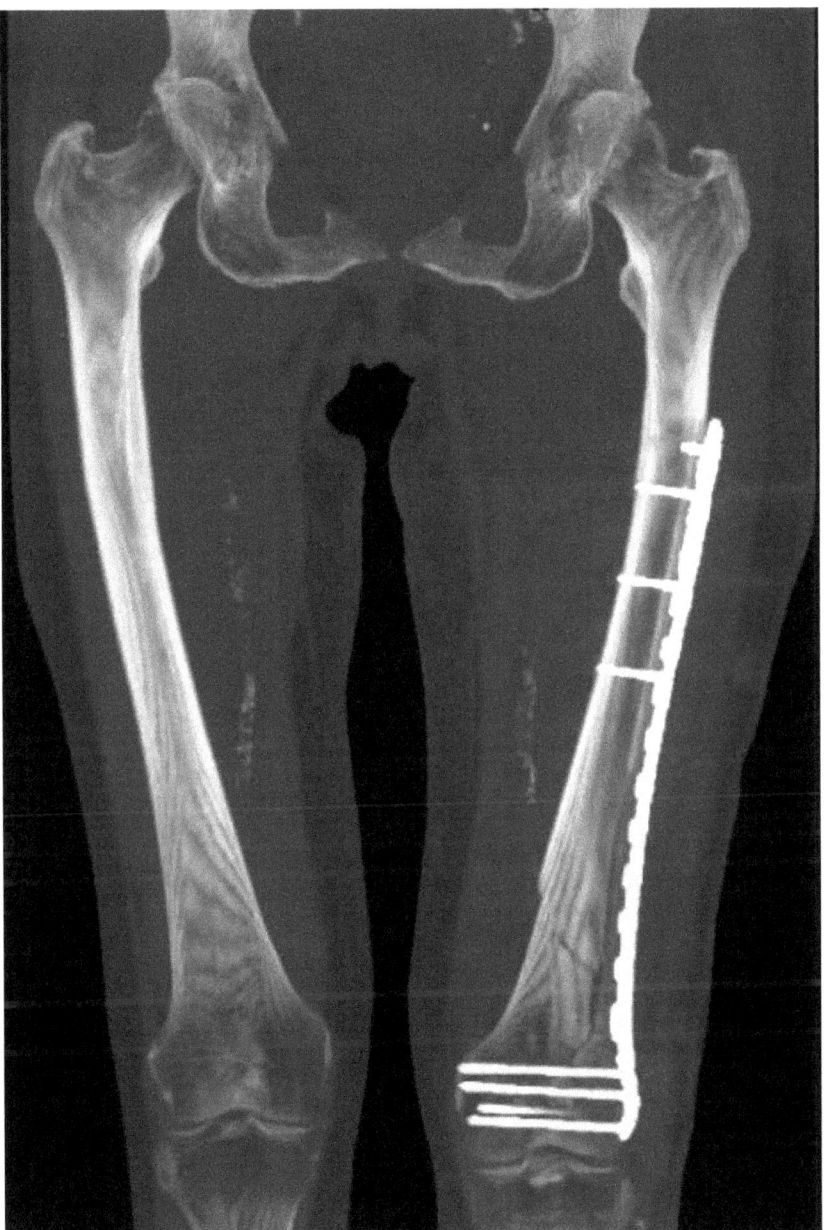

Figure 11. An image of a computed tomography scan of both femurs. The image was obtained by setting the slice thickness to 50 mm. This patient had a longer femur on the fractured side and no history of previous injuries. The fracture was reduced and fixated without elongation. Side-to-side variances in femoral shape are not uncommon [29].

4. Discussion

The results of this study show that, in a cohort of 25 elderly patients with distal femur fractures surgically treated with closed reduction on a traction table followed by MIPO fixation, "excellent" alignment was achieved in all patients, according to the Handolin et al. malalignment score [28]. Rotational malalignment of more than 15° was seen in only one patient, which is less frequent than previously published results [8–10]. We believe these results are clinically relevant, as improved postoperative alignment correlates with improved functional outcomes and decreased risk of non-union [13,14]. Improved rotational alignment also lowers the risk of articular cartilage shearing, negatively affecting knee function and promoting osteoarthritis [15–17].

Despite the advances in modern surgical techniques, postoperative malalignment is still being reported. In a recent multi-center RCT comparing nail and plate fixation in 126 distal femur fractures by Dunbar et al. [12], postoperative reduction was one of the outcomes assessed. The overall coronal postoperative malalignment (>5°) after MIPO fixation was found to be 32%. Valgus deformity was more common than varus deformity, at 27.4% and 4.8%, respectively, but no sagittal malalignment was found. Sagittal malalignment was, however, reported to be common in comminute periprosthetic distal femur fractures in a report by Sharma et al. [11]. In a report on pitfalls when applying lateral plates in distal femoral fractures, Collinge et al. [26] describes strategies for reducing displaced distal femur fractures with varus/valgus angulation and ante-/recurvatum angulation using fluoroscopy on a standard supine operating table. Rotational malalignment, however, is more challenging to assess and manage [26,30]. Buckley et al. [8], using CT, found a side-to-side rotational difference of 22.3–31.3° in 3 of 13 patients treated with MIPO fixation for a distal femur fracture. In a cohort study on rotational alignment of both distal femur fractures (38 patients) and femoral diaphyseal fractures (13 patients) after MIPO (on a traditional operating table), Kim et al. [9] concluded that, while the coronal and sagittal alignments were satisfactory in 96% of the patients, only 57% had satisfactory rotational alignment, using 8° as a threshold. However, the distribution of malrotation is not reported, and the results are, therefore, not presented in Table 3. Furthermore, Kim et al. referred to the grading of malrotation according to the Handolin et al. score. Still, the Handolin et al. score does not include a rotational malalignment component, as all scoring was performed on plain X-rays [28]. Lill et al. [10] concluded that the MIPO technique yielded significantly higher degrees of rotational malalignment (5 of 10 patients with >15°), typically external rotation, than open reduction and internal fixation (surgical setup not specified) using magnetic resonance imaging (MRI, Table 3).

Table 3. Studies on malrotation after surgery for distal femoral fractures using MIPO—minimally invasive plate osteosynthesis.

	Modality	Surgical Intervention	n	Mean Age (Min–Max)	Proportion RM 10–15°	Proportion RM > 15°
Buckley et al., 2011 [8]	CT	MIPO	13	38.1	15%	23%
Lill et al., 2016 [10]	MRI	MIPO + ORIF	10 + 10	44.8 (17–91)	20% + 20%	50% + 0%
Current study	CT	MIPO	25	81.4 (67–95)	12%	4%

CT; Computed Tomography, MRI; Magnetic Rensonace Imaging, RM; Rotational Malalignment, ORIF; Open Reduction Internal Fixation.

Compared to these previous studies, the traction table method used in the present study did provide an excellent reduction in all patients, according to the Handolin et al. criteria [28], and a better rotational alignment (Table 3).

To evaluate the result of the reduction, the contralateral unfractured femur is used as a reference, but the natural side-to-side rotational differences make its use somewhat unreliable [29,31,32]. Sutter et al. [33] compared unfractured femurs in 63 individuals, primarily investigating anatomical differences as a potential cause of hip symptoms using MRI. They found a significant average side-to-side difference of 4° of the femoral neck anteversion. Croom et al. [34] investigated both unfractured femurs in 164 patients with CT. Eighteen percent had an anteversion difference of over 10°, and 4% had over 15°. There is currently no evidence to specify a clinically relevant rotational malalignment threshold. However, Croom et al. suggested that the threshold for clinically relevant rotational malalignment should be 15°, considering natural side differences. Applied to the patients in the present study, only one of the 25 patients was fixed with remaining rotational malalignment.

Using a traction table has several advantages that could tribute to the beneficial outcome in the present study [20,35]. The traction table is the most commonly used setup for proximal and femoral shaft fractures; therefore, most orthopedic surgeons are familiar with its use. The setup allows for gross reduction without being hindered by draping or affecting sterility. Traction to reduce distal femur fractures is not a novel invention; traction was the most commonly used treatment before the era of open reduction and fixation with osteosynthesis. The treatment with traction until healing produced acceptable results [36]. By applying traction to the fractured leg, the reduction mechanism is caused by increasing the tension of the soft tissue (periosteum, muscles, and tendons). The ligamentotaxis self-aligns and, thereby, reduces the fracture [8]. Lowering the foot stand, combined with the dedicated dorsal support, neutralizes the pulling force of the gastrocnemius muscles and prevents apex-posterior malalignment (Figure 2). Sixteen of the 25 patients in the present study had a spiral fracture in the distal part of the shaft, fractures considered unstable and often with a rotational displacement [37]. The setup on the traction table, with the foot in a neutral forward position, is usually sufficient to reduce the fracture when traction is applied. Furthermore, the use of the traction table eliminates the need for the time-consuming visual recognition of rotational malalignment reference points [25], such as a bilateral frontal plane view of the lesser trochanter, which has been recommended to assess malrotation [30]. Lastly, the achieved reduction is maintained throughout the surgery. This eliminates the need for an assistant to maintain manual traction for reduction during the surgery. It also diminishes the need for an invasively applied external fixator or distractor.

The use of the MIPO technique in the fixation of distal femur fractures has been shown to be advantageous, with less violation of blood supply at the fracture site and, subsequently, a reported decrease of non-unions [3,4,38–44]. Obtaining a maximal contact area between the femoral bone surface and the plate reduces stress at the bone-implant interface. It reduces the risk of failure, especially in osteoporotic bone [45,46]. Using a long bridging plate with locking screws has also been shown to have biomechanical advantages [47–50], such as the lowest incidence of loss of fixation, more flexibility, and better capability to withstand permanent deformation in osteoporotic bone, compared to other fixation options [51–56]. The bridging plate concept used in the current study has also been reported to decrease the risk of non-unions [57–60].

There are, however, also limitations to the present study. Using the contralateral leg as a reference is standard practice, despite the inherent side-to-side variations. Thus, the contralateral leg may not accurately compare with the fractured femur. Differences may be amplified when the patients have had previous surgery, such as osteosynthesis or joint replacements. In addition, measurements of osteoporotic bone can be difficult.

Measurements of the sagittal alignment were challenging, reflected by the relatively low ICC. The combination of metal artifacts from total knee replacement, the proximity of screws from osteosynthesis, osteoporotic bone, and 3-mm thick CT slices did not allow angle measurements using Blumensaat's line for reference [61]. The method used for measuring sagittal angulation in the present study has not been validated, and the results should be interpreted with that in mind. However, the technique used for sagittal angulation measurements is rarely described in previous reports [9,11,28]. For measurements of the rotational alignment, we used the lesser trochanter and the center of the femoral medullary canal as the proximal reference. The main reason for choosing the lesser trochanter for reference was the high frequency of hip implants (total hip replacements and osteosynthesis). Previous studies have used the center of the femoral head, femoral neck, and greater trochanter, although they lie in different planes [8–10]. To our knowledge, using the lesser trochanter as a reference has not yet been validated.

The patients in the current study are typical for the elderly cohort who are most likely to sustain a distal femur fracture [1,2]. Although there were only 25 patients included in this study, which is slightly more than in most previous studies (Table 3), the limited number of patients could influence the external validity. Ideally, a larger cohort of patients would contribute to knowledge and external validity by comparing the two different surgical setups, traction table vs. traditional operating table.

One apparent strength is that the study is prospective. All the measurements were performed on full-length femur CT scans obtained within a week of operation before potential secondary displacement could occur. The reliability of the measurements showed a high ICC in rotation, length, and coronal plane but lower in the sagittal plane due to the lack of clear anatomic structures for measuring references in the sagittal plane.

5. Conclusions

The surgical setup technique for distal femur fractures with MIPO on a traction table with a dedicated femoral support provided an "excellent" result in all patients, according to the malalignment score by Handolin et al. [28]. Using the threshold for malrotation suggested by Croom et al. (15° side-to-side difference) [34], only 1/25 (18°) had malrotation, which is a lower rate of malrotation than previously published results on MIPO for distal femur fracture. The assessed surgical setup was easy to use and proved to be a valuable tool in the challenging task of reducing and fixating a distal femur fracture with MIPO. Further research with larger sample sizes comparing surgical results depending on a traditional operating table setup vs. a traction table setup would provide valuable knowledge on this topic.

Author Contributions: Conceptualization, M.P., C.E. and M.G.; methodology, all authors; writing—original draft preparation, M.P.; writing—review and editing, all authors. All authors have read and agreed to the published version of the manuscript.

Funding: This research received no external funding.

Institutional Review Board Statement: The study was conducted in accordance with the Declaration of Helsinki and approved by the Institutional Review Board in Gothenburg (registration number 008-12 approved 5 June 2012).

Informed Consent Statement: Informed consent was obtained from all subjects involved in the study.

Data Availability Statement: The data presented in this study are available on request from the corresponding author. The data are not publicly available due to national legislation.

Conflicts of Interest: The authors declare no conflict of interest.

References

1. Elsoe, R.; Ceccotti, A.A.; Larsen, P. Population-based epidemiology and incidence of distal femur fractures. *Int. Orthop.* **2018**, *42*, 191–196. [CrossRef] [PubMed]
2. Pietu, G.; Lebaron, M.; Flecher, X.; Hulet, C.; Vandenbussche, E. Epidemiology of distal femur fractures in France in 2011–12. *Orthop. Traumatol. Surg. Res.* **2014**, *100*, 545–548. [CrossRef]
3. Farouk, O.; Krettek, C.; Miclau, T.; Schandelmaier, P.; Guy, P.; Tscherne, H. Minimally invasive plate osteosynthesis and vascularity: Preliminary results of a cadaver injection study. *Injury* **1997**, *28* (Suppl. 1), A7–A12. [CrossRef]
4. Hoffmann, M.F.; Jones, C.B.; Sietsema, D.L.; Tornetta, P.; Koenig, S.J. Clinical outcomes of locked plating of distal femoral fractures in a retrospective cohort. *J. Orthop. Surg. Res.* **2013**, *8*, 43. [CrossRef] [PubMed]
5. Hake, M.E.; Davis, M.E.; Perdue, A.M.; Goulet, J.A. Modern Implant Options for the Treatment of Distal Femur Fractures. *J. Am. Acad. Orthop. Surg.* **2019**, *27*, e867–e875. [CrossRef]
6. Kregor, P.J.; Stannard, J.A.; Zlowodzki, M.; Cole, P.A. Treatment of distal femur fractures using the less invasive stabilization system: Surgical experience and early clinical results in 103 fractures. *J. Orthop. Trauma* **2004**, *18*, 509–520. [CrossRef]
7. Schutz, M.; Muller, M.; Regazzoni, P.; Hontzsch, D.; Krettek, C.; Van der Werken, C.; Haas, N. Use of the less invasive stabilization system (LISS) in patients with distal femoral (AO33) fractures: A prospective multicenter study. *Arch. Orthop. Trauma Surg.* **2005**, *125*, 102–108. [CrossRef]

8. Buckley, R.; Mohanty, K.; Malish, D. Lower limb malrotation following MIPO technique of distal femoral and proximal tibial fractures. *Injury* **2011**, *42*, 194–199. [CrossRef]
9. Kim, J.W.; Oh, C.W.; Oh, J.K.; Park, I.H.; Kyung, H.S.; Park, K.H.; Yoon, S.D.; Kim, S.M. Malalignment after minimally invasive plate osteosynthesis in distal femoral fractures. *Injury* **2017**, *48*, 751–757. [CrossRef] [PubMed]
10. Lill, M.; Attal, R.; Rudisch, A.; Wick, M.C.; Blauth, M.; Lutz, M. Does MIPO of fractures of the distal femur result in more rotational malalignment than ORIF? A retrospective study. *Eur. J. Trauma Emerg. Surg.* **2016**, *42*, 733–740. [CrossRef] [PubMed]
11. Sharma, V.; Laubach, L.K.; Krumme, J.W.; Satpathy, J. Comminuted periprosthetic distal femoral fractures have greater postoperative extension malalignment. *Knee* **2022**, *36*, 65–71. [CrossRef] [PubMed]
12. Dunbar, R.P.; Egol, K.A.; Jones, C.B.; Ertl, J.P.; Mullis, B.; Perez, E.; Collinge, C.A.; Ostrum, R.; Humphrey, C.; Gardner, M.J.; et al. Locked Lateral Plating Versus Retrograde Nailing for Distal Femur Fractures: A Multicenter Randomized Trial. *J. Orthop. Trauma* **2023**, *37*, 70–76. [CrossRef] [PubMed]
13. Kuwahara, Y.; Takegami, Y.; Tokutake, K.; Yamada, Y.; Komaki, K.; Ichikawa, T.; Imagama, S. How does intraoperative fracture malalignment affect postoperative function and bone healing following distal femoral fracture?: A retrospective multicentre study. *Bone Jt. Open.* **2022**, *3*, 165–172. [CrossRef]
14. Peschiera, V.; Staletti, L.; Cavanna, M.; Saporito, M.; Berlusconi, M. Predicting the failure in distal femur fractures. *Injury* **2018**, *49*, S2–S7. [CrossRef] [PubMed]
15. Yildirim, A.O.; Aksahin, E.; Sakman, B.; Kati, Y.A.; Akti, S.; Dogan, O.; Ucaner, A.; Bicimoglu, A. The effect of rotational deformity on patellofemoral parameters following the treatment of femoral shaft fracture. *Arch. Orthop. Trauma Surg.* **2013**, *133*, 641–648. [CrossRef] [PubMed]
16. Karaman, O.; Ayhan, E.; Kesmezacar, H.; Seker, A.; Unlu, M.C.; Aydingoz, O. Rotational malalignment after closed intramedullary nailing of femoral shaft fractures and its influence on daily life. *Eur. J. Orthop. Surg. Traumatol.* **2014**, *24*, 1243–1247. [CrossRef]
17. Gugenheim, J.J.; Probe, R.A.; Brinker, M.R. The effects of femoral shaft malrotation on lower extremity anatomy. *J. Orthop. Trauma* **2004**, *18*, 658–664. [CrossRef]
18. Wong, J.R.Y.; Tsamados, S.; Patel, A.; Jaiswal, P. Use of Traction Table for Reducing Complex Distal Femur Fractures: A Technical Trick. *Cureus* **2022**, *14*, e23889. [CrossRef]
19. Ehlinger, M.; Ducrot, G.; Adam, P.; Bonnomet, F. Distal femur fractures. Surgical techniques and a review of the literature. *Orthop. Traumatol. Surg. Res.* **2013**, *99*, 353–360. [CrossRef]
20. Ehlinger, M.; Adam, P.; Abane, L.; Arlettaz, Y.; Bonnomet, F. Minimally-invasive internal fixation of extra-articular distal femur fractures using a locking plate: Tricks of the trade. *Orthop. Traumatol. Surg. Res.* **2011**, *97*, 201–205. [CrossRef]
21. Paulsson, M.; Ekholm, C.; Jonsson, E.; Geijer, M.; Rolfson, O. Immediate full weight-bearing versus partial weight-bearing after plate fixation of distal femur fractures in elderly patients. A randomized controlled trial. *Geriatr. Orthop. Surg. Rehabil.* **2021**, *12*, 21514593211055889. [CrossRef] [PubMed]
22. Meinberg, E.G.; Agel, J.; Roberts, C.S.; Karam, M.D.; Kellam, J.F. Fracture and dislocation classification compendium-2018. *J. Orthop. Trauma* **2018**, *32* (Suppl. 1), S1–S170. [CrossRef] [PubMed]
23. Flierl, M.A.; Stahel, P.F.; Hak, D.J.; Morgan, S.J.; Smith, W.R. Traction table-related complications in orthopaedic surgery. *J. Am. Acad. Orthop. Surg.* **2010**, *18*, 668–675. [CrossRef] [PubMed]
24. Peyser, A.; Weil, Y.; Liebergall, M.; Mosheiff, R. Percutaneous compression plating for intertrochanteric fractures. Surgical technique, tips for surgery, and results. *Oper. Orthop. Traumatol.* **2005**, *17*, 158–177. [CrossRef]
25. Pietu, G.; Ehlinger, M. Minimally invasive internal fixation of distal femur fractures. *Orthop. Traumatol. Surg. Res.* **2017**, *103*, S161–S169. [CrossRef]
26. Collinge, C.A.; Gardner, M.J.; Crist, B.D. Pitfalls in the application of distal femur plates for fractures. *J. Orthop. Trauma* **2011**, *25*, 695–706. [CrossRef]
27. Koo, T.K.; Li, M.Y. A guideline of selecting and reporting intraclass correlation coefficients for reliability research. *J. Chiropr. Med.* **2016**, *15*, 155–163. [CrossRef]
28. Handolin, L.; Pajarinen, J.; Lindahl, J.; Hirvensalo, E. Retrograde intramedullary nailing in distal femoral fractures—Results in a series of 46 consecutive operations. *Injury* **2004**, *35*, 517–522. [CrossRef]
29. Dimitriou, D.; Tsai, T.Y.; Yue, B.; Rubash, H.E.; Kwon, Y.M.; Li, G. Side-to-side variation in normal femoral morphology: 3D CT analysis of 122 femurs. *Orthop. Traumatol. Surg. Res.* **2016**, *102*, 91–97. [CrossRef]
30. Marchand, L.S.; Jacobson, L.G.; Stuart, A.R.; Haller, J.M.; Higgins, T.F.; Rothberg, D.L. Assessing femoral rotation: A survey comparison of techniques. *J. Orthop. Trauma* **2020**, *34*, e96–e101. [CrossRef]
31. Laumonerie, P.; Ollivier, M.; LiArno, S.; Faizan, A.; Cavaignac, E.; Argenson, J.N. Which factors influence proximal femoral asymmetry?: A 3D CT analysis of 345 femoral pairs. *Bone Jt. J.* **2018**, *100*, 839–844. [CrossRef] [PubMed]
32. Reikeras, O.; Hoiseth, A.; Reigstad, A.; Fonstelien, E. Femoral neck angles: A specimen study with special regard to bilateral differences. *Acta Orthop. Scand.* **1982**, *53*, 775–779. [CrossRef] [PubMed]
33. Sutter, R.; Dietrich, T.J.; Zingg, P.O.; Pfirrmann, C.W. Femoral antetorsion: Comparing asymptomatic volunteers and patients with femoroacetabular impingement. *Radiology* **2012**, *263*, 475–483. [CrossRef] [PubMed]

34. Croom, W.P.; Lorenzana, D.J.; Auran, R.L.; Cavallero, M.J.; Heckmann, N.; Lee, J.; White, E.A. Is contralateral templating reliable for establishing rotational alignment during intramedullary stabilization of femoral shaft fractures? A study of individual bilateral differences in femoral version. *J. Orthop. Trauma* **2018**, *32*, 61–66. [CrossRef]
35. Shezar, A.; Rosenberg, N.; Soudry, M. Technique for closed reduction of femoral shaft fracture using an external support device. *Injury* **2005**, *36*, 450–453. [CrossRef]
36. Neer, C.S.I.; Grantham, S.A.; Shelton, M.L. Supracondylar Fracture of the Adult Femur: A study of one hundred and ten cases. *JBJS* **1967**, *49*, 591–613. [CrossRef]
37. Herrera, A.; Rosell, J.; Ibarz, E.; Albareda, J.; Gabarre, S.; Mateo, J.; Gracia, L. Biomechanical analysis of the stability of anterograde reamed intramedullary nails in femoral spiral fractures. *Injury* **2020**, *51* (Suppl. 1), S74–S79. [CrossRef]
38. Doshi, H.K.; Wenxian, P.; Burgula, M.V.; Murphy, D.P. Clinical Outcomes of Distal Femoral Fractures in the Geriatric Population Using Locking Plates With a Minimally Invasive Approach. *Geriatr. Orthop. Surg. Rehabil.* **2013**, *4*, 16–20. [CrossRef]
39. Grant, K.D.; Busse, E.C.; Park, D.K.; Baker, K.C. Internal Fixation of Osteoporotic Bone. *J. Am. Acad. Orthop. Surg.* **2018**, *26*, 166–174. [CrossRef]
40. Khursheed, O.; Wani, M.M.; Rashid, S.; Lone, A.H.; Manaan, Q.; Sultan, A.; Bhat, R.A.; Mir, B.A.; Halwai, M.A.; Akhter, N. Results of treatment of distal extra: Articular femur fractures with locking plates using minimally invasive approach—Experience with 25 consecutive geriatric patients. *Musculoskelet. Surg.* **2015**, *99*, 139–147. [CrossRef]
41. Kolb, W.; Guhlmann, H.; Windisch, C.; Marx, F.; Kolb, K.; Koller, H. Fixation of distal femoral fractures with the Less Invasive Stabilization System: A minimally invasive treatment with locked fixed-angle screws. *J. Trauma* **2008**, *65*, 1425–1434. [CrossRef] [PubMed]
42. Liu, F.; Tao, R.; Cao, Y.; Wang, Y.; Zhou, Z.; Wang, H.; Gu, Y. The role of LISS (less invasive stabilisation system) in the treatment of peri-knee fractures. *Injury* **2009**, *40*, 1187–1194. [CrossRef] [PubMed]
43. Abdelmonem, A.H.; Saber, A.Y.; El Sageir, M.; El-Malky, A. Evaluation of the Results of Minimally Invasive Plate Osteosynthesis Using a Locking Plate in the Treatment of Distal Femur Fractures. *Cureus* **2022**, *14*, e23617. [CrossRef] [PubMed]
44. Borade, A.; Sanchez, D.; Kempegowda, H.; Maniar, H.; Pesantez, R.F.; Suk, M.; Horwitz, D.S. Minimally Invasive Plate Osteosynthesis for Periprosthetic and Interprosthetic Fractures Associated with Knee Arthroplasty: Surgical Technique and Review of Current Literature. *J. Knee Surg.* **2019**, *32*, 392–402. [CrossRef] [PubMed]
45. Cornell, C.N.; Ayalon, O. Evidence for success with locking plates for fragility fractures. *HSS J.* **2011**, *7*, 164–169. [CrossRef]
46. von Rüden, C.; Augat, P. Failure of fracture fixation in osteoporotic bone. *Injury* **2016**, *47*, S3–S10. [CrossRef]
47. Beltran, M.J.; Collinge, C.A.; Gardner, M.J. Stress Modulation of Fracture Fixation Implants. *J. Am. Acad. Orthop. Surg.* **2016**, *24*, 711–719. [CrossRef]
48. Miranda, M.A. Locking plate technology and its role in osteoporotic fractures. *Injury* **2007**, *38* (Suppl. 3), S35–S39. [CrossRef]
49. Beltran, M.J.; Gary, J.L.; Collinge, C.A. Management of distal femur fractures with modern plates and nails: State of the art. *J. Orthop. Trauma* **2015**, *29*, 165–172. [CrossRef]
50. Bottlang, M.; Fitzpatrick, D.C.; Sheerin, D.; Kubiak, E.; Gellman, R.; Zandschulp, C.V.; Doornink, J.; Earley, K.; Madey, S.M. Dynamic Fixation of Distal Femur Fractures Using Far Cortical Locking Screws: A Prospective Observational Study. *J. Orthop. Trauma* **2014**, *28*, 181–188. [CrossRef]
51. Zlowodzki, M.; Williamson, S.; Cole, P.A.; Zardiackas, L.D.; Kregor, P.J. Biomechanical evaluation of the less invasive stabilization system, angled blade plate, and retrograde intramedullary nail for the internal fixation of distal femur fractures. *J. Orthop. Trauma* **2004**, *18*, 494–502. [CrossRef] [PubMed]
52. Duffy, P.; Trask, K.; Hennigar, A.; Barron, L.; Leighton, R.K.; Dunbar, M.J. Assessment of fragment micromotion in distal femur fracture fixation with RSA. *Clin. Orthop. Relat. Res.* **2006**, *448*, 105–113. [CrossRef] [PubMed]
53. Bogunovic, L.; Cherney, S.M.; Rothermich, M.A.; Gardner, M.J. Biomechanical considerations for surgical stabilization of osteoporotic fractures. *Orthop. Clin. N. Am.* **2013**, *44*, 183–200. [CrossRef]
54. Yaacobi, E.; Sanchez, D.; Maniar, H.; Horwitz, D.S. Surgical treatment of osteoporotic fractures: An update on the principles of management. *Injury* **2017**, *48* (Suppl. 7), S34–S40. [CrossRef]
55. Perren, S.M.; Linke, B.; Schwieger, K.; Wahl, D.; Schneider, E. Aspects of internal fixation of fractures in porotic bone. Principles, technologies and procedures using locked plate screws. *Acta Chir. Orthop. Traumatol. Cechoslov.* **2005**, *72*, 89–97.
56. Du, Y.R.; Ma, J.X.; Wang, S.; Sun, L.; Wang, Y.; Lu, B.; Bai, H.H.; Hu, Y.C.; Ma, X.L. Comparison of Less Invasive Stabilization System Plate and Retrograde Intramedullary Nail in the Fixation of Femoral Supracondylar Fractures in the Elderly: A Biomechanical Study. *Orthop. Surg.* **2019**, *11*, 311–317. [CrossRef]
57. Adams, J.D., Jr.; Tanner, S.L.; Jeray, K.J. Far cortical locking screws in distal femur fractures. *Orthopedics* **2015**, *38*, e153–e156. [CrossRef]
58. Rodriguez, E.K.; Zurakowski, D.; Herder, L.; Hall, A.; Walley, K.C.; Weaver, M.J.; Appleton, P.T.; Vrahas, M. Mechanical Construct Characteristics Predisposing to Non-union After Locked Lateral Plating of Distal Femur Fractures. *J. Orthop. Trauma* **2016**, *30*, 403–408. [CrossRef]
59. Henderson, C.E.; Lujan, T.J.; Kuhl, L.L.; Bottlang, M.; Fitzpatrick, D.C.; Marsh, J.L. 2010 Mid-America Orthopaedic Association Physician in Training Award: Healing Complications Are Common After Locked Plating for Distal Femur Fractures. *Clin. Orthop. Relat. Res.* **2011**, *469*, 1757–1765. [CrossRef] [PubMed]

60. Kim, S.-M.; Yeom, J.-W.; Song, H.K.; Hwang, K.-T.; Hwang, J.-H.; Yoo, J.-H. Lateral locked plating for distal femur fractures by low-energy trauma: What makes a difference in healing? *Int. Orthop.* **2018**, *42*, 2907–2914. [CrossRef]
61. Yazdi, H.; Akbari Aghdam, H.; Motaghi, P.; Mohammadpour, M.; Bahari, M.; Ghahfarokhi, S.G.; Ghaderi, M.T. Using Blumensaat's line to determine the sagittal alignment of the distal femur. *Eur. J. Orthop. Surg. Traumatol.* **2022**, *33*, 1031–1035. [CrossRef] [PubMed]

Disclaimer/Publisher's Note: The statements, opinions and data contained in all publications are solely those of the individual author(s) and contributor(s) and not of MDPI and/or the editor(s). MDPI and/or the editor(s) disclaim responsibility for any injury to people or property resulting from any ideas, methods, instructions or products referred to in the content.

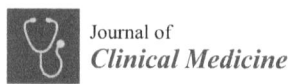

Article

Mismatch between Clinical–Functional and Radiological Outcome in Tibial Plateau Fractures: A Retrospective Study

Markus Bormann [1,*], David Bitschi [1], Claas Neidlein [1], Daniel P. Berthold [1], Maximilian Jörgens [1], Robert Pätzold [2], Julius Watrinet [2], Wolfgang Böcker [1], Boris Michael Holzapfel [1] and Julian Fürmetz [1,2]

1. Department of Orthopedics and Trauma Surgery, Musculoskeletal University Center Munich (MUM), University Hospital, LMU Munich, 81377 Munich, Germany
2. Department of Trauma Surgery, Trauma Center Murnau, 82418 Murnau, Germany
* Correspondence: markus.bormann@med.uni-muenchen.de

Abstract: Background: The evaluation of tibial plateau fractures (TPF) encompasses the assessment of clinical–functional and radiological parameters. In this study, the authors aimed to investigate the potential correlation between these parameters by utilizing both the clinical–functional and the modified radiological Rasmussen score. Methods: In this retrospective monocentric study conducted at a level-I trauma center, patients who underwent surgery between January 2014 and December 2019 due to a TPF were included. The clinical–functional Rasmussen score prior to the injury, at 1-year postoperatively, and during the last follow-up (minimum 18 months) was assessed using a standardized questionnaire. Additionally, the modified radiological Rasmussen score was determined at the 1-year postoperative mark using conventional radiographs in two planes. Results: A total of 50 patients were included in this study, comprising 40% (n = 20) men, and 60% (n = 30) women, with an average age of 47 ± 11.8 years (range 26–73 years old). Among them, 52% (n = 26) had simple fractures (classified according to Schatzker I–III), while 48% (n = 24; according to Schatzker IV–VI) had complex fractures. The mean follow-up was 3.9 ± 1.6 years (range 1.6–7.5 years). The functional Rasmussen score assessed before the injury and at follow-up showed an "excellent" average result. However, there was a significant difference in the values of complex fractures compared to before the injury. One year postoperatively, both the clinical–functional score and the modified radiological score demonstrated a "good" average result. The "excellent" category was more frequently observed in the functional score, while the "fair" category was more common in the radiological score. There was no agreement between the categories in both scores in 66% of the cases. Conclusions: The data from this retrospective study demonstrated that patients with TPF are able to achieve a nearly equivalent functional level in the medium-term after a prolonged recovery period, comparable to their pre-injury state. However, it is important to note that the correlation between clinical–functional and radiological parameters is limited. Consequently, in order to create prospective outcome scores, it becomes crucial to objectively assess the multifaceted nature of TPF injuries in more detail, both clinically and radiologically.

Keywords: tibial plateau fracture (TPF); Rasmussen score; clinical outcomes; radiological outcomes

1. Introduction

The incidence of tibial plateau fractures (TPF) has increased significantly over the past decade [1]. Consequently, the treatment strategies for this complex injury have undergone changes. Nowadays, computer tomography (CT) imaging is considered the gold standard for diagnostics [2], leading to the development of novel classification systems [3] and the establishment of a 360° operative treatment [4,5].

The fundamental principles of osteosynthetic treatment aim to achieve the most accurate possible joint surface reduction and anatomical reconstruction of both the width of the tibial head, joint angles, and limb alignment. In 1973, Rasmussen described how

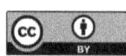

these parameters significantly impact patient outcomes [6], a finding that was subsequently validated by Kraus et al. and Beisemann et al. in the past years [5,7]. Additionally, Rasmussen developed a clinical–functional outcome score that is not reliant on radiological parameters [6]. As both scores were shown to be reliable and reproducible, they are still used today to assess the outcome in patients following TPF [8–11].

In the current literature, short- to medium-term outcomes following osteosynthesis of TPF are described as good to excellent [7,11–13]. However, in the long term, the functional scores tend to be lower on average, and the athletic level is reduced compared to pre-injury levels [5,14]. The rate of post-traumatic arthritis (PTA) following TPFs is reported to be between 13 and 83%, which may be higher in patients with articular sided complex fractures. Consequently, approximately 7% of the patients require a secondary total knee arthroplasty (TKA) within 10 years post-fracture [14–16]. However, there remains a scarcity in the literature reporting on functional outcomes and their correlation to fracture morphology.

The aim of this study is (1) to report on functional outcomes in patients following TPF and (2) to correlate them with the radiological outcomes. Hypothesis (1) was that after TPF, patients would achieve functional values equivalent to their pre-injury functional values and hypothesis (2) was that there is a correlation between functional outcomes, fracture morphology, and anatomical reconstruction.

2. Materials and Methods

2.1. Patient Selection

A retrospective chart review was performed on all patients at a German level-I trauma center, who underwent surgery for TPF between January 2014 and December 2019. Institutional review board approval was obtained before the initiation of the study. Patients were included if they had confirmed intra-articular TPF during pre-operative CT scans, if they were aged > 18 years, and if they had detailed documentation about trauma mechanism and information on demographics such as gender and age. Furthermore, radiographic imaging (X-ray in anteroposterior and lateral view) 12 months after surgery was required. Minimum follow-up was set at 18 months. Patients were excluded if they had extraarticular fractures (AO/OTA 41-A), other fractures than TPF, tibial shaft fractures, as well as inconsistent documentation.

2.2. Surgical Technique

Patients with TPF were operated on either by open reduction and internal fixation (ORIF) or by arthroscopically assisted closed reduction and internal fixation (CRIF).

2.3. Postoperative Rehabilitation

All patients were treated with a standardized, clinic-specific postoperative protocol. This includes an 8-week partial load-bearing period as well as a hard frame orthesis with flexion limitation at 60 degrees for 6 weeks.

2.4. Clinical Analysis

Outcome analysis included the clinical–functional Rasmussen score (Table 1). This score was collected for the period directly before sustaining TPF, 1 year postoperatively, as well as for the minimum follow-up. Additionally, at final follow-up, all patients were assessed for passive and active range of motion and clinical laxity testing.

2.5. Radiographic Analysis

The fractures were classified using the established systems of Schatzker, AO/OTA, and Moore by the first and senior author (Consultant and head of department, respectively) as well as by 2 scientific assistants on CT scans. Discrepancies in classifications between the raters were solved by discussion. The modified radiological Rasmussen score was determined at 1 year postoperatively using conventional X-rays in two planes by the same research group (Table 1). Fractures were classified as simple fractures when they had a confirmed TPF according to Schatzker I-III. In contrast, fractures were classified as complex fractures when they had a confirmed TPF according to Schatzker IV-VI and/or radiological evidence of knee dislocation according to Moore [17,18].

2.6. Statistical Analysis

Descriptive statistics were summarized as means and standard deviations for quantitative variables and counts and frequencies for categorical variables. The significance of differences in means and frequencies of continuous and categorical variables was examined. For this purpose, the Mann–Whitney, Wilcoxon, and McNemar tests, and the Spearmen correlation coefficient were used. Statistical significance for all comparisons was set at $p < 0.05$. All analyses were performed with SPSS Statistics 26.0 (IBM Corp., Armonk, NY 10504, USA). The graphical representation was performed using SPSS Statistics 26.0 (IBM Corp., Armonk, NY 10504, USA) and Microsoft Excel 365 MSO Version 2207 (Microsoft Corp., Redmond, WA, USA).

2.7. Rasmussen Scores

Table 1. Rasmussen scores—criteria and evaluation.

Radiological Score		Pts	Clinical–Functional Score		Pts
Depression	None	6	Pain	No pain	6
	<5 mm	4		Occasional pain	5
	5–10 mm	2		Stabbing pain in certain positions	4
	>10 mm	0		Constant pain after activity	2
Condylar widening	None	6		Significant rest pain	0
	<5 mm	4	Walking capacity	Normal for age	6
	5–10 mm	2		Outdoor > 1 h	4
	>10 mm	0		Outdoor > 15 min	2
Angulation (varus/valgus)	None	6		Only indoors	1
	<10°	4		Immobile	0
	10–20°	2	Extension	Normal	6
	>20°	0		Lack of extension < 10°	4
				Lack of extension > 10°	2
			Range of motion	>140°	6
				>120°	5
				>90°	4
				>60°	2
				>30°	1
				>0°	0
			Stability	Normal stability	6
				Instability in 20° flexion	5
				Instability in extension <10°	4
				Instability in extension >10°	2

Table 1. *Cont.*

Radiological Score	Clinical–Functional Score	Evaluation
18 points	27–30 points	excellent
12–17	20–26	good
6–11	10–19	fair
0–5	4–9	poor

3. Results

3.1. Participants

In this monocentric study, 319 patients were treated for TPF between January 2014 and December 2019. Of these patients, 50 were eligible for inclusion in the study (Figure 1).

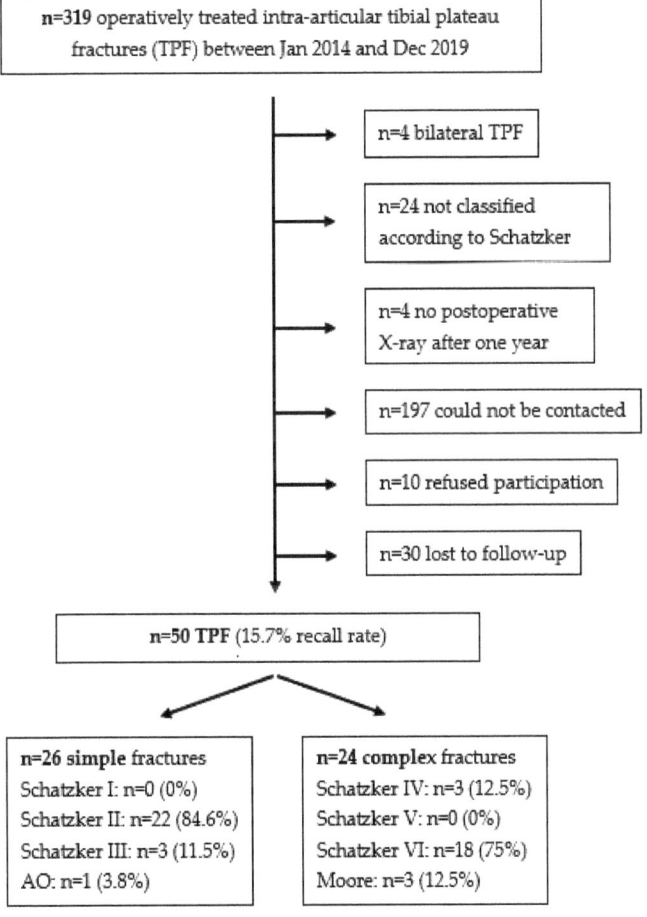

Figure 1. Flow chart patient selection.

The mean age of the patients was 47 ± 11.8 years, with a range between 26 and 73 years old. The mean follow-up was 3.9 ± 1.6 years, with a range between 1.6 and 7.5 years. Overall, 26 patients could be assigned to simple fractures (according to Schatzker I–III), while 24 patients were diagnosed with complex fractures (according to Schatzker IV–VI). The patient-specific data are presented in Table 2.

Table 2. Patient-specific data total collective.

Criteria	Total Collective (n = 50)	p-Value
Men vs. women	40% (n = 20) vs. 60% (n = 30)	
Mean age	47 ± 11.8 years (range 26-73 years old)	
Mean follow-up	3.9 ± 1.6 years (range 1.6-7.5 years)	
Mean BMI at surgery BMI at final follow-up Difference	24.4 ± 3.5 25.2 ± 3.6 +0.8	0.001

Schatzker (n) I
              II
              III
              IV
              V
              VI
              AO/Moore
	0 (0%)
	22 (44%)
	3 (6%)
	3 (6%)
	0 (0%)
	18 (36%)
	4 (8%)	

Surgical technique - Knee arthroscopy - ORIF	 3 (6%) 47 (94%)	

3.2. Surgical Technique

A total of 94% (n = 47) of patients were treated by ORIF, while 6% (n = 3) received arthroscopic-assisted CRIF with screw osteosynthesis. Of these 47 ORIF patients, 76.6% (n = 36) were treated by a single approach, most frequently anterolateral (66%, n = 31), while 23.4% (n = 11) received combined approaches. Single plate osteosynthesis was performed in 70.2% (n = 33, most common anterolateral—84.8%, n = 28) and 29.8% (n = 14) received combined osteosynthesis (double/triple plate, plate + screws). A total of 17% (n = 8) of patients treated by ORIF also received additional knee fracturoscopy.

Furthermore, in 36% (n = 18) of patients concomitant meniscal and/or ligamentous injury were treated in addition to osteosynthesis. The injuries treated were anterior/posterior cruciate ligament (ACL/PCL) refixations, meniscus sutures and collateral ligament refixations.

3.3. Clinical Outcomes

Table 3 shows the values of the Rasmussen scores at the different survey time points, compares the simple and complex fractures according to Schatzker, and lists the most frequent variant for each assessment category (pain, walking capacity, extension, etc.).

Table 3. Rasmussen scores—simple vs. complex—most common assessment category.

Criteria	Total Collective (n = 50)	p-Value

Rasmussen functional before injury
simple vs. complex
  -Pain
  -Walking capacity
  -Extension
  -Range of motion
  -Stability
	28.84 ± 0.37 (excellent)
	28.77 vs. 28.92
	84% (n = 42) no pain
	100% (n = 50) normal
	100% (n = 50) normal
	100% (n = 50) >120°
	100% (n = 50) normal
		0.16

Rasmussen functional 1a postoperative
simple vs. complex
  -Pain
  -Walking capacity
  -Extension
  -Range of motion
  -Stability
	24.68 ± 3.61 (good)
	25.69 vs. 23.58
	76% (n = 38) occasional
	44% (n = 22) normal
	54% (n = 27) normal
	66% (n = 33) >120°
	88% (n = 44) normal
		0.052

Table 3. Cont.

Criteria	Total Collective (n = 50)	p-Value
Rasmussen functional at follow-up	28.0 ± 2.17 (excellent)	
simple vs. complex	28.35 vs. 27.63	0.489
-Pain	80% (n = 40) no pain	
-Walking capacity	88% (n = 44) normal	
-Extension	88% (n = 44) normal	
-Range of motion	90% (n = 45) >120°	
-Stability	94% (n = 47) normal	
Rasmussen radiological 1a postoperative	13.44 ± 3.64 (good)	
simple vs. complex	14.0 vs. 12.83	0.447
-Depression	38% (n = 19) None	
-Condylar widening	46% (n = 23) None	
-Angulation	54% (n = 27) None	
Rasmussen functional vs. radiological 1a postoperative	Spearman-Rho = 0.075	0.605

In the clinical–functional Rasmussen score, patients achieve an average score before injury, which corresponds to an "excellent" result according to Rasmussen. One-year post-surgery the mean score corresponds to a "good" value for both simple and complex fractures. However, it is significantly worse in both groups ($p < 0.001$) compared to the pre-injury scores. Although the difference between the groups is measurable at this point, it is not statistically significant ($p = 0.052$). As the follow-up progresses, both groups demonstrate an increase in the average score, eventually reaching an "excellent" score. However, the value achieved for complex fractures remains significantly worse ($p < 0.01$) than before the injury. Otherwise, there is no significant difference ($p = 0.071$) for the simple fractures at the final follow-up.

The modified radiological Rasmussen score, one year after surgery, indicates a "good" result for both simple and complex fractures. The difference between the groups is not significant at this point ($p = 0.447$).

Figure 2 shows the number of patients in each result group. One year after surgery, more patients in the clinical–functional score group showed an "excellent" result compared to the modified radiological score group ($p = 0.189$). Notably, there are significantly more patients rated as "poor/fair" radiologically (n = 12) than clinical–functional (n = 3) at this time ($p = 0.035$).

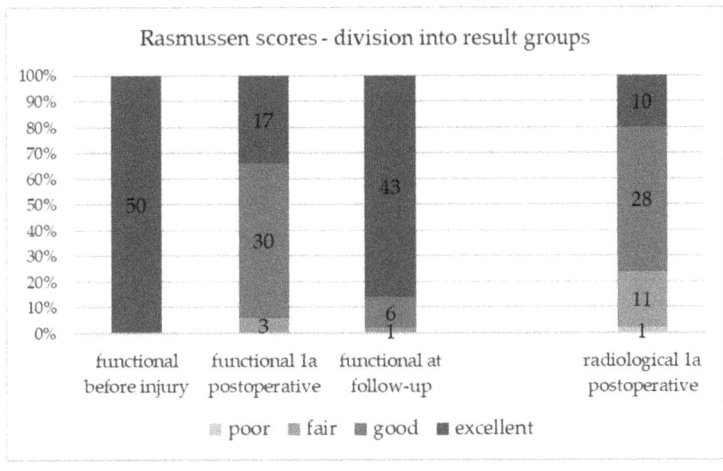

Figure 2. Rasmussen scores—division into result groups.

Figure 3 shows that the position of the median for both scores is within the "good" outcomes group 1-year postoperatively. In each case, the median is located above the arithmetic mean. Additionally, there is a noticeable reduction in scatter for the clinical–functional score leading up to the follow-up.

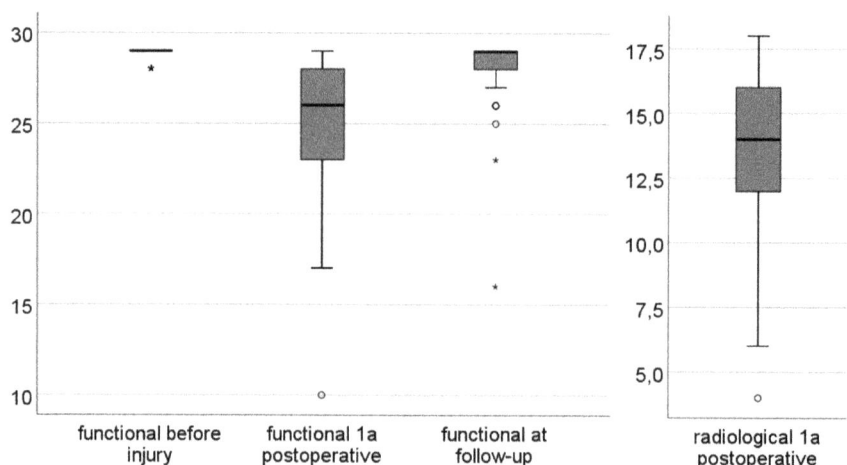

Figure 3. Dispersion of Rasmussen scores with median position. * = values with an interquartile range more than 3.

Table 4 shows the clinical–functional and radiological Rasmussen score after one year in a cross-tabulation.

Table 4. Cross-tabulation Rasmussen scores 1-year postoperatively.

		Rasmussen Radiological 1a Postoperative				In Total
		Excellent	Good	Fair	Poor	
Rasmussen functional 1a postoperative	excellent	3	13	1	0	17
	good	5	14	10	1	30
	fair	2	1	0	0	3
In total		10	28	11	1	50

When analyzing the assignment of patients to their respective outcome groups (poor, fair, good, excellent) based on the clinical–functional and modified radiological score after one year, it was found that 66% (n = 33) of the 50 cases had no match. Thereby, 50% (n = 25) of the patients had a lower rating in the radiological score compared to the clinical–functional score, while 16% (n = 8) showed a higher rating in the radiological score. The Spearman correlation coefficient shows no relevant correlation for the two scores (Rho = 0.075).

In the subgroup of patients who scored "moderate," there was entirely no agreement (in 100% of the cases) with the other score. Regarding patients rated as "good" in the clinical–functional score, 53.3% (n = 16) had no radiological match, and within this group 68.8% (n = 11) displayed a worse radiological score. On the other hand, among patients rated as "good" radiologically, 50% (n = 14) did not exhibit a corresponding result in the clinical–functional score, and within this group 92.9% (n = 13) had a better clinical–functional rating.

Interestingly, three patients with a clinical–functional rating of "fair" achieved an "excellent" radiological score twice and a "good" score once simultaneously. In the patient with a "good" rating, only a depression in the articular surface of < 5 mm was observed radiologically. These three patients shared the characteristic of exhibiting instability, in addition to individual differences in the clinical–functional score.

Among the twelve patients rated as "poor" or "fair" (Figure 2) in the radiological score, they either showed a significant depression exceeding 10 mm and/or a condylar widening ranging from 6 to 10 mm. In contrast, eleven patients achieved a "good" rating, while one patient achieved an "excellent" rating in the clinical–functional score.

Figure 4 shows the X-ray in two planes of a 31-year-old female patient 1 year postoperatively with a poor radiological Rasmussen and a good functional Rasmussen score.

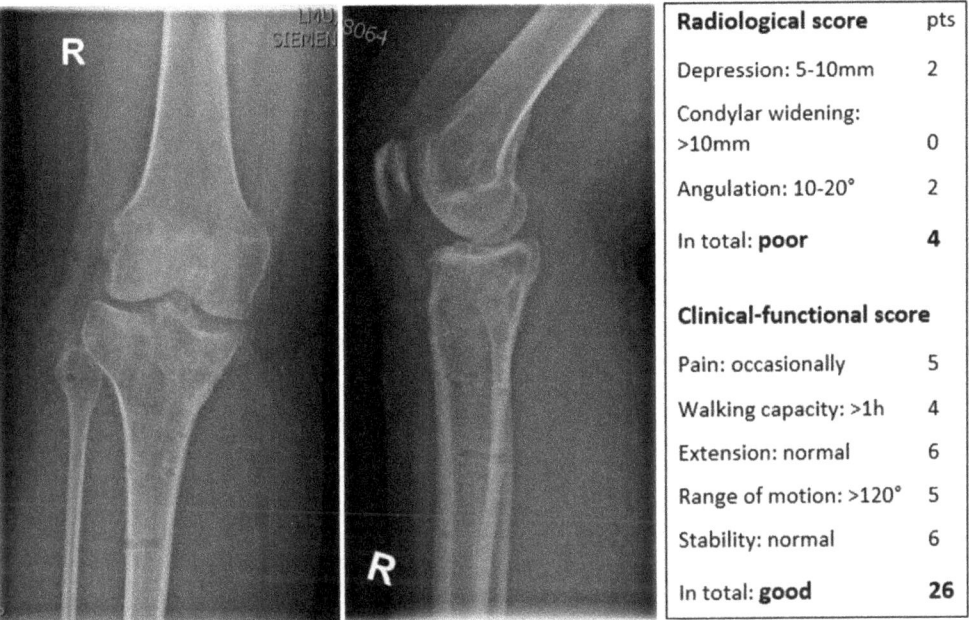

Figure 4. X-ray in two planes of a right (R) knee with the scores of a 31-year-old female patient.

4. Discussion

The most important finding of this study was that patients with TPF demonstrated an "excellent" outcome at a mean of 3.9 (+1.6) years post-surgery, as measured by the clinical–functional Rasmussen score. This outcome was observed regardless of the severity of the bony injury, according to the Schatzker classification. However, it is noteworthy that the clinical–functional scores were significantly worse after one year, but gradually improved during the subsequent observation period, indicating a prolonged recovery.

One year postoperatively, the patients achieve an average "good" score on both the clinical–functional and modified radiological Rasmussen score. However, this work also demonstrated that the different outcome groups (poor, fair, good, excellent) do not match in most of the cases, especially in the worse results. This underlines the importance of accurately assessing clinical function independently of postoperative radiographic findings for further treatment recommendations. Additionally, this once again proves that TPF is a complex joint injury that extends beyond just a fracture.

Previous research has reported a conversion rate of 3–7% for TKA within the first five years following osteosynthetic treatment of TPF [15,19,20], with the highest risk occurring within the initial two years [21–23]. Therefore, when discussing the possibility of secondary TKA with patients, it is crucial to consider the extended recovery period and the individual knee function independently of the X-ray. Moreover, it is important to note that TKA outcomes for patients with post-traumatic arthritis (PTA) are inferior, and the complication rates are higher compared to primary gonarthrosis cases [24,25].

In 1973, Rasmussen introduced his clinical–functional score [6]. The subjectively assessed parameters such as pain, walking capacity, and instability outweigh the objectively recorded ones like extension and range of motion, which is notably a limitation of the clinical–functional Rasmussen score. In particular, instability, which has been identified as a significant factor in the development of post-traumatic osteoarthritis [16], can also be evaluated through a clinical–apparative examination [26]. The fact that this study's patients showed an increase in BMI and a decrease in activity level during the recovery period suggests that the subjectively perceived excellent outcome may not be objectively substantiated. As demonstrated in this case for complex fractures, a statistically significant decrease in score (when comparing pre-injury to post-injury) does not necessarily result in a change in the scoring category. Hence, it is crucial to question this categorization.

Rasmussen's radiological score was also first described in 1973 [6]. Since then, significant advancements have occurred in radiological diagnostics for TPF, pre-, intra-, and postoperatively. Preoperative CT imaging is now considered the gold standard, and postoperative CT imaging is widely used for reposition control [2,27]. CT imaging provides more accurate visualization of the parameters used in the Rasmussen score, including depression, angulation, and widening of the tibial plateau [28–30]. This has led to well-defined limits for angulation and widening of the tibial plateau [2,6,31–33]. Different threshold values exist for the joint step, depending on whether it is in the load-bearing and/or meniscus-covered part. However, the current threshold values discussed are significantly lower than the gradations defined by Rasmussen [6,7,31,34–38].

In recent years, several clinical/functional outcome scores have been established, such as KOOS, Tegner, and IKDC, some of which are more comprehensive than the score developed by Rasmussen [39–42]. These scores mostly rely on subjective parameters [39–42]. However, apart from the modified Rasmussen score, no other radiological score has been widely adopted. Consequently, both Rasmussen scores are still frequently used in the current literature [8–10].

The lack of clear recommendations for MRI imaging in TPF indicates that the focus of radiological imaging continues to be the assessment of bony injury [2].

With the improved understanding of TPF as a complex joint injury in recent years, it has become more evident that, in addition to the bony and functional parameters defined by Rasmussen, meniscus, cartilage, and soft tissue lesions, and measurable instabilities contribute to the development of PTA and the overall outcome after TPF [31,43–45]. Extended imaging techniques (CT and MRI) and instrument-based diagnostics, including dynamic assessment, can help objectify these parameters. It is necessary to develop a scoring system based on comprehensive data that accurately represent the current and future outcomes after TPF.

5. Limitations

This study has several limitations. First, the data retrieved from this study are of retrospective nature, which could create selection bias. Second, the follow-up was only 18 months, as no long-term data were available. Third, no control group was available. However, all patients included in this study were indicated for surgery. Fourth, as mentioned above, apart from the modified Rasmussen score, no other radiological score has been widely adopted to date. Consequently, both Rasmussen scores are still frequently used in the current literature. Fifth, knee joint laxity was not measured in this study using dynamic reproducible methods. Lastly, no postoperative MRI was available to assess for progression of osteoarthritis or cartilage defects.

6. Conclusions

The data from this retrospective study demonstrated that patients with TPF are able to achieve a nearly equivalent functional level in the medium-term after a prolonged recovery period, comparable to their pre-injury state. However, it is important to note that the correlation between clinical–functional and radiological parameters is limited. Consequently, in order to create prospective outcome scores, it becomes crucial to objectively assess the multifaceted nature of TPF injuries in more detail, both clinically and radiologically.

Author Contributions: Conceptualization, D.B., J.F., and M.B.; methodology, D.B., M.B., R.P., and J.W.; data curation, C.N., M.J. and M.B.; writing—original draft preparation, D.B., M.B., J.F., and D.P.B.; visualization, D.B. and M.B.; supervision, J.F., B.M.H., and W.B.; project administration, M.B. All authors have read and agreed to the published version of the manuscript.

Funding: This research received no external funding.

Institutional Review Board Statement: The study was conducted in accordance with the Declaration of Helsinki and approved by the Institutional Ethics Committee of LMU Munich (21-0559, 18 June 2021).

Informed Consent Statement: Informed consent was obtained from all subjects involved in the study.

Data Availability Statement: Not applicable.

Conflicts of Interest: The authors declare no conflict of interest.

Abbreviations

TPF: tibial plateau fracture; 1a: 1 annus = 1 year; CT: computer tomography; MRI: magnetic resonance imaging; BMI: Body mass index; PTA: post-traumatic arthritis; TKA: total knee arthroplasty; ORIF: open reduction and internal fixation; CRIF: closed reduction and internal fixation; ACL/PCL: anterior/posterior cruciate ligament; KOOS: Knee injury and Osteoarthritis Outcome Score; IKDC: International Knee Documentation Committee; AO: Arbeitsgemeinschaft für Osteosynthesefragen; OTA: Orthopaedic Trauma Association.

References

1. Bormann, M.; Neidlein, C.; Gassner, C.; Keppler, A.M.; Bogner-Flatz, V.; Ehrnthaller, C.; Prall, W.C.; Böcker, W.; Fürmetz, J. Changing patterns in the epidemiology of tibial plateau fractures: A 10-year review at a level-I trauma center. *Eur. J. Trauma Emerg. Surg.* **2022**, *49*, 401–409. [CrossRef]
2. Deutsche Gesellschaft für Orthopädie und Unfallchirurgie e.V. (DGOU). Tibial Head Fractures. Version 1.0 (29 October2021). 2022. Available online: https://www.awmf.org/uploads/tx_szleitlinien/187-042l_S2k_Tibiakopffrakturen_2022-07.pdf (accessed on 3 October 2022).
3. Krause, M.; Preiss, A.; Müller, G.; Madert, J.; Fehske, K.; Neumann, M.V.; Domnick, C.; Raschke, M.; Südkamp, N.; Frosch, K.-H. Intra-articular tibial plateau fracture characteristics according to the "Ten segment classification". *Injury* **2016**, *47*, 2551–2557. [CrossRef] [PubMed]
4. Krause, M.; Frosch, K.-H. Change in the treatment of tibial plateau fractures. *Unfallchirurgie* **2022**, *125*, 527–534. [CrossRef]
5. Kraus, T.M.; Freude, T.; Stöckle, U.; Stuby, F.M. Pearls and pitfalls for the treatment of tibial head fractures. *Orthopade* **2016**, *45*, 24–31. [CrossRef] [PubMed]
6. Rasmussen, P.S. Tibial condylar fractures. Impairment of knee joint stability as an indication for surgical treatment. *J. Bone Joint Surg. Am.* **1973**, *55*, 1331–1350. [CrossRef]
7. Beisemann, N.; Vetter, S.Y.; Keil, H.; Swartman, B.; Schnetzke, M.; Franke, J.; Grützner, P.A.; Privalov, M. Influence of reduction quality on functional outcome and quality of life in the surgical treatment of tibial plateau fractures: A retrospective cohort study. *Orthop. Traumatol. Surg. Res.* **2021**, *108*, 102922. [CrossRef]
8. Krause, M.; The "Fracture committee" of the German Knee Society; Alm, L.; Berninger, M.; Domnick, C.; Fehske, K.; Frosch, K.-H.; Herbst, E.; Korthaus, A.; Raschke, M.; et al. Bone metabolism is a key factor for clinical outcome of tibial plateau fractures. *Eur. J. Trauma Emerg. Surg.* **2020**, *46*, 1227–1237. [CrossRef]
9. Prall, W.; Rieger, M.; Fürmetz, J.; Haasters, F.; Mayr, H.; Böcker, W.; Kusmenkov, T. Schatzker II tibial plateau fractures: Anatomically precontoured locking compression plates seem to improve radiological and clinical outcomes. *Injury* **2020**, *51*, 2295–2301. [CrossRef]
10. Rohra, N.; Suri, H.S.; Gangrade, K. Functional and Radiological Outcome of Schatzker type V and VI Tibial Plateau Fracture Treatment with Dual Plates with Minimum 3 years follow-up: A Prospective Study. *J. Clin. Diagn. Res.* **2016**, *10*, RC05-10. [CrossRef]
11. Elabjer, E.; Benčić, I.; Ćuti, T.; Cerovečki, T.; Ćurić, S.; Vidović, D. Tibial plateau fracture management: Arthroscopically-assisted versus ORIF procedure—Clinical and radiological comparison. *Injury* **2017**, *48*, S61–S64. [CrossRef]

12. Chen, H.-W.; Liu, G.-D.; Wu, L.-J. Clinical and radiological outcomes following arthroscopic-assisted management of tibial plateau fractures: A systematic review. *Knee Surg. Sports Traumatol. Arthrosc.* **2015**, *23*, 3464–3472. [CrossRef] [PubMed]
13. Rudran, B.; Little, C.; Wiik, A.; Logishetty, K. Tibial plateau fracture: Anatomy, diagnosis and management. *Br. J. Hosp. Med.* **2020**, *81*, 1–9. [CrossRef] [PubMed]
14. van Dreumel, R.; van Wunnik, B.; Janssen, L.; Simons, P.; Janzing, H. Mid- to long-term functional outcome after open reduction and internal fixation of tibial plateau fractures. *Injury* **2015**, *46*, 1608–1612. [CrossRef]
15. Elsoe, R.; Johansen, M.B.; Larsen, P. Tibial plateau fractures are associated with a long-lasting increased risk of total knee arthroplasty a matched cohort study of 7950 tibial plateau fractures. *Osteoarthr. Cartil.* **2019**, *27*, 805–809. [CrossRef]
16. Parkkinen, M.; Lindahl, J.; Mäkinen, T.J.; Koskinen, S.K.; Mustonen, A.; Madanat, R. Predictors of osteoarthritis following operative treatment of medial tibial plateau fractures. *Injury* **2018**, *49*, 370–375. [CrossRef] [PubMed]
17. Schatzker, J.; McBroom, R.; Bruce, D. The tibial plateau fracture. The Toronto experience 1968–1975. *Clin. Orthop. Relat. Res.* **1979**, *138*, 94–104.
18. Moore, T.M. Fracture-dislocation of the knee. *Clin. Orthop. Relat. Res.* **1981**, *156*, 128–140. [CrossRef]
19. Wasserstein, D.; Henry, P.; Paterson, J.M.; Kreder, H.J.; Jenkinson, R. Risk of total knee arthroplasty after operatively treated tibial plateau fracture: A matched-population-based cohort study. *J. Bone Joint Surg. Am.* **2014**, *96*, 144–150. [CrossRef]
20. Scott, C.E.H.; Davidson, E.; MacDonald, D.J.; White, T.O.; Keating, J.F. Total knee arthroplasty following tibial plateau fracture: A matched cohort study. *Bone Joint J.* **2015**, *97-B*, 532–538. [CrossRef]
21. Hansen, L.; Larsen, P.; Elsoe, R. Characteristics of patients requiring early total knee replacement after surgically treated lateral tibial plateau fractures—A comparative cohort study. *Eur. J. Orthop. Surg. Traumatol.* **2022**, *32*, 1097–1103. [CrossRef]
22. Scott, B.L.; Lee, C.S.; Strelzow, J.A. Five-Year Risk of Conversion to Total Knee Arthroplasty After Operatively Treated Periarticular Knee Fractures in Patients Over 40 Years of Age. *J. Arthroplast.* **2020**, *35*, 2084–2089. [CrossRef] [PubMed]
23. Tapper, V.S.; Pamilo, K.J.; Haapakoski, J.J.; Toom, A.; Paloneva, J. Risk of total knee replacement after proximal tibia fracture: A register-based study of 7,841 patients. *Acta Orthop.* **2022**, *93*, 179–184. [CrossRef]
24. Stevenson, I.; McMillan, T.E.; Baliga, S.; Schemitsch, E.H. Primary and Secondary Total Knee Arthroplasty for Tibial Plateau Fractures. *J. Am. Acad. Orthop. Surg.* **2018**, *26*, 386–395. [CrossRef]
25. Putman, S.; Argenson, J.-N.; Bonnevialle, P.; Ehlinger, M.; Vie, P.; Leclercq, S.; Bizot, P.; Lustig, S.; Parratte, S.; Ramdane, N.; et al. Ten-year survival and complications of total knee arthroplasty for osteoarthritis secondary to trauma or surgery: A French multicentre study of 263 patients. *Orthop. Traumatol. Surg. Res.* **2018**, *104*, 161–164. [CrossRef] [PubMed]
26. Mayr, H.O.; Hoell, A.; Bernstein, A.; Hube, R.; Zeiler, C.; Kalteis, T.; Suedkamp, N.P.; Stoehr, A. Validation of a Measurement Device for Instrumented Quantification of Anterior Translation and Rotational Assessment of the Knee. *Arthrosc. J. Arthrosc. Relat. Surg.* **2011**, *27*, 1096–1104. [CrossRef]
27. Milani, L.; Ferrari, S. Importance of CT Scan in Predicting the Outcomes of Tibial Plateau Fractures: A Retrospective Study of 216 Patients over 10 Years' Time. *Indian J. Orthop.* **2022**, *56*, 377–385. [CrossRef] [PubMed]
28. Vetter, S.Y.; Euler, F.; von Recum, J.; Wendl, K.; Grützner, P.A.; Franke, J. Impact of Intraoperative Cone Beam Computed Tomography on Reduction Quality and Implant Position in Treatment of Tibial Plafond Fractures. *Foot Ankle Int.* **2016**, *37*, 977–982. [CrossRef] [PubMed]
29. Beisemann, N.; Keil, H.; Swartman, B.; Schnetzke, M.; Franke, J.; Grützner, P.A.; Vetter, S.Y. Intraoperative 3D imaging leads to substantial revision rate in management of tibial plateau fractures in 559 cases. *J. Orthop. Surg. Res.* **2019**, *14*, 236. [CrossRef]
30. Gösling, T.; Klingler, K.; Geerling, J.; Shin, H.; Fehr, M.; Krettek, C.; Hüfner, T. Improved intra-operative reduction control using a three-dimensional mobile image intensifier—A proximal tibia cadaver study. *Knee* **2009**, *16*, 58–63. [CrossRef]
31. Davis, J.T.; Rudloff, M.I. Posttraumatic Arthritis After Intra-Articular Distal Femur and Proximal Tibia Fractures. *Orthop. Clin. N. Am.* **2019**, *50*, 445–459. [CrossRef]
32. Barei, D.P.; Nork, S.E.; Mills, W.J.; Coles, C.P.; Henley, M.B.; Benirschke, S.K. Functional Outcomes of Severe Bicondylar Tibial Plateau Fractures Treated with Dual Incisions and Medial and Lateral Plates. *J. Bone Jt. Surg.* **2006**, *88*, 1713–1721. [CrossRef]
33. Honkonen, S.E. Indications for Surgical Treatment of Tibial Condyle Fractures. *Clin. Orthop. Relat. Res.* **1994**, *302*, 199–205. [CrossRef]
34. Bai, B.; Kummer, F.J.; Sala, D.A.; Koval, K.J.; Wolinsky, P.R. Effect of Articular Step-off and Meniscectomy on Joint Alignment and Contact Pressures for Fractures of the Lateral Tibial Plateau. *J. Orthop. Trauma* **2001**, *15*, 101–106. [CrossRef]
35. Brown, T.D.; Anderson, D.D.; Nepola, J.V.; Singerman, R.J.; Pedersen, D.R.; Brand, R.A. Contact stress aberrations following imprecise reduction of simple tibial plateau fractures. *J. Orthop. Res.* **1988**, *6*, 851–862. [CrossRef] [PubMed]
36. Oeckenpöhler, S.; Domnick, C.; Raschke, M.; Müller, M.; Wähnert, D.; Kösters, C. A lateral fracture step-off of 2mm increases intra-articular pressure following tibial plateau fracture. *Injury* **2022**, *53*, 1254–1259. [CrossRef] [PubMed]
37. Singleton, N.; Sahakian, V.; Muir, D. Outcome After Tibial Plateau Fracture: How Important Is Restoration of Articular Congruity? *J. Orthop. Trauma* **2017**, *31*, 158–163. [CrossRef] [PubMed]
38. Giannoudis, P.V.; Tzioupis, C.; Papathanassopoulos, A.; Obakponovwe, O.; Roberts, C. Articular step-off and risk of post-traumatic osteoarthritis. Evidence today. *Injury* **2010**, *41*, 986–995. [CrossRef] [PubMed]
39. Roos, E.M.; Roos, H.P.; Lohmander, S.; Ekdahl, C.; Beynnon, B.D. Knee Injury and Osteoarthritis Outcome Score (KOOS)—Development of a Self-Administered Outcome Measure. *J. Orthop. Sports Phys. Ther.* **1998**, *28*, 88–96. [CrossRef]

40. Kessler, S.; Lang, S.; Puhl, W.; Stöve, J. The Knee Injury and Osteoarthritis Outcome Score—A multifunctional questionnaire to measure outcome in knee arthroplasty. *Z. Orthop. Grenzgeb.* **2003**, *141*, 277–282. [CrossRef]
41. Tegner, Y.; Lysholm, J. Rating systems in the evaluation of knee ligament injuries. *Clin. Orthop. Relat. Res.* **1985**, *198*, 42–49. [CrossRef]
42. Hefti, E.; Müller, W.; Jakob, R.P.; Stäubli, H.U. Evaluation of knee ligament injuries with the IKDC form. *Knee Surg. Sports Traumatol. Arthrosc.* **1993**, *1*, 226–234. [CrossRef] [PubMed]
43. Schenker, M.L.; Mauck, R.L.; Ahn, J.; Mehta, S. Pathogenesis and Prevention of Posttraumatic Osteoarthritis After Intra-articular Fracture. *J. Am. Acad. Orthop. Surg.* **2014**, *22*, 20–28. [CrossRef] [PubMed]
44. Papagelopoulos, P.J.; Partsinevelos, A.A.; Themistocleous, G.S.; Mavrogenis, A.F.; Korres, D.S.; Soucacos, P.N. Complications after tibia plateau fracture surgery. *Injury* **2006**, *37*, 475–484. [CrossRef] [PubMed]
45. Adams, J.D.J.; Loeffler, M.F. Soft Tissue Injury Considerations in the Treatment of Tibial Plateau Fractures. *Orthop. Clin. N. Am.* **2020**, *51*, 471–479. [CrossRef] [PubMed]

Disclaimer/Publisher's Note: The statements, opinions and data contained in all publications are solely those of the individual author(s) and contributor(s) and not of MDPI and/or the editor(s). MDPI and/or the editor(s) disclaim responsibility for any injury to people or property resulting from any ideas, methods, instructions or products referred to in the content.

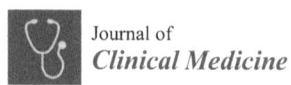

Article

Treatment of Plantar Fasciitis in Patients with Calcaneal Spurs: Radiofrequency Thermal Ablation or Extracorporeal Shock Wave Therapy?

Nevsun Pihtili Tas [1,*] and Oğuz Kaya [2]

[1] Department of Physical Medicine and Rehabilitation, Health Sciences University Elazig Fethi Sekin City Hospital, Elazig 23280, Turkey
[2] Department of Orthopedics and Traumatology, Elazig Fethi Sekin City Hospital, Elazig 23280, Turkey; oguzkayamd@gmail.com
* Correspondence: nevsunpihtili@gmail.com

Abstract: Background and Objectives: We aimed to compare the effectiveness of ESWT (Extracorporeal Shock Wave Therapy) and RFA (Radiofrequency Thermal Ablation) on pain, disability, and activity limitation in the treatment of plantar fasciitis in patients with calcaneal spurs. Materials and Methods: Patients who apply to Orthopedics and Traumatology and Physical Medicine and Rehabilitation departments with a complaint of heel pain are included in this retrospective study. We included patients diagnosed with calcaneal spurs who received treatment with ESWT ($n = 80$) and RFA ($n = 79$) between 1 August 2021 and 1 September 2022. All patients were evaluated using the Visual Analog Scale (VAS), Foot Function Index (FFI), and the Roles and Maudsley score (RM) before and after treatment. An evaluation was performed on average 6 months after treatment. Results: This study included 79 RFA patients (34 females and 45 males) with a mean age of 55.8 ± 9.6 years and 80 ESWT patients (20 females and 60 males) with a mean age of 49.1 ± 9.5 years. There was a significant decrease in VAS scores after treatment in both the RFA and ESWT groups (z: -4.98, z: -5.18, respectively, $p < 0.001$). The reductions in FFI pain, FFI activity restriction, FFI disability, and RM scores were significant in both groups, although the scores after treatment were lower in the RFA group. Conclusions: This study demonstrates that ESWT and RFA significantly reduced pain, disability, and activity restriction in the treatment of plantar fasciitis in patients with calcaneal spurs. ESWT proved particularly effective in alleviating pain, whereas RFA had more pronounced effects on reducing disability and activity limitations. The choice of treatment should be based on the patient's specific complaints.

Keywords: heel spur; extracorporeal shockwave therapy; radiofrequency ablation; visual analog scale; foot function index; the Roles and Maudsley score

1. Introduction

There are many causes of heel pain. Heel pain occurs as a result of systemic diseases or as a result of diseases that concern the bone, soft tissue, and nervous system. Among the causes of heel pain are tendonitis, bursitis, tarsal tunnel syndrome, neuroma, peripheral nervous system diseases, fractures, benign and malignant tumors of the bone, bone cysts, osteomyelitis, and systemic and rheumatological diseases [1,2]. Plantar fasciitis (PF) is the most common cause of heel pain [3]. High rates of calcaneal spurs (CSs) have been detected in patients with PF [4]. Right in front of the medial of the calcaneal tuberculin are fibrocartilaginous triangular protrusions of different sizes [5]. This condition affects 15–20% of the general population [5]. Pain can affect adults of all ages, regardless of an active or sedentary lifestyle [6]. However, as the age increases, the incidence of a CS increases due to the shortening of the length of the step and the contact of the middle foot and heel to more relative places [7].

Many factors are proposed in the etiology of CSs. These factors include age, sex, obesity, excessive exercise, foot structure and biomechanics, foot injuries, rheumatoid arthritis, diabetes, osteoarthritis, and gout, which can also be considered as contributing to plantar fasciitis [8]. A physical exam and the patient's medical history are used to make the diagnosis. In some cases, there may be no clinical evidence [9]. The classic symptom is moderate to high heel pain. Pain is felt when awakened from sleep. Reduces as you walk. The medial calcaneus in examination is sensitive and painful with palpation. Some patients experience pain during ankle dorsiflexion [10]. Direct graphs support diagnosis with symptoms and examination [11]. Although magnetic resonance imaging (MRI) and ultrasonography (US) have advantages in directly evaluating plantar fascia, radiographs allow the evaluation of conditions such as tumors, fractures, and calcaneal spurs [12,13].

Conservative methods are the first step of treatment. Rest, soft shoes, insoles, exercises, and non-steroidal anti-inflammatory drugs are conservative methods used for treatment. In patients who do not respond to conservative treatment, methods like steroid or PRP (platelet-rich plasma) injections, physical therapy modalities, ESWT (Extracorporeal Shock Wave Therapy), and RFA (Radiofrequency Thermal Ablation) are commonly used. In cases resistant to conservative and minimally invasive methods, surgical methods can be used. Surgical treatment can lead to complications and is not a definitive method of treatment [2,14,15]. The main goal of treatment is to reduce pain and improve quality of life.

Extracorporeal shock wave therapy (ESWT), which has been shown to be an effective and safe treatment for CS, has been widely used recently [16]. ESWT has been found to significantly reduce pain in patients with symptomatic calcaneal spurs [17]. ESWT is also used for shock waves, painful symptoms, and calcific accumulation. Low-energy ESWT is used in the treatment of enthesopathy and local painful conditions of the musculoskeletal system [18,19]. ESWT is a non-invasive method that stimulates micro-vascularization by creating controlled microtrauma through sound waves to the tissue. It also induces the release of enzymes that affect nociceptors and provides localized analgesia [17]. ESWT has been shown to be effective in reducing PF pain due to CSs [20].

Radiofrequency ablation (RFA) is a symptomatic, pain-relieving treatment option. RFA administration is used in the management of many painful conditions that require ablation of different nerve settlements, such as trigeminal neuralgia, complex regional pain syndrome, chronic postoperative pain, cancer pain, hyperhidrosis, facet joint pain, and knee osteoarthritis [21,22]. It is considered a safe and effective treatment for these types of heel pain [21,22]. In this procedure, a constant high-frequency, high-temperature electric current is applied to the target tissue [23].

In our study, we compared the effects of RFA and ESWT methods, of plantar fasciitis in patients with calcaneal spurs on pain and quality of life. In our literature review, we did not come across any other studies comparing the effectiveness of ESWT and RFA in the treatment of plantar fasciitis in patients with calcaneal spurs

2. Materials and Methods

This retrospective study was conducted on patients who complained of heel pain, received ESWT treatment at the Physical Medicine and Rehabilitation Clinic (FTR), and received RFA treatment at the Orthopedics and Traumatology clinic between August 2021 and September 2022. As a result of clinical examination and direct X-ray films patients with calcaneal spur were included. Patients who have not benefited from conservative treatments involving oral anti-inflammatory medication, insoles, and corticosteroid injection have not been treated for any medical treatment, injection, physical therapy, or surgical treatment, and RFA and ESWT have been selected for the past four weeks. Patients for whom pre-and/or post-treatment records, direct X-ray radiographic images, and historical data could not be fully obtained were excluded from this study. Data from 395 patients were evaluated, and 236 patients were not included in this study. This study consisted of

79 patients from the RFA group and 80 patients from the ESWT group. This study was agreed to by the Fırat University Ethics Committee.

There were two groups of patients. The ESWT group was selected from patients who were presented to the FTR clinic with plantar fasciitis pain due to calcaneal spurs, did not respond to conservative treatment, and did not receive RFA. The first group was treated with ESWT (Chattanooga Intelect® RPW 2 (DJO LLC CA, Vista, CA, USA) in the physiotherapy unit, with 3 weekly sessions repeated over 3 weeks, each consisting of a maximum of 2000 pulses at a frequency of 10 Hz. ESWT pressure was adjusted according to the patient's pain resistance. The applicator was placed over the maximum sensitivity point. Local or regional anesthesia was not applied. The treatment was performed with a cold gel. The second group was selected from patients who attended the Orthopedics and Traumatology clinic with plantar fasciitis pain due to calcaneal spurs, did not respond to conservative treatment, and did not undergo ESWT. The second group was treated with radiofrequency ablation (RFA). After the heel area was sterilized in the patient supine position, pain localization was detected by palpation, and local anesthesia was provided to the heel medial site with 1 mL %2 Lidocaine. In the desired location, a 10 mm needle cannula was inserted. The needle of the cannula was removed, and a 100 mm long, 22-gauge RFA (radiofrequency ablation) needle (JK2, NeuroTherm, Wilmington, MA, USA) was inserted into the cannula. First, patients were provided with a 1.5 V stimulus, and it was observed that there was no motor stimulation, such as fasciculation or movement of the toes. It was confirmed that the impedance was between 300 and 500. Thermal RFA was applied for 120 s at 60–80 °C, with the temperature increasing up to 80 °C. Thermal RFA was applied for a total of 180 s, with an additional 60 s while monitoring the impedance. In patients who reported severe pain at 80 °C, the temperature was lowered to 60 °C. Considering that patients may experience mild pain (at a tolerable level for the patient) if they do not feel any pain below 60 °C, the procedure was continued between 60 °C and 80 °C. Thus, the effectiveness of the procedure was monitored in communication with the patient. RFA is applied to patients who have not been relieved by conservative or steroid treatment. An evaluation was performed on average 6 months after the treatment.

In this study, Visual Analog Scale (VAS) scores with a range of 100 mm were used to assess pain intensity, and Foot Function Index (FFI) and Roles and Maudsley score (RM) scores were used to assess foot pain, disability, and activity limitation.

Visual Analog Scale (VAS): A table used for digitizing values that cannot be measured numerically. The patient's condition is marked in a 100 mm line. It is a common, reliable test and can be applied easily.

Foot Function Index (FFI): Created to assess the impact of foot pathology on function in terms of pain, disability, and activity limitation. FFI is an index of 23 items divided into 3 subscales. The FFI has been reviewed for test reliability [24].

The Roles and Maudsley score (RM): A subjective evaluation of the patient's pain and activity limitations: (1 = excellent result with no symptoms after treatment; 2 = significant improvement compared to before treatment; 3 = some improvement in the patient; and 4 = weak, the symptoms are the same as or worse than before treatment) [25].

No complications (soft tissue infection, symptomatic hematoma, nerve damage, or plantar fascia rupture) were observed with RFA and ESWT.

This study was approved by the local ethics committee (decision date: 27 May 2021; decision number: 10 July 2021).

The accession numbers will be provided during the review.

The Statistical Analysis

The data were analyzed using the statistical package for social sciences (SPSS), version 22 (SPSS Inc., Chicago, IL, USA). Quantitative data are expressed as average ± standard deviation (SD), while qualitative data are expressed as numbers. The Shapiro–Wilk test was used for normality distribution. The distribution of the normality was checked using the independent T-test. In the univariate analysis of the variables in the study, the Kruskal–Wallis and Wilcoxon tests were used according to the variable type and the assumptions. The differences between the categories of the observations in the categorical variables were tested using the chi-squared test Wilcoxon test in the analysis of dependent data, which was applied. A *p*-value of <0.05 was considered statistically significant.

3. Results

This study included 79 RFA patients (34 females and 45 males) with a mean age of 55.8 ± 9.6 years and 80 ESWT patients (20 females and 60 males) with a mean age of 49.1 ± 9.5 years. The mean BMI values were 28.52 ± 3.8 in the RFA group and 28.7 ± 2.6 in the ESWT group. Regarding age and BMI, there were no significant differences between the patient groups (*p*: 0.095, *p*: 0.795). The results are shown in Table 1.

Table 1. Results of patient groups.

	RFA (*n*: 79)	ESWT (*n*: 80)	*p*
BMI (kg/m^2)	28.52 ± 3.8	28.7 ± 2.6	0.795
Age (year)	55.8 ± 9.6	49.1 ± 9.5	0.095
Visual Analog Scale			
Before treatment	7.26	7.34	0.838
End of treatment	2.6	1.15	0.025
FFI pain			
Before treatment	55.43	52.31	0.229
End of treatment	2.86	9.05	0.038
FFI disability			
Before treatment	15.86	27	0.005
End of treatment	1.24	4.62	0.02
FFI activity restriction			
Before treatment	55.76	40.79	<0.001
End of treatment	1.8	10.72	0.072

FFI: Foot Function Index; ESWT: Extracorporeal Shock Wave Therapy; RFA: Radiofrequency Ablation; BMI; Body Mass Index.

There was a significant decrease in VAS scores after treatment in both the RFA and ESWT groups (z: −4.98, z: −5.18, respectively, *p*: 0.00). The decreases in FFI pain, FFI activity restriction, FFI disability, and RM scores were significant in both groups, but the scores after treatment were lower in the RFA group. The before and after treatment measurement values for the patient groups are given in Table 2.

Table 2. Patient groups before and after measurement values.

	RFA Min–Max (Median)	ESWT Min–Max (Median)
Visual Analog Scale		
Before treatment	2–10 (7.26)	0–10 (7.3)
End of treatment	0–10 (2.6)	0–8 (1.15)
Change according to BT *p*	0.00 (z: −4.98)	0.00 (z: −5.18)
FFI pain		
Before treatment	36–81 (55.4)	20–76 (52.31)
End of treatment	0–40 (2.8)	0–60 (9.05)
Change according to BT *p*	0.00 (z: −5.64)	0.00 (z: −5.16)
FFI disability		
Before treatment	2–69 (15.86)	0–81(27)
End of treatment	0–20 (1.24)	0–27(4.62)
Change according to BT *p*	0.00 (z: −5.58)	0.00 (z: −5.12)
FFI activity restriction		
Before treatment	21–79 (55.76)	0–76(40.79)
End of treatment	0–40 (1.8)	0–59 (10.72)
Change according to BT *p*	0.00 (z: −5.64)	0.00 (z: −5.14)
RM		
Before treatment	3–4 (3.64)	2–4 (3.34)
End of treatment	1–2(1.05)	1–3(1.29)
Change according to BT *p*	0.00 (z: −5.84)	0.00 (z: −5.14)

VAS: Visual Analog Scale; RM: The Roles and Maudsley score; FFI: Foot Function Index; ESWT: Extracorporeal Shock Wave Therapy; RFA: Radiofrequency Ablation; BT: Before treatment.

4. Discussion

In this study, we compared the effectiveness of ESWT and RFA in the treatment of calcaneal spurs. Although many methods have been suggested for the treatment of CSs, there is still limited evidence. The study investigating the efficacy of ESWT and RFA has not been identified in the literature, so we believe that our study adds to the literature on CS treatment. It was observed that both treatment methods were effective in reducing pain, and although the FFI disability and activity limitation scores of patients in the RFA group were higher, the post-treatment scores were significantly reduced compared to ESWT. The BMI values of our patients (p: 0.795), as well as the pre-treatment VAS, FFI pain, and RM scores, were similar in both groups (p: 0.83, p: 0.22, $p < 0.01$, respectively). Similar improvements in pain scores were observed in both the ESWT and RFA groups.

One of the methods used in the treatment of plantar fasciitis is ESWT, which uses high- or low-energy shock waves to treat the interface between calcaneus and plantar fascia. Although the mechanism of this method in reducing pain is not known precisely, various mechanisms have been proposed. The air gaps developing in the tissues are thought to physically separate the plantar fascia from the calcaneus as a result of ESWT administration, causing transdermal release. It has not been clearly demonstrated that the reduction in pain after ESWT administration may be the result of calcaneal nerve damage and whether this effect is temporary or permanent [26]. Numerous clinical trials have been conducted on ESWT efficacy in plantar fasciitis in patients with calcaneal spur detection. A useful method in symptomatic patients resistant to conservative treatment. Weil et al. found satisfactory results in 82% of patients treated with ESWT [27,28].

Our study showed statistically significant effects of ESWT on pain and FFI scores. Improvements in VAS scores were higher in the ESWT group than RFA. Improvement in VAS scores with ESWT and RFA was parallel with the literature [29,30].

We observed significant improvements in daily life activities in the treatment group with RFA compared to the ESWT group. The improvements in VAS, FFI, and RM scores were significant in the RFA treatment group. Although the activity limitation scores of patients were higher in the RFA group, it was observed that there was a significant decrease in the score after treatment. Our data support the notion that patients who suffer from more restraint in their daily activities may prefer RFA over ESWT. There are studies demonstrating that the reduction in pain with RFA begins in the first month and continues into the 12th month. In patients who underwent RFA treatment, statistically significant improvements were observed in VAS and ankle-heel scoring in evaluations conducted at 1 and 6 months [31]. There are also publications showing that the pain-relieving feature of ESWT varies between 6 and 12 months [32]. This study found significant improvements in VAS and FFI scores in our patients during the sixth month of evaluation. Pain reduction was more significant with ESWT.

An electrode, ultrasound (USG), or fluoroscopy can be used during the procedure. However, successful results have also been reported without the use of USG or fluoroscopy [33]. In this study, we did not use USG or fluoroscopy during the procedure. We repositioned the probes on the heel in foot or foot movements to prevent possible neurological injuries. No complications were seen in any of our patients.

According to our results, RFA is especially in patients with severe pain and limited daily activity, who do not respond to conservative treatment can be a useful alternative to surgery or ESWT. Erken et al. suggested that RFA is an effective alternative treatment option for patients with resistant plantar fasciitis who do not respond to other conservative treatments [34]. Similarly, Landsman et al. [35] showed that RFA is an effective method of treating plantar fasciitis. Despite being invasive, RFA can also prevent certain associated complications, such as local hematoma and neuropathic pain. Local hematoma and neuropathic pain were not seen in our study. RFA is also useful for patients who have failed conservative treatment and ESWT but do not want to risk traditional surgery. It has the advantage of fewer complications and a faster recovery time compared to surgery.

In patients with calcaneal spurs, PF causes pain and difficulty in daily work. ESWT and RFA are preferable methods for patients who do not benefit from conservative methods of treatment. Our study's strength is that it is the first to evaluate RFA and ESWT in calcaneal spurs. The RFA patient group had higher VAS and FFI scores. Therefore, we could not clarify which method could be more useful. Studies comparing the two methods should be made between groups with the same VAS and FFI scores. Our work is retrospective. We should also say that the follow-up time is short, and different results can be achieved in long-term follow-up.

According to our results, both methods are beneficial, and the choice of treatment should be based on the patient's complaints and needs. Our results have shown that, according to RFA, ESWT also showed a significant reduction in pain. ESWT, a non-invasive technique, can be selected for patients with pain at the forefront. On the other hand, RFA can be preferred by patients with more physical activity limitations. We think that the improvement in functional scores in RFA is a safe method that is preferable to ESWT in patients with physical activity limitations.

5. Conclusions

As a result, ESWT appears more effective in VAS scores, and RFA appears more effective in functional scores.

Author Contributions: N.P.T. and O.K. analyzed the cases and designed this study. N.P.T. and O.K. provided several cases. N.P.T. wrote the draft manuscript. All authors have read and agreed to the published version of the manuscript.

Funding: This research received no external funding.

Institutional Review Board Statement: This observational study was approved by the Firat University Ethics Committee (10 July 2021) and conducted in accordance with the Declaration of Helsinki and Good Clinical Practice. A written informed consent form was obtained from each patient.

Informed Consent Statement: Informed consent was obtained from all subjects involved in this study.

Data Availability Statement: The accession numbers will be provided during the review.

Conflicts of Interest: The authors declare no conflict of interest.

References

1. Brown, C. A review of subcalcaneal heel pain and plantar fasciitis. *Aust. Fam. Physician* **1996**, *25*, 875–881.
2. Luffy, L.; Grosel, J.; Thomas, R.; So, E. Plantar fasciitis. *J. Am. Acad. Physician Assist.* **2018**, *31*, 20–24. [CrossRef]
3. Rompe, J.D. Plantar Fasciopathy. *Sports Med. Arthrosc.* **2009**, *17*, 100–104. [CrossRef] [PubMed]
4. Johal, K.S.; Milner, S.A. Plantar fasciitis and the calcaneal spur: Fact or fiction? *Foot Ankle Surg.* **2012**, *18*, 39–41. [CrossRef] [PubMed]
5. McPoil, T.G.; Martin, R.L.; Cornwall, M.W.; Wukich, D.K.; Irrgang, J.J.; Godges, J.J. Heel Pain—Plantar Fasciitis. *J. Orthop. Sport. Phys. Ther.* **2008**, *38*, A1–A18. [CrossRef] [PubMed]
6. Xu, D.; Jiang, W.; Huang, D.; Hu, X.; Wang, Y.; Li, H.; Zhou, S.; Gan, K.; Ma, W. Comparison Between Extracorporeal Shock Wave Therapy and Local Corticosteroid Injection for Plantar Fasciitis. *Foot Ankle Int.* **2020**, *19*, 200–205. [CrossRef] [PubMed]
7. Kirkpatrick, J.; Yassaie, O.; Mirjalili, S.A. The plantar calcaneal spur: A review of anatomy, histology, etiology and key associations. *J. Anat.* **2017**, *230*, 743–751. [CrossRef]
8. Duran, E.; Bilgin, E.; Ertenli, A.İ.; Kalyoncu, U. The frequency of Achilles and plantar calcaneal spurs in gout patients. *Turk. J. Med. Sci.* **2021**, *51*, 1841–1848. [CrossRef] [PubMed]
9. Beytemür, O.; Öncü, M. The age dependent change in the incidence of calcaneal spur. *Acta Orthop. Traumatol. Turc.* **2018**, *52*, 367–371. [CrossRef]
10. Yi, T.I.; Lee, G.E.; Seo, I.S.; Huh, W.S.; Yoon, T.H.; Kim, B.R. Clinical Characteristics of the Causes of Plantar Heel Pain. *Ann. Rehabil. Med.* **2011**, *35*, 507. [CrossRef] [PubMed]
11. McMillan, A.M.; Landorf, K.B.; Barrett, J.T.; Menz, H.B.; Bird, A.R. Diagnostic imaging for chronic plantar heel pain: A systematic review and meta-analysis. *J. Foot Ankle Res.* **2009**, *2*, 32. [CrossRef]
12. Ahmad, J.; Karim, A.; Daniel, J.N. Relationship and Classification of Plantar Heel Spurs in Patients with Plantar Fasciitis. *Foot Ankle Int.* **2016**, *37*, 994–1000. [CrossRef]
13. Lareau, C.R.; Sawyer, G.A.; Wang, J.H.; DiGiovanni, C.W. Plantar and Medial Heel Pain. *J. Am. Acad. Orthop. Surg.* **2014**, *22*, 372–380. [CrossRef] [PubMed]

14. Hasegawa, M.; Urits, I.; Orhurhu, V.; Orhurhu, M.S.; Brinkman, J.; Giacomazzi, S.; Foster, L.; Manchikanti, L.; Kaye, A.D.; Kaye, R.J.; et al. Current Concepts of Minimally Invasive Treatment Options for Plantar Fasciitis: A Comprehensive Review. *Curr. Pain. Headache Rep.* **2020**, *24*, 55. [CrossRef] [PubMed]
15. Young, C.C.; Rutherford, D.S.; Niedfeldt, M.W. Treatment of plantar fasciitis. *Am. Fam. Physician* **2001**, *63*, 467–474. [PubMed]
16. Mishra, B.N.; Poudel, R.R.; Banskota, B.; Shrestha, B.K.; Banskota, A.K. Effectiveness of extra-corporeal shock wave therapy (ESWT) vs. methylprednisolone injections in plantar fasciitis. *J. Clin. Orthop. Trauma* **2019**, *10*, 401–405. [CrossRef] [PubMed]
17. Hayta, E.; Salk, I.; Gumus, C.; Tuncay, M.S.; Cetin, A. Extracorporeal shock-wave therapy effectively reduces calcaneal spur length and spur-related pain in overweight and obese patients. *J. Back. Musculoskelet. Rehabil.* **2016**, *30*, 17–22. [CrossRef] [PubMed]
18. Rompe, J.D.; Hopf, C.; Nafe, B.; Burger, R. Low-energy extracorporeal shock wave therapy for painful heel: A prospective controlled single-blind study. *Arch. Orthop. Trauma Surg.* **1996**, *115*, 75–79. [CrossRef] [PubMed]
19. Maier, M.; Steinborn, M.; Schmitz, C.; Stäbler, A.; Köhler, S.; Pfahler, M.; Dürr, H.R.; Refior, H.J. Extracorporeal shock wave application for chronic plantar fasciitis associated with heel spurs: Prediction of outcome by magnetic resonance imaging. *J. Rheumatol.* **2000**, *27*, 2455–2462. [PubMed]
20. Yalcin, E.; Keskin Akca, A.; Selcuk, B.; Kurtaran, A.; Akyuz, M. Effects of extracorporal shock wave therapy on symptomatic heel spurs: A correlation between clinical outcome and radiologic changes. *Rheumatol. Int.* **2012**, *32*, 343–347. [CrossRef]
21. Chua, N.H.L.; Vissers, K.C.; Sluijter, M.E. Pulsed radiofrequency treatment in interventional pain management: Mechanisms and potential indications—A review. *Acta Neurochir.* **2011**, *153*, 763–771. [CrossRef] [PubMed]
22. Jain, S.K.; Suprashant, K.; Kumar, S.; Yadav, A.; Kearns, S.R. Comparison of Plantar Fasciitis Injected With Platelet-Rich Plasma vs. Corticosteroids. *Foot Ankle Int.* **2018**, *39*, 780–786. [CrossRef]
23. Deniz, S.; Baka, O.; Inangil, G. Application of Radiofrequency in Pain Management. In *Pain Management*; IntechOpen: London, UK, 2016.
24. Budiman-Mak, E.; Conrad, K.J.; Roach, K.E. The foot function index: A measure of foot pain and disability. *J. Clin. Epidemiol.* **1991**, *44*, 561–570. [CrossRef]
25. Roles, N.C.; Maudsley, R.H. Radial tunnel syndrome: Resistant tennis elbow as a nerve entrapment. *J. Bone Jt. Surg. Br.* **1972**, *54*, 499–508. [CrossRef]
26. Kurtoglu, A.; Kochai, A.; Inanmaz, M.E.; Sukur, E.; Keskin, D.; Türker, M.; Sen, Z.; Daldal, I.; Avan, L.Y. Effectiveness of radiofrequency ablation for treatment of plantar fasciitis. *Medicine* **2022**, *101*, e29142. [CrossRef] [PubMed]
27. Weil, L.S.; Roukis, T.S.; Weil, L.S.; Borrelli, A.H. Extracorporeal shock wave therapy for the treatment of chronic plantar fasciitis: Indications, protocol, intermediate results, and a comparison of results to fasciotomy. *J. Foot Ankle Surg.* **2002**, *41*, 166–172. [CrossRef] [PubMed]
28. Rompe, J.D.; Furia, J.; Weil, L.; Maffulli, N. Shock wave therapy for chronic plantar fasciopathy. *Br. Med. Bull.* **2007**, *81–82*, 183–208. [CrossRef]
29. Zhou, B.; Zhou, Y.; Tao, X.; Yuan, C.; Tang, K. Classification of Calcaneal Spurs and Their Relationship With Plantar Fasciitis. *J. Foot Ankle Surg.* **2015**, *54*, 594–600. [CrossRef] [PubMed]
30. Erden, T.; Toker, B.; Cengiz, O.; Ince, B.; Asci, S.; Toprak, A. Outcome of Corticosteroid Injections, Extracorporeal Shock Wave Therapy, and Radiofrequency Thermal Lesioning for Chronic Plantar Fasciitis. *Foot Ankle Int.* **2021**, *42*, 69–75. [CrossRef] [PubMed]
31. Eke, I.; Akcal, M.A.; Sayrac, A.V.; Iyetin, Y. Effects of intralesional pulsed radiofrequency treatment on pain in patients with calcaneal spur: Results of 460 patients. *BMC Musculoskelet. Disord.* **2021**, *22*, 1033. [CrossRef] [PubMed]
32. Ryskalin, L.; Morucci, G.; Natale, G.; Soldani, P.; Gesi, M. Molecular Mechanisms Underlying the Pain-Relieving Effects of Extracorporeal Shock Wave Therapy: A Focus on Fascia Nociceptors. *Life* **2022**, *12*, 743. [CrossRef] [PubMed]
33. Wu, P.T.; Lee, J.S.; Wu, K.C.; Wu, T.T.; Shao, C.J.; Liang, F.W.; Chern, T.C.; Su, F.C.; Jou, I.M. Ultrasound-Guided Percutaneous Radiofrequency Lesioning When Treating Recalcitrant Plantar Fasciitis: Clinical Results. *Ultraschall Med. Eur. J. Ultrasound* **2014**, *37*, 56–62. [CrossRef] [PubMed]
34. Erken, H.Y.; Ayanoglu, S.; Akmaz, I.; Erler, K.; Kiral, A. Prospective Study of Percutaneous Radiofrequency Nerve Ablation for Chronic Plantar Fasciitis. *Foot Ankle Int.* **2014**, *35*, 95–103. [CrossRef]
35. Landsman, A.S.; Catanese, D.J.; Wiener, S.N.; Richie, D.H., Jr.; Hanft, J.R. A Prospective, Randomized, Double-blinded Study with Crossover to Determine the Efficacy of Radio-frequency Nerve Ablation for the Treatment of Heel Pain. *J. Am. Podiatr. Med. Assoc.* **2013**, *103*, 8–15. [PubMed]

Disclaimer/Publisher's Note: The statements, opinions and data contained in all publications are solely those of the individual author(s) and contributor(s) and not of MDPI and/or the editor(s). MDPI and/or the editor(s) disclaim responsibility for any injury to people or property resulting from any ideas, methods, instructions or products referred to in the content.

Article

Gluteal Muscle Fatty Atrophy: An Independent Risk Factor for Surgical Treatment in Elderly Patients Diagnosed with Type-III Fragility Fractures of the Pelvis

Christoph Linhart [1], Dirk Mehrens [2], Luca Maximilian Gellert [1], Christian Ehrnthaller [1], Johannes Gleich [1], Christopher Lampert [1], Maximilian Lerchenberger [1], Wolfgang Böcker [1], Carl Neuerburg [1] and Yunjie Zhang [1,*]

1 Department of Orthopaedics and Trauma Surgery, Musculoskeletal University Center Munich (MUM), University Hospital, LMU Munich, 81377 Munich, Germany; christoph.linhart@med.uni-muenchen.de (C.L.); luca.gellert@med.uni-muenchen.de (L.M.G.); christian.ehrnthaller@med.uni-muenchen.de (C.E.); johannes.gleich@med.uni-muenchen.de (J.G.); christopher.lampert@med.uni-muenchen.de (C.L.); maximilian.lerchenberger@med.uni-muenchen.de (M.L.); direktion-unfall@med.uni-muenchen.de (W.B.); carl.neuerburg@med.uni-muenchen.de (C.N.)
2 Department of Radiology, University Hospital, LMU Munich, 81377 Munich, Germany; dirk.mehrens@med.uni-muenchen.de
* Correspondence: yunjie.zhang@med.uni-muenchen.de

Abstract: Background: Gluteal muscle fatty atrophy (gMFA) might impair pelvic stability and negatively influence remobilization in patients with fragility fractures of the pelvis (FFP). This study aimed to investigate the association between gMFA and surgical indication in patients with FFP. Methods and materials: A retrospective analysis of 429 patients (age ≥80) diagnosed with FFP was performed. gMFA of the gluteus maximus, medius, and minimus was evaluated using a standard scoring system based on computer tomography images. Results: No significant difference was found in gMFA between genders or among FFP types. The severity of gMFA did not correlate with age. The severity of gMFA in the gluteus medius was significantly greater than in the gluteus maximus, whereas the most profound gMFA was found in the gluteus minimus. gMFA was significantly more severe in patients who underwent an operation than in conservatively treated patients with type-III FFP, and an independent correlation to surgical indication was found using logistic regression. Conclusion: Our findings imply that gMFA is an independent factor for surgical treatment in patients with type-III FFP. Besides focusing on the fracture pattern, the further evaluation of gMFA could be a feasible parameter for decision making toward either conservative or surgical treatment of type-III FFP.

Keywords: muscle fatty atrophy; FFP; geriatric trauma

1. Introduction

Fragility fractures of the pelvis (FFP) are amongst the most common low-energy traumatic fractures in elderly patients, particularly those over 80 years [1,2]. The three-year mortality in patients suffering from FFP was reported to be about 14%, and 17% in those hospitalized [3]. Pelvic fractures constitute 7% of all fractures related to osteoporosis in individuals aged over 50 in the United States, contributing to 5% of the overall cost burden [4]. The main goals of using either conservative or operative treatment in patients with FFP are to relieve pain and restore mobility and self-independency [5].

Muscle fatty atrophy (MFA), also known as muscle fat infiltration or myosteatosis, is characterized by fat accumulation within skeletal muscle tissue [6]. MFA tends to increase with age, contributing to a decline in muscle strength and function in older adults [7]. The biological mechanism of MFA is still unclear. The diagnosis of MFA often involves imaging techniques such as magnetic resonance imaging or computer tomography (CT), where the extent of fat infiltration within muscle tissue can be visualized [8].

The gluteal muscles, including the gluteus maximus, medius, and minimus, play a fundamental role in stabilizing the pelvis. They are the main stabilizers of the pelvis throughout the stride phase and facilitate the abduction and extension of the thigh [9,10]. They also contribute to balance, posture, and hip joint stability [11]. Daguet et al. reported that gluteal muscle fatty atrophy (gMFA) is associated with poorer physical performance, like chair rising [12]. The fatty atrophy of the gluteus minimus and medius might predispose the elderly to fall-related fractures [13]. The hip abductive strength was proven to be essential to the success of rehabilitation in hip-fractured patients [14,15]. Pelvic fractures like FFP disrupt the normal biomechanics of the pelvis. The atrophied gluteal muscle can result in difficulty with remobilization and pelvic instability in patients with FFP [13,16].

The surgical indication is partially dependent on the classification of the FFP according to the therapy recommendation by Rommens et al. [5,17,18]. A consensus about the optimal treatment regimen for patients with FFP has not been achieved. This is because the general condition of geriatric patients greatly affects the decision because their physiological reserve might be largely limited [19]. It is a multidisciplinary play between biomechanics and geriatric medicine. Fast remobilization could reduce complications such as deep venous thrombosis, pulmonary embolism, pressure ulcers, pneumonia, and decreased muscle strength [20]. Every extra day with immobilization in the hospital is accompanied by a drastically increased mortality rate. Consequently, the early identification of elderly patients with the indication for surgical therapy due to FFP might benefit remobilization and reduce the mortality rate.

Currently, the connection between MFA and fracture in geriatric patients has drawn more attention. Yerli et al. reported that fatty atrophy in the psoas muscle in elderly patients could influence the type of hip fractures [15]. Lee et al. demonstrated that the spinal fracture risk was increased by multifidus muscle fatty infiltration [21]. However, the influence of gMFA on the management of patients with FFP has rarely been discussed. Therefore, we aim to investigate the clinical significance of gMFA in elderly patients (age $\geq$ 80) with FFP. We hypothesized that gMFA was associated with a surgical indication in elderly patients with FFP. The clinical significance of the current study is the exploration of a potentially new factor, gMFA, which can be easily evaluated preoperatively from CT images so that surgical decisions can be made more accurately for elderly patients with FFP.

2. Methods and Materials

The current study protocol was approved and registered by the local ethics committee (Registration No. 518-18). The study was a retrospective observational single-center study. Patients (age $\geq$ 80) diagnosed with FFP and consecutively admitted to our university teaching hospital from January 2003 to December 2019 were enrolled. The exclusion criteria were pathological fracture, high-energy trauma, and patients with an established palliative concept. Informed consent was obtained from all study participants or their legal representatives. The patient data were retrieved from the inpatient database of our hospital and irreversibly anonymized before analysis in a confidential database (Microsoft Excel 2018, Microsoft Corporation, Redmond, WA, USA). Demographic data, including age and gender, were collected. Preoperative comorbidities, such as chronic kidney disease, cardiac insufficiency, and coronary artery disease, were collected.

Multidisciplinary geriatric co-management was carried out in our center for the clinical management of this patient group. A surgical indication was decided based on the fracture morphology/classification and, more importantly, on general conditions and basic illnesses that could have substantial effects on operative risk and outcomes of the patients, such as heart failure, kidney failure, or age. Surgeries were performed by a senior trauma surgeon in our center with minimally invasive techniques. Open reduction and internal fixations were performed only by necessity. If conservative treatment was indicated, patients received standardized pain management according to WHO (World Health Organization) guidelines. Physiotherapy was initiated as soon as possible with weight-bearing as-tolerated. An operation would be indicated and performed when early mobilization failed after 5 days. No follow-up was conducted after the surgery because it was considered irrelevant to the hypothesis.

The FFP classification used in the current study was first described by Rommens and Hofmann [17]. Briefly, type I was featured with an isolated anterior ring fracture. In type II, the posterior pelvic ring was fractured without displacement. Type III was characterized by unilateral fracture displacement on the posterior pelvic ring. When the fracture displacement was bilateral on the posterior pelvic ring, the fracture was rated as type IV. The classification was documented as the diagnosis of each patient and controlled by senior orthopedic and radiologic consultants.

Pelvic CT was performed for all patients as a clinical routine for pelvic fracture. Intravenous contrast fluid was administered if indicated. The CT scan included sections at least from the level of the lesser trochanter of the femur to the level of the iliac crest. The axial reconstruction of the pelvis at the level of the anterior inferior iliac spine was defined as a standard plane for scoring. This was because it provided a clear view of the muscle bellies of the gluteus maximus, medius, and minimus, which were approximately centered at this particular level. The coronal plane was used secondarily for evaluation if needed.

The classification system based on CT was first established by Goutallier et al. [22]. Score 0 was defined as normal muscle without obvious fatty infiltration, score 1 for minimal atrophy with minor fatty streaks, score 2 for mild atrophy with a lower volume of fatty infiltration than muscle, score 3 for moderate atrophy with an equal amount of fatty infiltration to the muscle, and score 4 for severe atrophy, by which the volume of fatty infiltration was greater than the volume of muscle tissue (Figure 1).

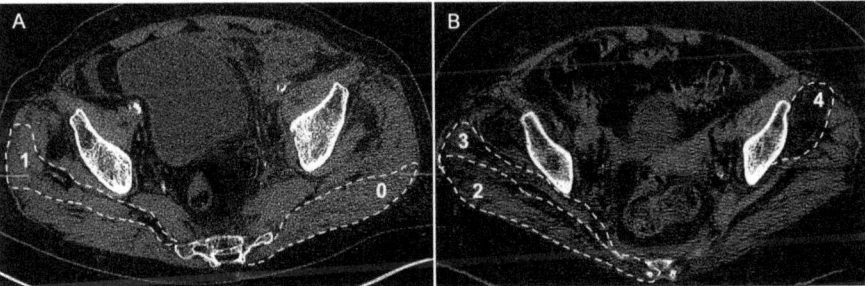

Figure 1. Examples of gMFA with different severities according to Goutallier grading scores based on CT pelvis images. (**A**) The area marked with 0 is an example of a score of 0 with no fat in the gluteus maximus, which was rare in the investigated population. The gluteus medius marked with 1 represented a score of 1 with intramuscular fatty steaks. (**B**) The area marked with 2 exemplified a score of 2 in gluteus maximus with mild atrophy, in which the proportion of fat infiltration was less than that of muscle. Nearby, an exaggerated fat infiltration could be found in the gluteus medius, marked by 3, where the proportion of fat and muscle were subjectively equal. The gluteus minimus, marked by 4, showed the most profound fat infiltration, where fat infiltration exceeded in quantity.

The primary scoring was performed by an orthopedic surgeon with three years of experience and then examined by an orthopedic surgeon with eight years of experience. Ambiguous cases were re-scored by consensus. Fifty cases were randomly selected and were rated separately by a musculoskeletal radiologist with six years of experience, and the intraclass correlation coefficient (ICC) was examined to ensure the reliability and reproducibility of the current method.

SPSS version 27.0 (SPSS Inc., Chicago, IL, USA) was used for statistical analysis. The ICC was calculated using Kendall's tau method with ordinal data. For parametric data, the Kolmogorov–Smirnov test was performed to verify the normality. If normality was confirmed, a 2-sided t-test was used to determine the difference between the two groups; if not, the 2-sided Mann–Whitney U test was applied. For non-parametric data, the 2–sided Mann–Whitney U test was used. The Kruskal–Wallis test, followed by the Student–Newman–Keuls method, was performed to estimate stochastic probability in the intergroup comparison among three or more groups. The Pearson correlation coefficient (r) was used to identify the strength of the correlation. Multivariate logistic regression was performed to investigate the association of different potentially confounding variables such as sex, age, cardiac illness (heart failure or coronary artery disease), or renal insufficiency to the surgical treatment. A p-value of <0.05 was considered statistically significant.

3. Results

An overview of the included population in the current study is summarized in Table 1. A total of 429 patients ≥80 years diagnosed with FFP were investigated, from which the number of females was about 3.7 times the number of males. No difference was found in the rate of operation between genders. The rate of operation increased, confronting the severity of the fracture.

Table 1. Baseline clinical data.

			n = 429	%	Operation, n	%	Age, Mean ± SD
Gender	Male		91	21.21%	14	15.38%	86.85 ± 4.49
	Female		338	78.79%	49	14.50%	87.42 ± 4.54
Classification	I		55		1	1.82%	87.60 ± 4.02
		Ia	52	94.55%	0	0.00%	87.77 ± 4.00
		Ib	3	5.45%	1	33.33%	84.70 ± 3.92
	II		286		29	10.14%	87.16 ± 4.45
		IIa	56	19.65%	4	7.14%	86.78 ± 5.68
		IIb	37	12.98%	6	16.22%	86.64 ± 4.37
		IIc	193	67.72%	19	9.84%	87.36 ± 4.25
	III		68		20	29.41%	88.26 ± 4.95
		IIIa	14	19.72%	1	7.14%	89.85 ± 6.09
		IIIb	22	30.99%	8	36.36%	88.24 ± 4.23
		IIIc	32	45.07%	11	34.38%	87.57 ± 4.87
	IV		20		13	65.00%	85.78 ± 5.19
		IVa	7	33.33%	4	57.14%	88.49 ± 6.22
		IVb	6	28.57%	5	83.33%	83.41 ± 2.64
		IVc	7	33.33%	4	57.14%	85.11 ± 5.00

SD: standard deviation.

Kendall's Tau test was performed to validate the reliability and reproducibility of the scoring method used in this study. Kendall's coefficient value was 0.70 based on a subset of 50 randomly selected subjects, which was considered a strong interobserver agreement.

There was no significant difference in the total score of gMFA between genders (male 12.70 ± 4.27, female 13.44 ± 4.05, p = 0.23, Figure 2). The severity of each component of the gluteal muscles was evaluated (Figure 3). The score of gMFA was significantly higher (p < 0.001) in the gluteus medius (left: 2.34 ± 0.89, right 2.33 ± 0.97) compared to the score of gluteus maximus (left: 1.44 ± 0.65, right: 1.52 ± 0.76). The severest gMFA was found in the gluteus minimus (left: 2.87 ± 1.01, right: 2.79 ± 1.02, p < 0.001). No difference was found between the two sides.

The correlation between age and gMFA in patients over 80 with FFP was analyzed, and no significant correlation was found (y = 0.04 x + 9.36, p = 0.30, r^2 = 0.002, Figure 4). No significant intraclass difference in the total fatty atrophy score was found among type-I to type-IV FFP (Figure 5).

The gMFA was significantly more severe in patients diagnosed with type-III FFP receiving operative treatment than those receiving non-operative treatment (15.50 ± 2.61 and 12.90 ± 4.25, respectively, p = 0.01, Figure 6). The mean total score of gMFA in the patients receiving surgery was higher than those receiving non-operative treatment diagnosed with type-II (13.03 ± 4.27 and 12.78 ± 4.12, respectively, p = 0.80) and type-IV FFP (15.92 ± 2.90 and 12.57 ± 2.94, respectively, p = 0.06) though both were without statistical significance. The analysis of type I was not performed because there was only one operated case.

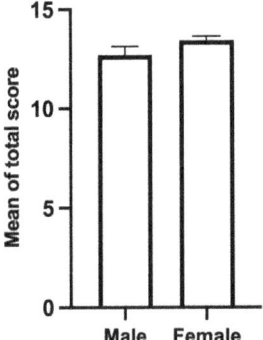

Figure 2. Mean comparison of gMFA using the total score between genders. Mean ± standard error of the mean. No significant difference was found in the overall score of gluteal fatty atrophy between genders.

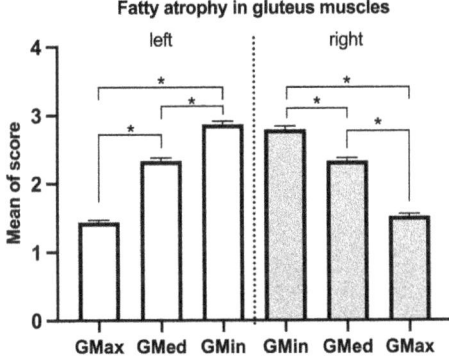

Figure 3. Average score of fatty atrophy in different gluteal muscles. Mean ± standard error of the mean. The score for fatty atrophy exhibited a significant increase in the gluteus medius compared to the gluteus maximus score. The most severe fatty atrophy was observed in the gluteus minimus, with no significant differences detected between the two sides. GMax: gluteus maximus, GMed: gluteus medius, GMin: gluteus minimus. * $p < 0.001$.

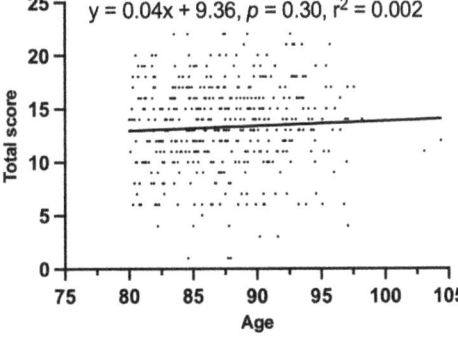

Figure 4. Correlation between age and gMFA.

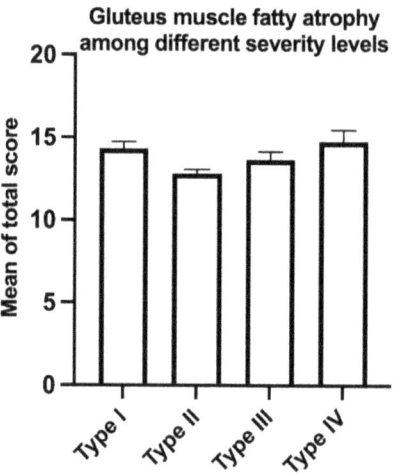

Figure 5. Mean comparison of gMFA using the total score among different FFP classifications. Mean ± standard error of the mean. There was no significant intraclass difference in the total fatty atrophy score observed across type-I to type-IV FFP.

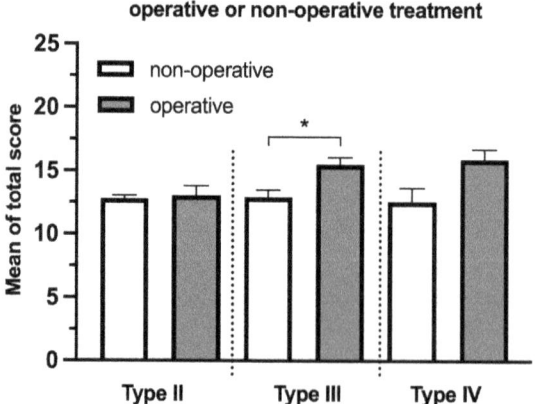

Figure 6. Mean comparison of gMFA using the total score between patients receiving operation and conservatively treated patients in type-II, type-III, and type-IV FFP. Mean ± standard error of the mean. Patients diagnosed with type-III FFP who underwent operative treatment exhibited significantly more pronounced gluteal fatty atrophy than those undergoing non-operative treatment. * $p < 0.05$. The analysis of type I was not performed because there was only 1 case operated.

Further, logistic regression was conducted to evaluate the association between gMFA and operative decisions in patients with type-III FFP. The total score of gMFA was significantly associated with the operative decision when other factors that could influence operability, such as age, cardiac illness (heart failure or coronary artery disease), or renal insufficiency, were also included (OR: 1.22, 95% CI: 1.01–1.47, $p < 0.05$, Table 2).

Table 2. Analysis of risk factors for operative indication in patients diagnosed with type-III FFP using logistic regression.

Factors	OR	95% CI	p-Value
Sex (male)	1.13	0.27–4.78	0.87
Age	0.93	0.83–1.05	0.26
Total score	1.22	1.01–1.47	0.04 *
HF or CAD	0.63	0.12–3.31	0.39
CKD	1.90	0.42–8.53	0.11

OR: odds ratio; CI: confidence interval; HF: heart failure; CAD: coronary artery disease; CKD: chronic kidney disease. * $p < 0.05$.

4. Discussion

The key finding of the current study is that the severity of gMFA could potentially be a factor for surgical indication in geriatric patients with type-III FFP. The early determination of potential surgical candidates with the help of possible factors, independent from fracture classification in orthogeriatric patients with FFP, could prompt the remobilization and reduce complications due to immobilization and prolonged hospital stays.

So far, there is no gold standard for the treatment of patients with FFP. Surgical treatments are often first indicated after the failure of conservative treatment due to the patient's frailty, causing a relatively higher intraoperative and postoperative risk for bleeding, postoperative infection, postoperative delirium, and cardiovascular and renal complications [23]. A steep increase in incidence and economic burden caused by FFP in the elderly population, especially those above the age of 80, has been reported in many countries like the USA, Germany, and Finland [1,4,24]. This is associated with demographic change, leading to a growth in the geriatric population [25]. To the author's knowledge, the current study is the first effort to discuss the impact of gMFA on the management of very elderly patients with FFP.

Aging is recognized as an important factor for gMFA [26]. However, the positive correlation between aging and gMFA did not exist in the current study population, where all patients were older than 80. Our result showed that the biological status of the muscle did not match the real age in this patient group. One of our previous works found that the speed of postoperative remobilization in the geriatric population with pertrochanteric fracture was significantly quicker in patients with better nutrition status and was also independent of age [27]. This finding implies that age is no longer a reliable reference in managing a very elderly population. A more comprehensive evaluation should be given to determine the operability and patient's potential for remobilization.

In addition, unlike the incidence of osteoporosis, which was reported to be higher in females, the scale of gMFA did not differ between genders. No difference in gMFA was found among the four types of FFP. Thus, the severity of gMFA was not associated with the fracture complexity induced by trauma. Furthermore, the severity of gMFA was unequal among the gluteus maximus, medius, and minimus and was significantly more profound in the gluteus medius and minimus. This is possibly due to a decreased demand for hip abduction, supported by gluteus medius and minimus, in the daily activity of the elderly population. By contrast, the hip extension supported by the gluteus maximus is more frequently used, for example, in rising from chairs and stair climbing. Physiologically, the gluteus medius and minimus are critically involved during the stride to support the pelvic balance. Fatty atrophy in these two muscles could impair the mobility of the elderly in daily life and also remobilization after fractures like FFP [28,29]. Chi et al. reported that the gluteus medius and minimus fatty atrophy are associated with fall-related fractures [13]. These findings implied that functional training and active treatment due to the injury of gluteal muscle, especially gluteus medius and minimus, could be important for fall prevention and remobilization after a pelvic fracture [30].

Interestingly, the current study found that the total score of gMFA in patients undergoing surgeries with type-III FFP was significantly greater than in non-operated patients.

The posterior pelvic ring in type-III FFP was completely interrupted with dislocation. In this case, the additional stability provided by the gluteal muscle might be critical for the patient's mobilization after a fracture. Meanwhile, gMFA decreased muscle strength and impaired muscle function due to disrupting the normal contractile function of muscle fibers [31,32]. Patients suffering from type-III FFP with preclinical severe gMFA had generally weakened gluteal muscle function, which could negatively influence their baseline mobility. Our results indicate that these patients are more likely to need surgery to help them achieve remobilization. In the current patient group (age ≥ 80), comorbidities could also influence the operation decision. Logistic regression showed that gMFA is an independent factor associated with surgical treatment.

By contrast, gMFA played a less important role in FFP type II and IV. Although the total score was slightly higher, no significance was found in patients receiving surgical treatment compared with those conservatively treated. According to the classification and the anatomy, the bony posterior pelvic structure in type-II FFP was fractured but not dislocated with or without an anterior fracture. Being the largest subgroup with 289 patients, only about 10% of patients diagnosed with type-II FFP underwent an operation. In other words, type-II FFP is considered relatively stable, so the loss of muscle function seems less decisive in maintaining stability and does not affect the surgical indication. On the other hand, 20 patients with type-IV FFP were concluded in the current study with a 65% operation rate. This subtype of FFP was characterized by marked vertical instability on both sides of the posterior pelvis, for which surgical treatment was strongly recommended due to its instability [5]. In this context, the surgical indication is mainly induced by the high instability of the fracture. The gMFA, contrarily, might have only a limited impact.

Certain limitations must be recognized in the current study. First, it was a single-center retrospective study. The study design was controlled by using the STROBE checklist for observational study [33] (Supplementary Materials). The surgical indication might vary largely from center to center. Our hospital is a geriatric traumatology center. Working together with geriatrics, the surgical indication for these patients was decided in consensus and should be representative. The sample size for type-I, II, and IV FFP was relatively small due to the uneven distribution of the fracture types and, more importantly, the age threshold (≥ 80) of inclusion criteria. This caused limitations in the variables chosen to build the logistic regression model. Consequently, a multi-center study with more study objects should be conducted to examine the current hypotheses. Moreover, other factors like osteoporosis can also be associated with the tendency of surgical treatment. It would be interesting to include bone mineral density test results and to conduct future studies from a biomechanical perspective.

Taken together, gMFA was commonly found in very elderly patients with FFP without gender differences. The severity of gMFA did not correlate with age and was more profound in gluteus minimus and medius than maximus in those orthogeriatric patients. The gMFA was an independent factor for surgical indication in patients with type-III FFP.

Supplementary Materials: The following supporting information can be downloaded at: https://www.mdpi.com/article/10.3390/jcm12226966/s1, Figure S1: STROBE Statement—Checklist of items that should be included in reports of cohort studies.

Author Contributions: Conceptualization: Y.Z. and C.L. (Christoph Linhart); Methodology, D.M., Y.Z. and C.L. (Christoph Linhart); Software, Y.Z. and M.L.; Validation, M.L., C.E. and C.N.; Formal Analysis, Y.Z.; Resources, C.L. (Christoph Linhart), J.G. and W.B.; Data Curation, C.L. (Christopher Lampert) and L.M.G.; Writing—Original Draft Preparation, Y.Z.; Writing—Review and Editing, M.L., C.N. and W.B.; Supervision, C.E., W.B. and C.N. All authors have read and agreed to the published version of the manuscript.

Funding: This research received no external funding.

Institutional Review Board Statement: The study protocol was approved by the ethics committee of Ludwig Maximilian University of Munich, Munich, Germany (approval number: 518-18).

Informed Consent Statement: Written informed consent has been obtained from the patients to publish this paper.

Data Availability Statement: The data presented in this study are available on request from the corresponding author.

Conflicts of Interest: The authors declare no conflict of interest.

References

1. Kannus, P.; Parkkari, J.; Niemi, S.; Sievanen, H. Low-Trauma Pelvic Fractures in Elderly Finns in 1970–2013. *Calcif. Tissue Int.* **2015**, *97*, 577–580. [CrossRef] [PubMed]
2. Andrich, S.; Haastert, B.; Neuhaus, E.; Neidert, K.; Arend, W.; Ohmann, C.; Grebe, J.; Vogt, A.; Jungbluth, P.; Rosler, G.; et al. Epidemiology of Pelvic Fractures in Germany: Considerably High Incidence Rates among Older People. *PLoS ONE* **2015**, *10*, e0139078. [CrossRef] [PubMed]
3. Prieto-Alhambra, D.; Aviles, F.F.; Judge, A.; Van Staa, T.; Nogues, X.; Arden, N.K.; Diez-Perez, A.; Cooper, C.; Javaid, M.K. Burden of pelvis fracture: A population-based study of incidence, hospitalisation and mortality. *Osteoporos. Int.* **2012**, *23*, 2797–2803. [CrossRef] [PubMed]
4. Burge, R.; Dawson-Hughes, B.; Solomon, D.H.; Wong, J.B.; King, A.; Tosteson, A. Incidence and economic burden of osteoporosis-related fractures in the United States, 2005–2025. *J. Bone Miner. Res.* **2007**, *22*, 465–475. [CrossRef]
5. Rommens, P.M.; Arand, C.; Hofmann, A.; Wagner, D. When and How to Operate Fragility Fractures of the Pelvis? *Indian J. Orthop.* **2019**, *53*, 128–137. [CrossRef]
6. Al Saedi, A.; Debruin, D.A.; Hayes, A.; Hamrick, M. Lipid metabolism in sarcopenia. *Bone* **2022**, *164*, 116539. [CrossRef]
7. Eken, G.; Misir, A.; Tangay, C.; Atici, T.; Demirhan, N.; Sener, N. Effect of muscle atrophy and fatty infiltration on mid-term clinical, and functional outcomes after Achilles tendon repair. *Foot Ankle Surg.* **2021**, *27*, 730–735. [CrossRef]
8. McCrum, E. MR Imaging of the Rotator Cuff. *Magn. Reson. Imaging Clin. N. Am.* **2020**, *28*, 165–179. [CrossRef]
9. Sadler, S.; Cassidy, S.; Peterson, B.; Spink, M.; Chuter, V. Gluteus medius muscle function in people with and without low back pain: A systematic review. *BMC Musculoskelet. Disord.* **2019**, *20*, 463. [CrossRef]
10. Semciw, A.I.; Green, R.A.; Murley, G.S.; Pizzari, T. Gluteus minimus: An intramuscular EMG investigation of anterior and posterior segments during gait. *Gait Posture* **2014**, *39*, 822–826. [CrossRef]
11. Flack, N.A.; Nicholson, H.D.; Woodley, S.J. A review of the anatomy of the hip abductor muscles, gluteus medius, gluteus minimus, and tensor fascia lata. *Clin. Anat.* **2012**, *25*, 697–708. [CrossRef]
12. Daguet, E.; Jolivet, E.; Bousson, V.; Boutron, C.; Dahmen, N.; Bergot, C.; Vicaut, E.; Laredo, J.D. Fat content of hip muscles: An anteroposterior gradient. *J. Bone Jt. Surg.* **2011**, *93*, 1897–1905. [CrossRef] [PubMed]
13. Chi, A.S.; Long, S.S.; Zoga, A.C.; Parker, L.; Morrison, W.B. Association of Gluteus Medius and Minimus Muscle Atrophy and Fall-Related Hip Fracture in Older Individuals Using Computed Tomography. *J. Comput. Assist. Tomogr.* **2016**, *40*, 238–242. [CrossRef] [PubMed]
14. Stasi, S.; Papathanasiou, G.; Chronopoulos, E.; Dontas, I.A.; Baltopoulos, I.P.; Papaioannou, N.A. The Effect of Intensive Abductor Strengthening on Postoperative Muscle Efficiency and Functional Ability of Hip-Fractured Patients: A Randomized Controlled Trial. *Indian J. Orthop.* **2019**, *53*, 407–419. [CrossRef] [PubMed]
15. Yerli, M.; Yuce, A.; Ayaz, M.B.; Bayraktar, T.O.; Erkurt, N.; Dedeoglu, S.S.; Imren, Y.; Gurbuz, H. Effect of psoas and gluteus medius muscles attenuation on hip fracture type. *Hip Int.* **2023**, *33*, 952–957. [CrossRef] [PubMed]
16. Howard, E.E.; Pasiakos, S.M.; Fussell, M.A.; Rodriguez, N.R. Skeletal Muscle Disuse Atrophy and the Rehabilitative Role of Protein in Recovery from Musculoskeletal Injury. *Adv. Nutr.* **2020**, *11*, 989–1001. [CrossRef]
17. Rommens, P.M.; Hofmann, A. Comprehensive classification of fragility fractures of the pelvic ring: Recommendations for surgical treatment. *Injury* **2013**, *44*, 1733–1744. [CrossRef]
18. Rommens, P.M.; Wagner, D.; Hofmann, A. Fragility Fractures of the Pelvis. *JBJS Rev.* **2017**, *5*, e3. [CrossRef]
19. Lee, H.; Lee, E.; Jang, I.Y. Frailty and Comprehensive Geriatric Assessment. *J. Korean Med. Sci.* **2020**, *35*, e16. [CrossRef]
20. Babayev, M.; Lachmann, E.; Nagler, W. The controversy surrounding sacral insufficiency fractures: To ambulate or not to ambulate? *Am. J. Phys. Med. Rehabil.* **2000**, *79*, 404–409. [CrossRef]
21. Lee, D.G.; Bae, J.H. Fatty infiltration of the multifidus muscle independently increases osteoporotic vertebral compression fracture risk. *BMC Musculoskelet. Disord.* **2023**, *24*, 508. [CrossRef] [PubMed]
22. Goutallier, D.; Postel, J.M.; Bernageau, J.; Lavau, L.; Voisin, M.C. Fatty muscle degeneration in cuff ruptures. Pre- and postoperative evaluation by CT scan. *Clin. Orthop. Relat. Res.* **1994**, *304*, 78–83. [CrossRef]
23. Kong, C.; Zhang, Y.; Wang, C.; Wang, P.; Li, X.; Wang, W.; Wang, Y.; Shen, J.; Ren, X.; Wang, T.; et al. Comprehensive geriatric assessment for older orthopedic patients and analysis of risk factors for postoperative complications. *BMC Geriatr.* **2022**, *22*, 644. [CrossRef] [PubMed]
24. Hu, S.; Guo, J.; Zhu, B.; Dong, Y.; Li, F. Epidemiology and burden of pelvic fractures: Results from the Global Burden of Disease Study 2019. *Injury* **2023**, *54*, 589–597. [CrossRef] [PubMed]
25. Rau, C.S.; Lin, T.S.; Wu, S.C.; Yang, J.C.; Hsu, S.Y.; Cho, T.Y.; Hsieh, C.H. Geriatric hospitalizations in fall-related injuries. *Scand. J. Trauma Resusc. Emerg. Med.* **2014**, *22*, 63. [CrossRef] [PubMed]

26. Li, C.W.; Yu, K.; Shyh-Chang, N.; Jiang, Z.; Liu, T.; Ma, S.; Luo, L.; Guang, L.; Liang, K.; Ma, W.; et al. Pathogenesis of sarcopenia and the relationship with fat mass: Descriptive review. *J. Cachexia Sarcopenia Muscle* **2022**, *13*, 781–794. [CrossRef] [PubMed]
27. Faust, L.M.; Lerchenberger, M.; Gleich, J.; Linhart, C.; Keppler, A.M.; Schmidmaier, R.; Bocker, W.; Neuerburg, C.; Zhang, Y. Predictive Value of Prognostic Nutritional Index for Early Postoperative Mobility in Elderly Patients with Pertrochanteric Fracture Treated with Intramedullary Nail Osteosynthesis. *J. Clin. Med.* **2023**, *12*, 1792. [CrossRef]
28. Greco, A.J.; Vilella, R.C. *Anatomy, Bony Pelvis and Lower Limb, Gluteus Minimus Muscle*; StatPearls: Treasure Island, FL, USA, 2023.
29. Shah, A.; Bordoni, B. *Anatomy, Bony Pelvis and Lower Limb, Gluteus Medius Muscle*; StatPearls: Treasure Island, FL, USA, 2023.
30. Inacio, M.; Ryan, A.S.; Bair, W.N.; Prettyman, M.; Beamer, B.A.; Rogers, M.W. Gluteal muscle composition differentiates fallers from non-fallers in community dwelling older adults. *BMC Geriatr.* **2014**, *14*, 37. [CrossRef]
31. Lassche, S.; Rietveld, A.; Heerschap, A.; van Hees, H.W.; Hopman, M.T.; Voermans, N.C.; Saris, C.G.; van Engelen, B.G.; Ottenheijm, C.A. Muscle fiber dysfunction contributes to weakness in inclusion body myositis. *Neuromuscul. Disord.* **2019**, *29*, 468–476. [CrossRef]
32. Hamrick, M.W.; McGee-Lawrence, M.E.; Frechette, D.M. Fatty Infiltration of Skeletal Muscle: Mechanisms and Comparisons with Bone Marrow Adiposity. *Front. Endocrinol.* **2016**, *7*, 69. [CrossRef]
33. von Elm, E.; Altman, D.G.; Egger, M.; Pocock, S.J.; Gøtzsche, P.C. The Strengthening the Reporting of Observational Studies in Epidemiology (STROBE) statement: Guidelines for reporting observational studies. *J. Clin. Epidemiol.* **2008**, *61*, 344–349. [CrossRef]

Disclaimer/Publisher's Note: The statements, opinions and data contained in all publications are solely those of the individual author(s) and contributor(s) and not of MDPI and/or the editor(s). MDPI and/or the editor(s) disclaim responsibility for any injury to people or property resulting from any ideas, methods, instructions or products referred to in the content.

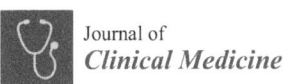

Article

Micro-Structural and Biomechanical Evaluation of Bioresorbable and Conventional Bone Cements for Augmentation of the Proximal Femoral Nail

Christoph Linhart *, Manuel Kistler, Maximilian Saller, Axel Greiner, Christopher Lampert, Matthias Kassube, Christopher A. Becker, Wolfgang Böcker and Christian Ehrnthaller

Department of Orthopaedics and Trauma Surgery, Musculoskeletal University Center Munich (MUM), University Hospital, LMU Munich, Marchioninistr. 15, 81377 Munich, Germany;
manuel.kistler@med.uni-muenchen.de (M.K.); maximilian.saller@med.uni-muenchen.de (M.S.);
axel.greiner@med.uni-muenchen.de (A.G.); christopher.lampert@med.uni-muenchen.de (C.L.);
matthias_kassube@hotmail.de (M.K.); christopher.becker@med.uni-muenchen.de (C.A.B.);
wolfgang.boecker@med.uni-muenchen.de (W.B.); christian.ehrnthaller@med.uni-muenchen.de (C.E.)
* Correspondence: christoph.linhart@med.uni-muenchen.de

Citation: Linhart, C.; Kistler, M.; Saller, M.; Greiner, A.; Lampert, C.; Kassube, M.; Becker, C.A.; Böcker, W.; Ehrnthaller, C. Micro-Structural and Biomechanical Evaluation of Bioresorbable and Conventional Bone Cements for Augmentation of the Proximal Femoral Nail. *J. Clin. Med.* **2023**, *12*, 7202. https://doi.org/10.3390/jcm12237202

Academic Editor: Wing Hoi Cheung

Received: 18 October 2023
Revised: 5 November 2023
Accepted: 18 November 2023
Published: 21 November 2023

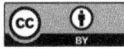

Copyright: © 2023 by the authors. Licensee MDPI, Basel, Switzerland. This article is an open access article distributed under the terms and conditions of the Creative Commons Attribution (CC BY) license (https://creativecommons.org/licenses/by/4.0/).

Abstract: Osteoporotic proximal femur fractures are on the rise due to demographic change. The most dominant surgical treatment option for per/subtrochanteric fractures is cephalomedullary nailing. As it has been shown to increase primary stability, cement augmentation has become increasingly popular in the treatment of osteoporotic per/subtrochanteric femur fractures. The ultimate goal is to achieve stable osteosynthesis, allowing for rapid full weight-bearing to reduce possible postoperative complications. In recent years, bioresorbable bone cements have been developed and are now mainly used to fill bone voids. The aim of this study was to evaluate the biomechanical stability as well as the micro-structural behaviour of bioresorbable bone cements compared to conventional polymethylmethacrylate (PMMA)-cements in a subtrochanteric femur fracture model. Biomechanical as well as micro-computed tomography morphology analysis revealed no significant differences in both bone cements, as they showed equal mechanical stability and tight interdigitation into the spongious bone of the femoral head. Given the positive risk/benefit ratio for bioresorbable bone cements, their utilisation should be evaluated in future clinical studies, making them a promising alternative to PMMA-bone cements.

Keywords: bone cement; PMMA; micro-computed tomography; biomechanics; proximal femur fracture; osteoporosis; cement augmentation; subtrochanteric fracture

1. Introduction

Due to the change in demographics, the incidence of proximal femur fractures will increase over the next few years and represent a major health care issue [1]. Elderly patients often present with multiple comorbidities, leading to a significant increase in perioperative and postoperative complications. As a result, proximal femur fractures are associated with a high one-year mortality rate of up to 30% [2]. The treatment goal of proximal femur fractures must therefore ensure the preservation of function and independence in orthogeriatric patients [3]. Among proximal femur fractures, the per/subtrochanteric fracture is most common, followed by femoral neck fractures [4]. Whereas femoral neck fractures are mostly treated with hip joint arthroplasty, joint-preserving osteosynthesis is the predominant surgical treatment for per/subtrochanteric fractures. Osteosynthesis in pertrochanteric fractures is either performed using a dynamic hip screw (DHS, DePuySynthes® Inc., Oberdorf, Switzerland) or a proximal femur nail with a hip component. The current evidence does not promote one solution, whereas a trend towards the use of intramedullary implants is observed [5–7]. This study focuses on reverse-oblique subtrochanteric fractures, especially

AO (Arbeitsgemeinschaft für Osteosynthesefragen) 31-A3. Being the most unstable fracture type among all proximal femur fractures, predominantly intramedullary implants are used.

As already mentioned, the most common treatment option for per/subtrochanteric femur fractures nowadays is nailing of the proximal femur. High initial stability due to intramedullary load distribution together with short duration of the surgical procedure have led to an increase in the use of the dynamic hip screw. Additionally, these fractures of the femur are predominantly associated with osteoporosis. Despite the reduced biomechanical bone stability and an increased perioperative risk in prevalent osteoporosis, a surgical procedure that allows rapid full weight-bearing mobilisation must be achieved [1], as a significant increase in mortality was observed when patients were treated with weight-bearing restrictions [8]. Cement augmentation with polymethylmethacrylate (PMMA) of proximal femoral nailing (PFNA) for the treatment of pertrochanteric femoral fractures is the most commonly used and standardised method to deal with that problem [3], as it has been shown to increase primary stability. The additional augmentation increases the contact area of the implant-bone interface. Biomechanical investigations were already able to demonstrate the higher stability of the cement-augmented PFNA for the treatment of osteoporosis-associated fractures when compared to the non-cemented control [9,10]. Prospective studies showed good functional results with no evidence of cement-associated complications for cement augmentation with PMMA of the PFNA in orthogeriatric patients [11–13]. Although augmentation of PFNA did not affect the walking ability in the early postoperative period, it led to significantly fewer implant failure- or migration-caused reoperations. This implicates a higher stability of the osteosynthesis construct, allowing a fast full weight-bearing mobilisation [13].

However, PMMA also faces some points of criticism, such as thermal injury to surrounding tissues [14], possible intraarticular leakage, and its failing ability for resorption and transformation into bone. Therefore, various surgeons deny cement augmentation, even though it would be possible [15].

To avoid these negative side effects, bioresorbable liquid bone substitutes with similar physical properties to PMMA and high mechanical strength due to curing processes were developed during the last few years. Bioresorbable bone cement consists of both α-CaS hemihydrates and hydroxyapatite (HA) [16]. The calcium sulphate will be resorbed and replaced by in-growing bone, whereas the hydroxyapatite component persists and functions as a matrix. Thereby, it combines the advantage of immediate stability with the osteoconductive characteristics of a bone substitute material [17,18].

In its first intention, bioresorbable bone cement was used as an alternative for autologous bone grafting in traumatic injuries with bone loss [19]. Moreover, several studies investigated its use for the filling of bone cysts [20], as well as balloon kyphoplasty, and verified the safety of the procedure [21]. In addition, clinical studies showed that bioresorbable bone cements could be used instead of PMMA in the treatment of osteoporotic and traumatic vertebral fractures [22]. However, so far, bioresorbable bone cements have never been tested as an alternative for augmentation of osteosynthesis implants, although the advantages of failing exothermal reactions and biodegradable properties are obvious. It has to be taken into account that bioresorbable bone cements represent a very heterogeneous group of substances that are commercially available from various manufacturers with different characteristics regarding application capability, strength, and resorption.

The aim of this study was to evaluate bioresorbable cement for the augmentation of PFNA in proximal femur fractures. We hypothesised comparable biomechanical as well as physical properties that will allow a safe use together with a proximal femur nail. Therefore, we compared cement augmentation with bioresorbable cement to cement augmentation with conventional, commercially used PMMA. In addition, biomechanical studies examining the primary stability of each type of cement, micro-structural properties (distance between trabecular structures and cement before and after loading) were analysed by micro-computed tomography (μCT). Since its introduction in the 1980s, μCT has become an essential tool in musculoskeletal research and plays a pivotal role in the evaluation of bone microarchitecture in small animal models ex vivo [23]. In our study, we were the first to use long human tubular bones to visualise the trabecular-cement interface in particular.

2. Materials and Methods

After ethical approval from the Human Research Ethics Committee of the University of Munich, LMU, Germany (No. 8-030), 10 fresh frozen human femora of female donors >75 years were commercially obtained from Science Care (Phoenix, AZ, USA). The 10 human femora were split up into two groups, each consisting of five specimens. The femora were frozen at −24 °C and thawed at room temperature for 24 h before experimental testing. To increase comparability and reduce bias, only pairs (both femora) from each donor were used. A short PFNA (L = 240 mm, D = 10 mm) (PFNA, DePuySynthes® Inc., West Chester, PA, USA) was implanted in each of these human specimens according to the official manufacturer's instructions. For the purpose of minimally invasive implantation and standardisation, the original manufacturer's instrumentation was used. The fracture was set standardised according to an AO 31-A3 fracture that is 50° oblique in terms of a "reverse-oblique" fracture. After successful implantation of the PFNA, the fracture was marked on the intact bone. The angle was determined by the shaft axis. The osteotomy was carefully performed with a hand saw without damaging the nail.

Afterwards, all specimens were tapered at the distal end and embedded under a 6° valgus position in metal pots using a polyurethane resin (RenCast® FC 52/53 Isocyanat; FC 53 Polyol, Huntsman Corporation, The Woodlands, TX, USA). Five specimens were augmented using classical PMMA-cement (Traumacem; DePuy Synthes® Inc., West Chester, PA, USA) and five using bioresorbable bone cement (Cerament; BoneSupport, Lund, Sweden). Augmentation for both cements was performed with an application instrument for the PMMA-cement under fluoroscopic control until a uniform distribution using 3–4 mL of cement in the femoral head was achieved. The function of the iliotibial tract was simulated with a 3 mm steel cable that becomes continuously stretched with increasing load. To measure the force characteristic of the simulated tractus iliotibialis during force application of the bone, a 5 kN load cell (8417–6005, Burster Praezisionsmesstechnik GmbH and Co. KG, Gernsbach, Germany) was implemented in the wire rope. A program was created in LabVIEW 2014 (Version 14.0.1, National Instruments, Austin, TX, USA) to calibrate the sensor and collect the force data. Sensor calibration was performed using the universal testing machine. Specified tensile and compressive forces in the range from −200 N (compressive force) to +1500 N (tensile force) were applied to the force sensor in 100 N increments. A 3D ultrasound system (Zebris CMS 20, Zebris Medical GmbH, Isny, Germany) was used to track the scope of 3D movement of the bone segments to measure the displacement of the fracture gap in three dimensions in millimeters. Depending on the application, the system has a resolution of 1/10 mm − 1/100 mm with a measurement error of 0.25%. These ultrasound markers were screwed in place by an additively manufactured holder or, in some special cases, directly to the bone with hot glue. All tests were performed on an electrodynamic universal testing machine (ElectroPulsTM E10000, Instron, Norwood, IL, USA). The simulated tractus iliotibialis was slightly preloaded before loading until an effective joint force of 50 N was applied on the testing machine. Afterwards, biomechanical testing of the instrumented specimens was performed under displacement-controlled force application at 10 mm/min up to effective joint loads of 200 N and 400 N without creating a failure. All load procedures were repeated three times to avoid possible settling of the implant. Biomechanical stability was assessed by measuring the amount of fracture displacement and axial stiffness of the bone construct (N/mm) of the instrumented specimen. Stiffness was defined as the resistance of the bone structure against elastic deformation in response to an applied load without considering the geometry of the cross section. Additionally, force distribution of the iliotibial tract (N) during force application of the bones was measured as a secondary parameter for dislocation due to the expected tension release following fragment dislocation. For the μCT, due to the size of the femora and the need to rotate the specimens, a special bone holder was made using a 3D printer (Ultimaker

2+ Extended, Ultimaker B.V., Utrecht, The Netherlands). This was achieved by creating a computer-aided 3D model (Catia V5, Dassault Systemes, Velizy-Villacoublay, France) based on the bone size.

To obtain high-resolution images of the trabecular-material interface, the femora were imaged with a custom-build research µCT (CT-Alpha, Procon X-Ray, Sarstedt, Germany), equipped with an nanofocus X-ray source (XWT-225-TCHE, X-Ray-Worx, Germany) set at 200 kV/240 mA (with a 1 mm aluminium filter) and a 75 µm pixel size CMOS flat panel detector (Dexela 2923, PerkinElmer, Santa Clara CA, USA) at a 2 × 2 binning. 1440 images with an exposure time of 250 ms and a two-time averaging were recorded over a full 360° rotation. All scans were performed both before and after biomechanical testing and cement application. The distance between trabecular structures and cement was measured in each of the 10 regions of interest (ROI). The acquired raw data was reconstructed with X-Aid (Mitos, Germany) after correction of geometrical errors and beam hardening.

After the computed tomography images were taken, the Dragonfly software (Object Research Systems (ORS) Inc, Montreal, QC, Canada, 2020) was used to analyse the images.

A region of interest was created for each plane and coloured through all the images of that plane to measure the progression between cement and trabeculae within a specimen, always at the same points.

For each of the three planes (axial, sagittal, longitudinal), a line of 9 mm length was then placed at the ROI. 10 measurements were taken, starting at 0 mm and with 1 mm between each measurement (Figure 1).

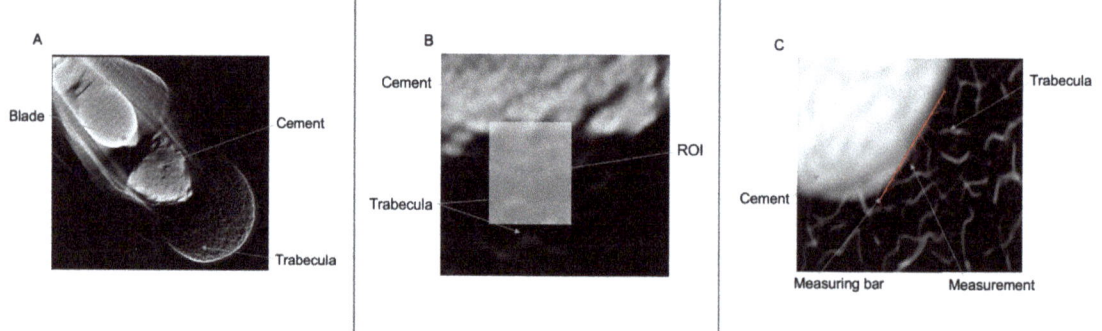

Figure 1. (**A**): Overview in micro-computed tomography of the cement-trabecular interphase of the proximal femur; (**B**): detail of the ROI; (**C**): schematic drawing of the ROI and the points of evaluation of the cement-trabecular interphase.

For each measurement, the distance between the cement and the nearest trabeculae was measured. Once 10 measurements were taken, the measurement procedure was performed again, five frames forward from the last one.

When cement was no longer visible in the ROI of a plane, the measurement was stopped and moved to the next plane.

Statistical Analysis

For data collection and analysis, the software SPSS (IBM Corp. Released 2021) was used. IBM SPSS Statistics for Macintosh, Version 28.0. Armon, NY, USA: IBM Corp) and Excel (Microsoft, released 2021, Microsoft Excel for Macintosh, Version 16.50) were used. All charts were created with Prism 9 (GraphPad Software, Inc., La Jolla, CA, USA).

To evaluate the data for homogeneity of variances, the Levene test was used. Normal distributed data was analysed using the *t*-test for paired or unpaired samples. For non-normally distributed data, the Wilcoxon test (paired) or the Mann-Whitney-U test (unpaired) were used. Differences with a *p*-value < 0.05 were defined as significantly different.

3. Results

3.1. Biomechanics

All results of the biomechanical testing (Table 1) were normally distributed and showed no significant difference between the two types of cement. In detail, the p-value of the dislocation in the fracture gap between the cements resulted at 200 N in a slightly reduced displacement of 9.8% for the bioresorbable cement group ($p = 0.65$) and at 400 N in an almost evenly distributed displacement (1.7% less in the bioresorbable cement group; $p = 0.89$). The axial stiffness of the bone construct revealed a non-significant ($p = 0.33$) reduction in the PMMA-cement group of 25.4% at 200 N and a 2.9% reduction at 400 N ($p = 0.67$). Additionally, the force of the iliotibial tract indicated no significant differences at 200 N ($p = 0.53$) and 400 N ($p = 0.10$).

Table 1. Results of the biomechanical tests between two bone cements at different test loads.

Test load	200 N		400 N	
Cement	PMMA	Bio-Cement	PMMA	Bio-Cement
Fracture displacement in mm	1.13 ± 0.39	1.02 ± 0.32	1.22 ± 0.31	1.20 ± 0.26
Axial bone stiffness in N/mm	31.13 ± 12.75	41.73 ± 16.66	30.16 ± 2.34	31.08 ± 3.60
Iliotibial tract force in N	345.00 ± 33.76	334.80 ± 8.03	740.80 ± 53.80	695.00 ± 13.45

3.1.1. PMMA-Cement

The average distance between the cement and the trabeculae in the PMMA-cement group before conducting the biomechanical test was 642 ± 13 (SEM) µm. After loading, the mean value in the PMMA-cement group increased up to 718 ± 20 (SEM) µm (Figure 2). Therefore, the distance between cement and trabeculae has increased by 12%. The statistical analysis showed no significant difference ($p = 0.87$).

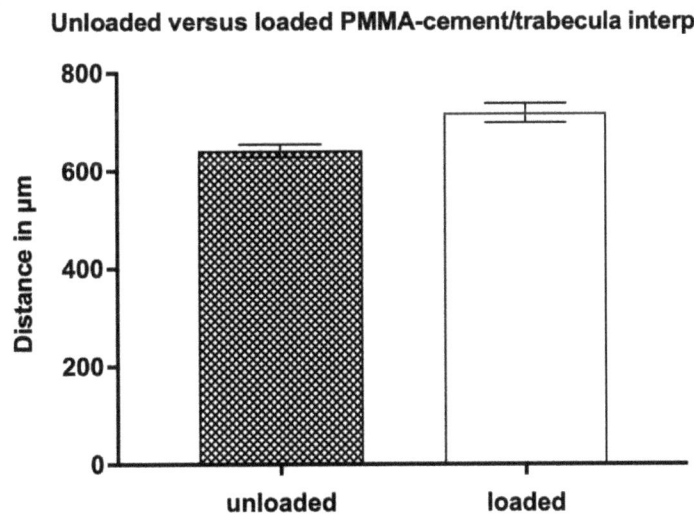

Figure 2. Cont.

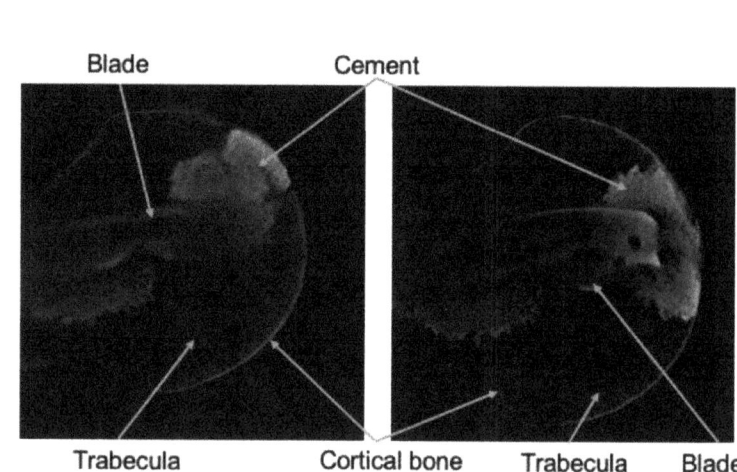

Figure 2. (**A**): Average distance (in micrometers) between unloaded versus loaded PMMA-cement and the closest trabecular structure. Data presented as mean ± SEM (standard error of the mean); (**B**): Unloaded (**left**) vs. loaded (**right**) PMMA-cement/trabecula interphase picture of the micro-CT. The specimen was treated with a proximal femur nail and augmented with PMMA-cement before a CT scan was taken.

3.1.2. Bioresorbable-Cement

In the bioresorbable cement group, the average distance between cement and trabeculae before the biomechanical test was 530 ± 15 (SEM) μm. After biomechanical loading, the average distance of the bioresorbable-cement group decreased to 485 ± 10 (SEM) μm (Figure 3). This difference of 8.5% was significantly different ($p = 0.03$).

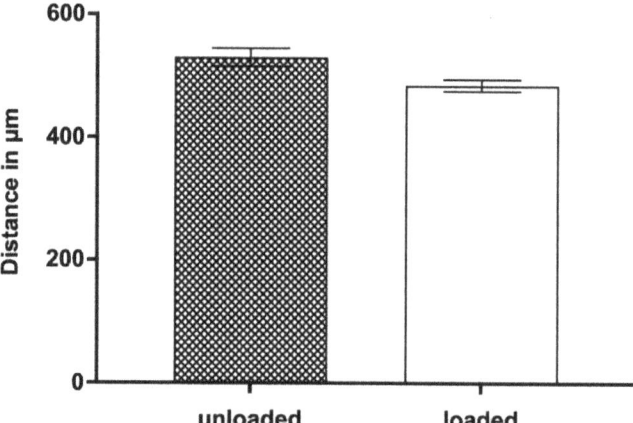

Figure 3. *Cont.*

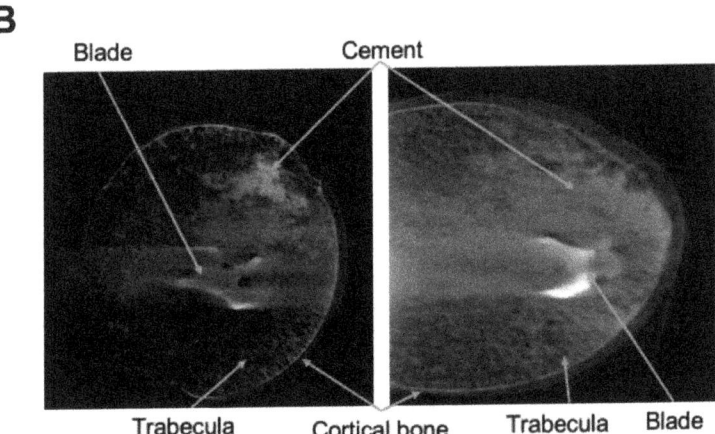

Figure 3. (**A**): Average distance (in micrometers) between unloaded versus loaded bioresorbable cement and the closest trabecula structure. Data presented as mean ± SEM (standard error of the mean); (**B**): Unloaded (**left**) vs. loaded (**right**) bioresorbable-cement/trabecula interphase picture of the 5 micro-CT. The specimen was treated with a proximal femur nail and augmented with bioresorbable cement before a CT scan was taken.

3.2. Micro-Computed Tomography

3.2.1. Unloaded PMMA-Cement vs. Bioresorbable-Cement

While comparing the two different types of cement before the biomechanical experiment, more profound differences were evaluated. The average cement-trabecular distance in the unloaded PMMA-cement group was 642 ± 13 (SEM) μm when compared to 530 ± 15 (SEM) μm in the group with bioresorbable cement (Figure 4). Statistical analysis showed a significant difference ($p \leq 0.0001$) between the two groups. It turns out that the cement-trabeculae interphase before loading has a 17% tighter structure than in the PMMA group before loading (Figure 4).

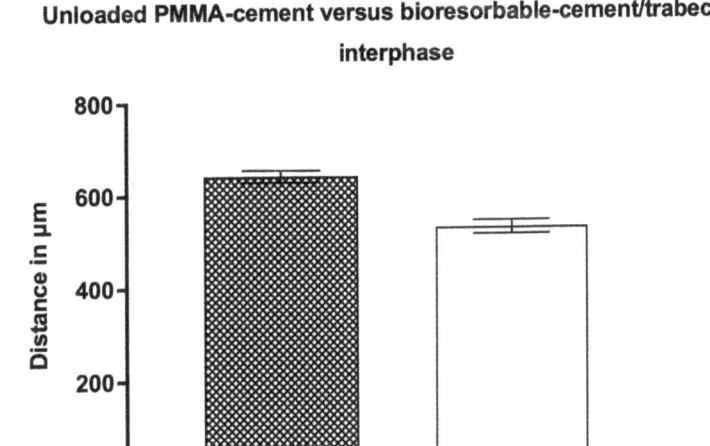

Figure 4. *Cont.*

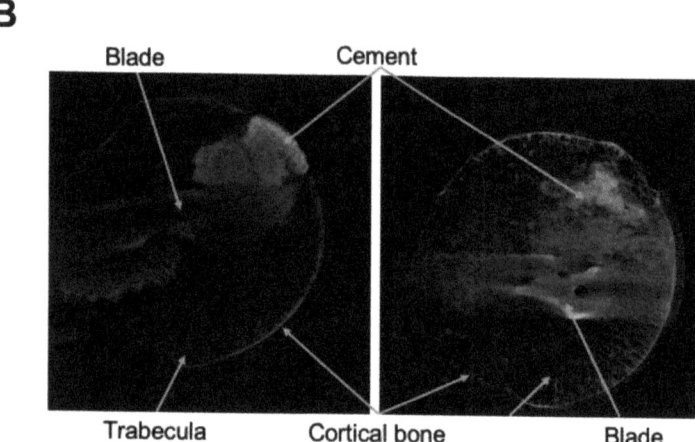

Figure 4. (**A**): Average distance (in micrometers) between unloaded PMMA-cement versus unloaded bioresorbable-cement and the closest trabecular structure. Data presented as mean ± SEM (standard error of the mean); (**B**): Unloaded PMMA (**left**) vs. unloaded (**right**) bioresorbable-cement/trabecula interphase picture of the micro-CT. The specimen was treated with a proximal femur nail and augmented with PMMA- or bioresorbable-cement before a CT scan was taken.

3.2.2. Loaded PMMA-Cement vs. Bioresorbable-Cement

Biomechanical loading of the specimens was able to confirm the trend towards higher indentation in the bioresorbable-cement group as seen before loading. While the average cement-trabecular distance in the PMMA-cement group was 718 ± 20 (SEM) μm, the bioresorbable-cement group showed values of 485 ± 10 (SEM) μm (Figure 5). There was a significant difference ($p \leq 0.0001$) between the two groups, which was reflected in a 32.5% tighter cement-trabeculae interphase in the structure of the bioresorbable cement.

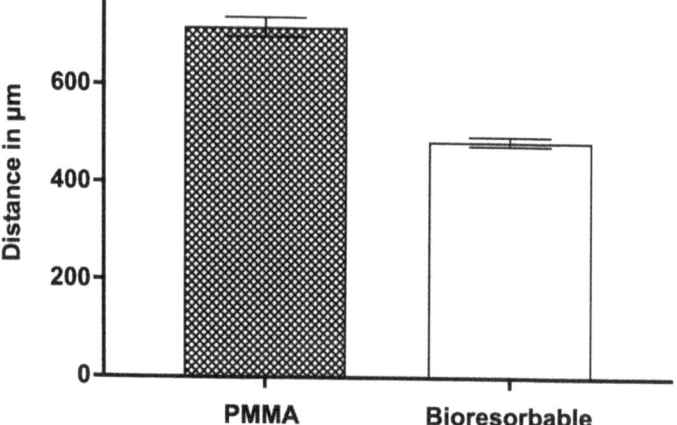

Figure 5. *Cont.*

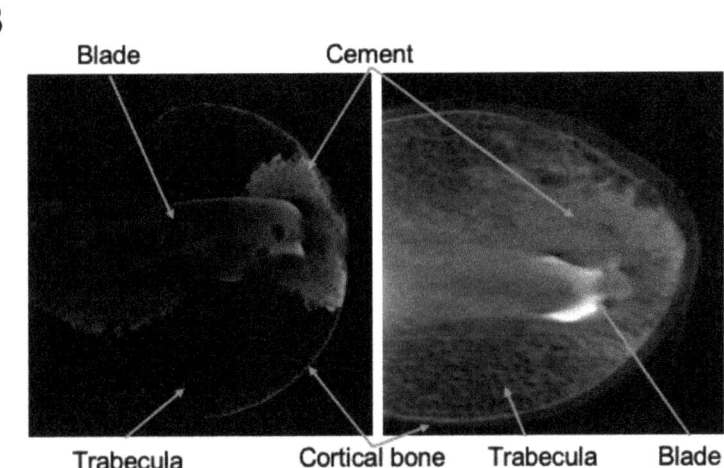

Figure 5. (**A**): Average distance (in micrometers) between loaded PMMA-cement versus loaded bioresorbable-cement and the closest trabecular structure. Data presented as mean ± SEM (standard error of the mean); (**B**): Loaded PMMA (**left**) vs. loaded (**right**) bioresorbable-cement/trabecula interphase picture of the micro-CT. The specimen was treated with a proximal femur nail and augmented with PMMA- or bioresorbable-cement before a CT scan was taken.

4. Discussion

In this study, the micro-structural and biomechanical properties of PMMA as well as bioresorbable bone cements used for augmentation of the femoral head were compared for the first time in a subtrochanteric fracture model.

We were able to demonstrate that the use of bioresorbable bone cement in an experimental unstable subtrochanteric femur fracture model resulted in a tight interaction of the injected cement with the surrounding trabecular bone with biomechanical properties similar to classic PMMA-bone cement after the conduction of a classical loading test.

During the last few years, the augmentation of implants used for osteosynthesis has become increasingly popular [13]. While this technique was used primarily in proximal femur fractures [24], its usage has been expanded to include other osteoporotic fractures such as proximal humerus, insufficiency fractures of the sacrum, and vertebral fractures [25,26]. Possible advantages include the increase of primary fixation strength [10] to prevent secondary dislocation and implant failure and, therefore, ultimately achieve mobilisation and weight-bearing as soon as possible. Various biomechanical studies were already able to demonstrate an increase in primary fixation strength compared to non-augmented proximal femoral nails [10]. A randomised clinical trial was able to demonstrate the safety of the augmentation of the femoral head with PMMA with comparable clinical outcomes and increased cost-effectiveness due to reduced implant failure rates [13,27].

Currently, PMMA bone cement is the only substance approved for augmentation of osteosynthesis implants. Special compositions from various manufacturers with favourable injection characteristics for their distinct type and application location were developed during the last few years to prevent possible risks during application. Although, in clinical studies, no augmentation-related negative side-effects have been reported so far [2,11,12] possible risks such as bone/cartilage necrosis due to the exothermic reaction while hardening as well as leakage (e.g., intraarticular in fractures close to joints), and intravasal (e.g., spinal vertebrae during vertebral kyphoplasty) are often mentioned and still raise concerns among orthopaedic surgeons. Only recently, a study focussing specifically on postoperative complications after augmentation of the femoral head in femur fractures was published. In addition, a small drop in blood pressure indicating a small systemic effect of the cement application, no significant alterations regarding postoperative complications such as infection, embolism, heart-attack, or mortality were seen [28].

With the intention of avoiding possible negative side-effects of PMMA and a hypothetical benefit of a biodegradable substance, the development of bioresorbable bone cements has been fostered throughout the last few years. These bone cements were initially developed to fill up bone voids as an alternative to autologous bone, which is limited in the amount that can be harvested [19].

Being a heterogeneous group of substances, bioresorbable bone cements have become increasingly sophisticated, being fluid in the application phase with uniform distribution and then becoming increasingly biomechanically stable after hardening [29]. In addition, being used as a bone void filler in the beginning, bioresorbable bone cements have become popular in vertebral compression fractures [21], osteomyelitis [30], and bone cysts [20]. The utilisation of bioresorbable bone cements in fractures with the need for bone grafting as an alternative to autologous bone has only recently been investigated and found to be similar in terms of outcome but superior in terms of blood loss and postoperative pain in comparison to autologous iliac crest bone grafting [19].

Just recently, a similar study to ours investigated the utilisation of a custom-made magnesium-based bioresorbable cement for its use in augmentation of the femoral head. In contrast to our study, the biomechanical stability of bioresorbable cement was inferior in comparison to PMMA. A possible explanation could be seen in the different characteristics of the used cement types [31]. In contrast to the commercially available CaS-based bone cement used in our study, implant augmentation was performed using an experimental custom-made magnesium-based cement. It is noteworthy, that the experimental setup differed greatly from ours, limiting comparability. Instead of testing the proximal femur during an experimental setup with axial load and additional simulation of the tractus iliotibialis, only a rotational test of the augmented femoral head implant was performed in the latter study. Therefore, it is tempting to speculate that a commercially available CaS-based bioresorbable bone cement seems to be more favourable for the use of implant augmentation.

Generally speaking, the advantageous characteristic properties of bioresorbable bone cement in comparison to classical PMMA-cement are obvious. They do not result in high temperatures during hardening with possible bone/cartilage damage, provide biomechanical stability, and are replaced by autologous bone over time [32].

As shown in this study, the application of bioresorbable bone cement through commonly used applicators for PMMA-cement was performed without any limitations and was safe. Microstructural evaluation showed a close interaction of the bioresorbable bone cement with the autologous trabecular bone structures. Objective evaluation showed an even closer indentation of bioresorbable cement in comparison to classical PMMA-cement by 21%.

Not only was the application of the bioresorbable cement safe, but it also led to a good distribution in the femoral head. Biomechanical evaluation with a non-destructive load test overall showed similar primary stability of the bioresorbable cement compared to PMMA-cement. At a closer look, the bioresorbable cement even showed a non-significantly higher stability of 25% at 200 N, which decreased to 3% at 400 N, possibly due to a settling effect.

Limitations of the Study

The major limitation of our study is the relatively small sample size. The true intergroup differences may have been more profound with a larger sample size.

Additional limitations arise from the chosen study design's cross-sectional character and the individual variability of donor specimens, with unknown underlying comorbidities possibly affecting the results.

The utilisation of human fresh frozen specimens may influence the distribution and reactivity of the injected bone cements. However, besides clinical application in humans, no superior study design exists for performing a feasibility study.

5. Conclusions

The reduced distance between trabecular bone and cement in the group of bioresorbable cement is an indication of better interlocking of the cement in the surrounding bone, which can be explained by the more fluid consistency of the bioresorbable cement. The fact that after loading, the cement/bone distance decreases in the bioresorbable-cement group but increases in the PMMA-group could be an expression of the different fatigue strength of PMMA-cement compared to the bioresorbable-cement. Whereas it can be suspected that PMMA-cement will not change its structure during loading, bioresorbable-cement might show some settling during loading, possibly explaining the closer indentation after loading. Although settling could be suspected with a decrease in biomechanical strength, no significant differences between PMMA-cement and bioresorbable-cement were observed in regard to dislocation of the fracture gap, axial stiffness, and the force curve of the tractus iliotibialis. Therefore, bioresorbable bone cement seems to inherit all the beneficial properties to be suitable for augmentation of osteosynthesis implants, and their use should be evaluated in a clinical study as the next step.

Author Contributions: Conceptualisation, C.L. (Christoph Linhart) and C.E.; methodology, C.L. (Christoph Linhart) and C.E.; investigation, M.K. (Matthias Kassube), M.S., C.L. (Christoph Linhart) and C.A.B.; resources, M.S. and A.G.; data curation, M.K. (Manuel Kistler), C.L. (Christoph Linhart), C.L. (Christopher Lampert) and C.A.B.; writing—original draft preparation, M.K. (Matthias Kassube) and C.L. (Christoph Linhart); writing—review and editing, C.L. (Christoph Linhart) and C.E.; visualization, M.K. (Matthias Kassube); supervision, W.B.; project administration, W.B.; funding acquisition, C.L. (Christoph Linhart). All authors have read and agreed to the published version of the manuscript.

Funding: This study was funded by FöFoLe-Grant Reg.-No. 1043 of Ludwig-Maximilians-University of Munich.

Institutional Review Board Statement: The study was conducted in accordance with the Declaration of Helsinki and approved by the Ethics Committee of the University of Munich, LMU, Germany (No. 8–030).

Informed Consent Statement: Not applicable.

Data Availability Statement: The data presented in this study are available on request from the corresponding author. The data are not publicly available due to privacy reasons.

Conflicts of Interest: The authors declare no conflict of interest. The funders had no role in the design of the study; in the collection, analyses, or interpretation of data; in the writing of the manuscript; or in the decision to publish the results.

References

1. Friedman, S.M.; Mendelson, D.A. Epidemiology of fragility fractures. *Clin. Geriatr. Med.* **2014**, *30*, 175–181. [CrossRef]
2. Kammerlander, C.; Gosch, M.; Kammerlander-Knauer, U.; Luger, T.J.; Blauth, M.; Roth, T. Long-term functional outcome in geriatric hip fracture patients. *Arch. Orthop. Trauma Surg.* **2011**, *131*, 1435–1444. [CrossRef]
3. Neuerburg, C.; Gosch, M.; Blauth, M.; Bocker, W.; Kammerlander, C. Augmentation techniques on the proximal femur. *Unfallchirurg* **2015**, *118*, 755–764. [CrossRef] [PubMed]
4. Vigano, M.; Pennestri, F.; Listorti, E.; Banfi, G. Proximal hip fractures in 71,920 elderly patients: Incidence, epidemiology, mortality and costs from a retrospective observational study. *BMC Public Health* **2023**, *23*, 1963. [CrossRef] [PubMed]
5. Zhu, Q.; Xu, X.; Yang, X.; Chen, X.; Wang, L.; Liu, C.; Lin, P. Intramedullary nails versus sliding hip screws for AO/OTA 31-A2 trochanteric fractures in adults: A meta-analysis. *Int. J. Surg.* **2017**, *43*, 67–74. [CrossRef]
6. Shen, L.; Zhang, Y.; Shen, Y.; Cui, Z. Antirotation proximal femoral nail versus dynamic hip screw for intertrochanteric fractures: A meta-analysis of randomized controlled studies. *Orthop. Traumatol. Surg. Res.* **2013**, *99*, 377–383. [CrossRef] [PubMed]
7. Guo, Q.; Shen, Y.; Zong, Z.; Zhao, Y.; Liu, H.; Hua, X.; Chen, H. Percutaneous compression plate versus proximal femoral nail anti-rotation in treating elderly patients with intertrochanteric fractures: A prospective randomized study. *J. Orthop. Sci.* **2013**, *18*, 977–986. [CrossRef] [PubMed]
8. Ariza-Vega, P.; Kristensen, M.T.; Martin-Martin, L.; Jimenez-Moleon, J.J. Predictors of long-term mortality in older people with hip fracture. *Arch. Phys. Med. Rehabil.* **2015**, *96*, 1215–1221. [CrossRef]

9. Fensky, F.; Nuchtern, J.V.; Kolb, J.P.; Huber, S.; Rupprecht, M.; Jauch, S.Y.; Sellenschloh, K.; Puschel, K.; Morlock, M.M.; Rueger, J.M.; et al. Cement augmentation of the proximal femoral nail antirotation for the treatment of osteoporotic pertrochanteric fractures--a biomechanical cadaver study. *Injury* **2013**, *44*, 802–807. [CrossRef]
10. Ehrnthaller, C.; Olivier, A.C.; Gebhard, F.; Durselen, L. The role of lesser trochanter fragment in unstable pertrochanteric A2 proximal femur fractures—Is refixation of the lesser trochanter worth the effort? *Clin. Biomech.* **2017**, *42*, 31–37. [CrossRef]
11. Kammerlander, C.; Doshi, H.; Gebhard, F.; Scola, A.; Meier, C.; Linhart, W.; Garcia-Alonso, M.; Nistal, J.; Blauth, M. Long-term results of the augmented PFNA: A prospective multicenter trial. *Arch. Orthop. Trauma Surg.* **2014**, *134*, 343–349. [CrossRef] [PubMed]
12. Kammerlander, C.; Gebhard, F.; Meier, C.; Lenich, A.; Linhart, W.; Clasbrummel, B.; Neubauer-Gartzke, T.; Garcia-Alonso, M.; Pavelka, T.; Blauth, M. Standardised cement augmentation of the PFNA using a perforated blade: A new technique and preliminary clinical results. A prospective multicentre trial. *Injury* **2011**, *42*, 1484–1490. [CrossRef] [PubMed]
13. Kammerlander, C.; Hem, E.S.; Klopfer, T.; Gebhard, F.; Sermon, A.; Dietrich, M.; Bach, O.; Weil, Y.; Babst, R.; Blauth, M. Cement augmentation of the Proximal Femoral Nail Antirotation (PFNA)—A multicentre randomized controlled trial. *Injury* **2018**, *49*, 1436–1444. [CrossRef]
14. Boner, V.; Kuhn, P.; Mendel, T.; Gisep, A. Temperature evaluation during PMMA screw augmentation in osteoporotic bone--an in vitro study about the risk of thermal necrosis in human femoral heads. *J. Biomed. Mater. Res. B Appl. Biomater.* **2009**, *90*, 842–848. [CrossRef] [PubMed]
15. Sermon, A.; Slock, C.; Coeckelberghs, E.; Seys, D.; Panella, M.; Bruyneel, L.; Nijs, S.; Akiki, A.; Castillon, P.; Chipperfield, A.; et al. Quality indicators in the treatment of geriatric hip fractures: Literature review and expert consensus. *Arch. Osteoporos.* **2021**, *16*, 152. [CrossRef]
16. Rauschmann, M.; Vogl, T.; Verheyden, A.; Pflugmacher, R.; Werba, T.; Schmidt, S.; Hierholzer, J. Bioceramic vertebral augmentation with a calcium sulphate/hydroxyapatite composite (Cerament SpineSupport): In vertebral compression fractures due to osteoporosis. *Eur. Spine J.* **2010**, *19*, 887–892. [CrossRef]
17. Abramo, A.; Geijer, M.; Kopylov, P.; Tagil, M. Osteotomy of distal radius fracture malunion using a fast remodeling bone substitute consisting of calcium sulphate and calcium phosphate. *J. Biomed. Mater. Res. B Appl. Biomater.* **2010**, *92*, 281–286. [CrossRef]
18. Nusselt, T.; Hofmann, A.; Wachtlin, D.; Gorbulev, S.; Rommens, P.M. CERAMENT treatment of fracture defects (CERTiFy): Protocol for a prospective, multicenter, randomized study investigating the use of CERAMENT™ BONE VOID FILLER in tibial plateau fractures. *Trials* **2014**, *15*, 75. [CrossRef]
19. Hofmann, A.; Gorbulev, S.; Guehring, T.; Schulz, A.P.; Schupfner, R.; Raschke, M.; Huber-Wagner, S.; Rommens, P.M.; Group, C.E.S. Autologous Iliac Bone Graft Compared with Biphasic Hydroxyapatite and Calcium Sulfate Cement for the Treatment of Bone Defects in Tibial Plateau Fractures: A Prospective, Randomized, Open-Label, Multicenter Study. *J. Bone Jt. Surg. Am.* **2020**, *102*, 179–193. [CrossRef]
20. Dong, C.; Klimek, P.; Abacherli, C.; De Rosa, V.; Krieg, A.H. Percutaneous cyst aspiration with injection of two different bioresorbable bone cements in treatment of simple bone cyst. *J. Child. Orthop.* **2020**, *14*, 76–84. [CrossRef]
21. Masala, S.; Nano, G.; Marcia, S.; Muto, M.; Fucci, F.P.; Simonetti, G. Osteoporotic vertebral compression fracture augmentation by injectable partly resorbable ceramic bone substitute (Cerament I SPINESUPPORT): A prospective nonrandomized study. *Neuroradiology* **2012**, *54*, 1245–1251. [CrossRef]
22. Marcia, S.; Boi, C.; Dragani, M.; Marini, S.; Marras, M.; Piras, E.; Anselmetti, G.C.; Masala, S. Effectiveness of a bone substitute (CERAMENT™) as an alternative to PMMA in percutaneous vertebroplasty: 1-year follow-up on clinical outcome. *Eur. Spine J.* **2012**, *21* (Suppl. 1), S112–S118. [CrossRef] [PubMed]
23. Bouxsein, M.L.; Boyd, S.K.; Christiansen, B.A.; Guldberg, R.E.; Jepsen, K.J.; Muller, R. Guidelines for assessment of bone microstructure in rodents using micro-computed tomography. *J. Bone Min. Res.* **2010**, *25*, 1468–1486. [CrossRef] [PubMed]
24. Yamamoto, N.; Ogawa, T.; Banno, M.; Watanabe, J.; Noda, T.; Schermann, H.; Ozaki, T. Cement augmentation of internal fixation for trochanteric fracture: A systematic review and meta-analysis. *Eur. J. Trauma Emerg. Surg.* **2022**, *48*, 1699–1709. [CrossRef] [PubMed]
25. Schuetze, K.; Eickhoff, A.; Roderer, G.; Gebhard, F.; Richter, P.H. Osteoporotic Bone: When and How to Use Augmentation? *J. Orthop. Trauma* **2019**, *33* (Suppl. 8), S21–S26. [CrossRef]
26. Mattie, R.; Brar, N.; Tram, J.T.; McCormick, Z.L.; Beall, D.P.; Fox, A.; Saltychev, M. Vertebral Augmentation of Cancer-Related Spinal Compression Fractures: A Systematic Review and Meta-Analysis. *Spine* **2021**, *46*, 1729–1737. [CrossRef]
27. Joeris, A.; Kabiri, M.; Galvain, T.; Vanderkarr, M.; Holy, C.E.; Plaza, J.Q.; Tien, S.; Schneller, J.; Kammerlander, C. Cost-Effectiveness of Cement Augmentation Versus No Augmentation for the Fixation of Unstable Trochanteric Fractures. *J. Bone Jt. Surg. Am.* **2022**, *104*, 2026–2034. [CrossRef]
28. Schuetze, K.; Ehinger, S.; Eickhoff, A.; Dehner, C.; Gebhard, F.; Richter, P.H. Cement augmentation of the proximal femur nail antirotation: Is it safe? *Arch. Orthop. Trauma Surg.* **2021**, *141*, 803–811. [CrossRef]
29. Nilsson, M.; Zheng, M.H.; Tagil, M. The composite of hydroxyapatite and calcium sulphate: A review of preclinical evaluation and clinical applications. *Expert. Rev. Med. Devices* **2013**, *10*, 675–684. [CrossRef]
30. Pesch, S.; Hanschen, M.; Greve, F.; Zyskowski, M.; Seidl, F.; Kirchhoff, C.; Biberthaler, P.; Huber-Wagner, S. Treatment of fracture-related infection of the lower extremity with antibiotic-eluting ceramic bone substitutes: Case series of 35 patients and literature review. *Infection* **2020**, *48*, 333–344. [CrossRef]

31. Hoelscher-Doht, S.; Heilig, M.; von Hertzberg-Boelch, S.P.; Jordan, M.C.; Gbureck, U.; Meffert, R.H.; Heilig, P. Experimental magnesium phosphate cement paste increases torque of trochanteric fixation nail advanced blades in human femoral heads. *Clin. Biomech.* **2023**, *109*, 106088. [CrossRef] [PubMed]
32. Hettwer, W.; Horstmann, P.F.; Bischoff, S.; Gullmar, D.; Reichenbach, J.R.; Poh, P.S.P.; van Griensven, M.; Gras, F.; Diefenbeck, M. Establishment and effects of allograft and synthetic bone graft substitute treatment of a critical size metaphyseal bone defect model in the sheep femur. *APMIS* **2019**, *127*, 53–63. [CrossRef] [PubMed]

Disclaimer/Publisher's Note: The statements, opinions and data contained in all publications are solely those of the individual author(s) and contributor(s) and not of MDPI and/or the editor(s). MDPI and/or the editor(s) disclaim responsibility for any injury to people or property resulting from any ideas, methods, instructions or products referred to in the content.

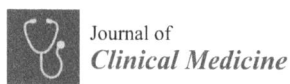

Article

The Outcome of under 10 mm Single-Incision Surgery Using a Non-Specialized Volar Plate in Distal Radius Fractures: A Retrospective Comparative Study

Chang-Yu Huang [1,2], Chia-Che Lee [1], Chih-Wei Chen [1], Ming-Hsiao Hu [1], Kuan-Wen Wu [1], Ting-Ming Wang [1], Jyh-Horng Wang [1] and Tzu-Hao Tseng [1,*]

1 Department of Orthopaedic Surgery, National Taiwan University Hospital, Taipei City 100225, Taiwan
2 Department of Orthopaedic Surgery, En Chu Kong Hospital, New Taipei City 237, Taiwan
* Correspondence: b92401004@gmail.com; Tel.: +886-2-23123456 (ext. 65228)

Abstract: Background: The distal radius fracture is a common orthopedic injury. We aimed to share the surgical steps and investigate the outcomes of treating distal radius fractures with wounds ≤ 10 mm using a globally accessible locking plate. Methods: We collected 46 patients who underwent surgery via a <10 mm wound, with a control group consisting of 40 patients who underwent conventional procedures. Both groups were treated using the same volar plate. We compared the radiographic reduction quality, including volar tilt angle, radial inclination angle, and ulna variance. Additionally, clinical outcomes, such as pain assessed using VAS, Q-Dash score, and PRWE, were evaluated. Patient satisfaction with the wound was also analyzed. The follow-up time for the clinical outcomes was 24.2 ± 13.47 months. Results: There were no differences in the quality of reduction in parameters such as the volar tilt angle ($p = 0.762$), radial inclination angle ($p = 0.986$), and ulna variance ($p = 0.166$). Both groups exhibited comparable results in pain VAS ($p = 0.684$), Q-Dash score ($p = 0.08$), and PRWE ($p = 0.134$). The ≤10 mm incision group displayed an increase in satisfaction with the wound ($p < 0.001$). Conclusions: Treating distal radius fractures with a <10 mm wound using a non-specialized locking plate is a feasible approach. It does not compromise the quality of fracture reduction or functional scores and improves wound satisfaction.

Keywords: distal radius fracture; open reduction and internal fixation; minimally invasive; functional outcome; radiographic outcome

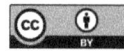

Citation: Huang, C.-Y.; Lee, C.-C.; Chen, C.-W.; Hu, M.-H.; Wu, K.-W.; Wang, T.-M.; Wang, J.-H.; Tseng, T.-H. The Outcome of under 10 mm Single-Incision Surgery Using a Non-Specialized Volar Plate in Distal Radius Fractures: A Retrospective Comparative Study. *J. Clin. Med.* 2023, 12, 7670. https://doi.org/10.3390/jcm12247670

Academic Editors: Christian Ehrnthaller and Yuji Uchio

Received: 16 November 2023
Revised: 6 December 2023
Accepted: 12 December 2023
Published: 14 December 2023

Copyright: © 2023 by the authors. Licensee MDPI, Basel, Switzerland. This article is an open access article distributed under the terms and conditions of the Creative Commons Attribution (CC BY) license (https://creativecommons.org/licenses/by/4.0/).

1. Introduction

Distal radius fractures are common orthopedic injuries, frequently resulting from falls or accidents and affecting individuals of all age groups [1]. Treatment options vary based on the fracture's severity, including casting [2,3] or surgery [4,5]. These fractures can lead to pain, reduced wrist function, and potential complications, imposing healthcare costs, impacting workforce productivity, and straining the healthcare system [6–9]. Effective diagnosis, treatment, and rehabilitation are vital to mitigate their overall impact on patients and society.

Surgical treatment for distal radius fractures offers advantages for people with higher functional demand requiring a faster recovery [10]. It enables the precise realignment of fractured bones, reducing the risk of malunion. Surgery often involves the use of internal fixation devices, such as locking plates and screws, to provide stable support during the healing process [11–13]. This approach is the prevailing trend in distal radius fracture surgery, maintaining alignment, enhancing stability, and facilitating early mobilization and wrist function recovery [12,13]. Locking plate systems are increasingly favored by orthopedic surgeons for their reliability and effectiveness in addressing complex fractures, leading to improved patient outcomes.

Minimally invasive surgery for distal radius fractures is currently a popular trend, typically defined by incisions smaller than three centimeters [14]. Patient satisfaction is more closely related to whether the fracture is properly aligned, while the size of the wound only affects aesthetics. However, due to advancements in surgical techniques and implant development, surgeons aspire to achieve equivalent treatment outcomes with smaller incisions, thereby minimizing the wound size to 1–1.5 cm [14–18]. Nonetheless, there are still some limitations, with certain studies requiring two incisions [14] or specially designed plates [14,15]. Most reports did not compare these smaller incisions to conventional techniques [14,17,18], making it challenging to assess their impact on fracture reduction and patient satisfaction regarding function and aesthetics.

This study aimed to overcome these limitations by performing distal radius fracture surgery with an ultimate small incision smaller than or equal to one centimeter. We utilized widely available locking plates instead of specially designed ones and compared the outcomes to conventional surgery. Our objectives were to assess the impact on fracture reduction, patient functional outcomes, and satisfaction with the incision. This study also details the surgical procedures, demonstrating how to perform distal radius fracture surgery with incisions smaller than or equal to one centimeter using non-specialized locking plates.

2. Materials and Methods

2.1. Patients

We conducted a retrospective cohort study in the corresponding author's hospital. The study was approved by the hospital's Ethics Committee, and a waiver of informed consent for the retrospective use of patient data (approval number: 202308080RIND) was obtained. We investigated 46 consecutive patients who underwent ultimate mini-incision surgery using a 2.4 mm Variable-Angle LCP Two-Column Volar Distal Radius Plate (Depuy Synthes, Oberdorf, Switzerland) for a distal radius fracture between August 2019 and January 2023. The ultimate mini-incision surgeries were all performed using THT. The indication for ultimate incision surgery was AO/OTA classification type 23A1, 23A2, 23A3, 23B3, and 23C1 adult fractures with one of the following fracture displacements: (1) step-off more than 2 mm, (2) dorsal tilt more than 15 degrees, (3) radial inclination less than 15 degrees, or (4) radial shortening more than 5 mm. Fracture types other than AO/OTA classification types 23A1, 23A2, 23A3, 23B3, and 23C1 for distal radius fractures were excluded. We collected another group of patients as the control group. These were 40 consecutive patients who underwent conventional incision surgery using the same locking plate, with the same surgical indications in the same period mentioned above. The conventional incision surgeries were performed by the co-authors, including CCL, CWC, MHH, KWW, and TMW. Figure 1 shows the flowchart of this study. The higher number of surgeons using conventional incisions despite a lower total number of patients is not indicative of these surgeons having less experience. The reason lies in the fact that in our hospital, younger surgeons have a higher frequency of on-call duties. In the years 2019–2023, THT had more on-call duties, resulting in a greater volume of fracture surgeries. On the other hand, more senior surgeons, such as those using conventional incisions, having already gone through stages with increased on-call responsibilities, contribute to this pattern. The follow-up time for clinical outcomes was 24.2 ± 13.47 months (ranging from 9 to 50 months).

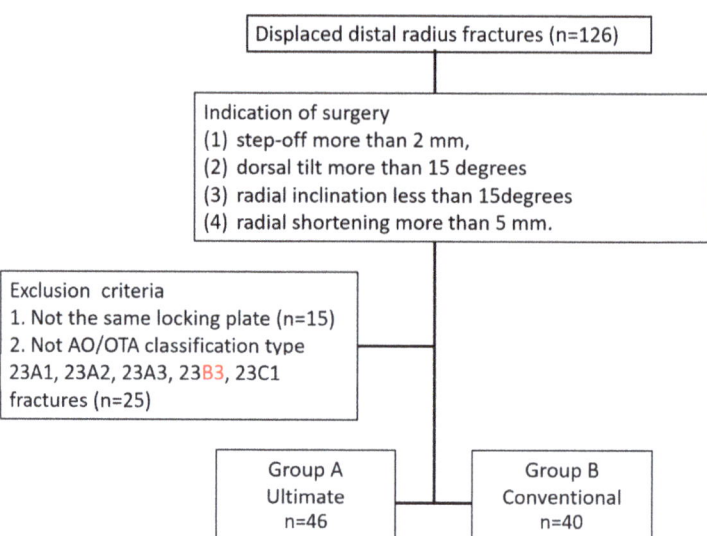

Figure 1. Flowchart of the study.

2.2. Surgical Techniques of Ultimate Incision Surgery

For the ultimate mini-incision surgery, the surgical technique was primarily based on a previous publication with modifications [18]. A pneumatic tourniquet is used at a pressure of 250 mmHg. A vertical incision between 8 and 10 mm was made at the radial border of the flexor carpi radialis (FCR). The distal end of the incision is about 25–30 mm proximal to the distal wrist crease (Figure 2). In general, if the pre-operative X-ray indicates that the main fracture line is within 2 cm of the joint, the surgical incision will start from the proximal 25 mm of the wrist crease. Conversely, if it is beyond 2 cm, it will start from 30 mm. The subcutaneous tissue and the superficial tendon sheath are incised using scissors as long as possible. When incising the proximal sheath, flexion of the wrist can help increase the incised length (Figure 3). After retracting the FCR tendon ulnarly, the deep tendon sheath is incised in the same manner.

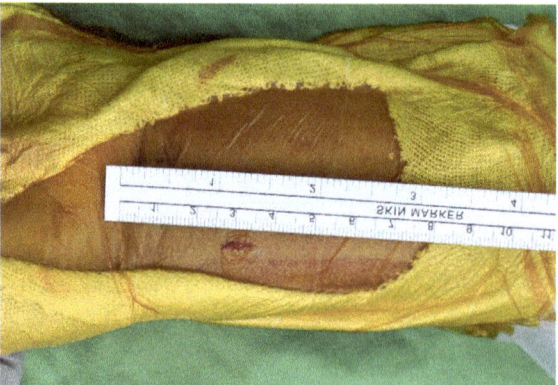

Figure 2. The distal end of the incision was about 25–30 mm proximal to the distal wrist crease. The length of the incision was about 8–10 mm.

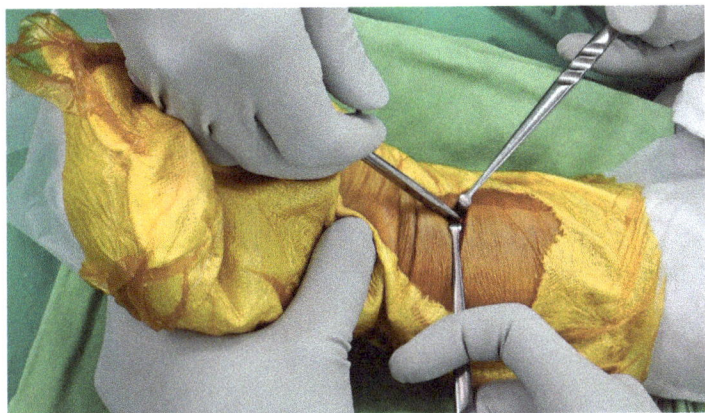

Figure 3. Flexion of the wrist can help increase the incised length of the proximal subcutaneous tissue and tendon sheath.

In our experience, in such a small incision, deliberately preserving the pronator quadratus muscle can actually make this muscle more susceptible to injury during the surgical procedure and harder to repair. Therefore, we vertically incise the distal half of the pronator quadratus during surgery, preserving approximately 3 mm of the muscle on the radial side to facilitate subsequent repair.

Subsequently, we begin by reducing the displaced fracture. If the volar cortex is still in contact, the fracture can typically be realigned through a simple manipulation. For instance, one finger can be inserted into the wound to support the volar cortex of the proximal fragment, while the other four fingers push the distal fragment towards the volar side to assist in reduction. Alternatively, with the fracture site as the pivot point, a bone elevator can also be used to elevate the distal fragment displaced towards the dorsal side back to its original position. In cases where there is a significant dorsal tilt, the Kapandji technique with a K-wire in the dorsal fracture may be necessary to aid in restoring volar tilt. Additionally, since we exclude comminuted joint fractures, such as type C2 and C3 fractures, and only include simple articular fractures (type C1), simply reducing the fracture line extending from the joint to the volar cortex allows joint reduction. An example of a type C1 fracture is shown in Figure 4. If managing comminuted joint fractures, the use of the ultimate incision is not recommended.

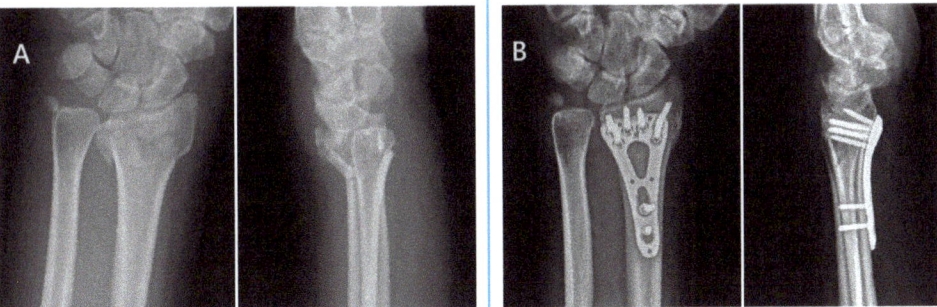

Figure 4. Type C1 fracture. (**A**) Pre-operative X-ray and (**B**) post-operative X-ray.

After reducing the fracture, we typically start by temporarily stabilizing it with a K-wire, followed by inserting the locking plate into the wound. We utilize a 2.4 mm variable-angle LCP two-column volar distal radius plate (Depuy Synthes). In terms of plate length, we select a plate with two shaft holes, and the choice between the narrow design and the standard design is made based on the size of the bone. When inserting the plate, it's essential to be mindful that the plate should be oriented perpendicular to the skin, allowing one distal corner of the plate to enter the wound first (Figure 5). Attempting to use a retractor to open the wound at this stage is not beneficial and may lead to increased wound tearing or exacerbation of the skin condition. Once the plate is inserted, it is important to ensure that the pronator quadratus is not beneath the plate. We then check the plate position with an image intensifier.

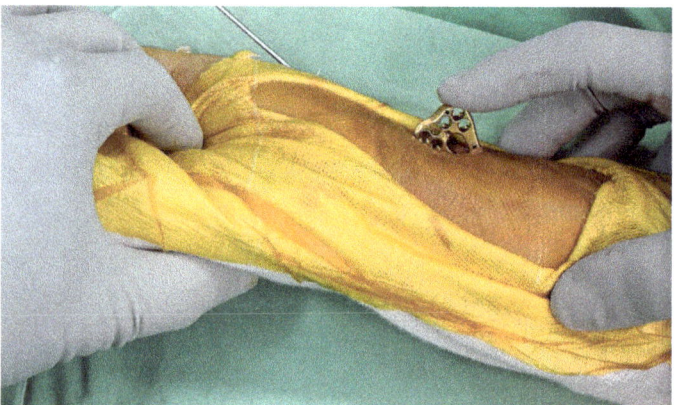

Figure 5. Insert the plate into the surgical wound. The plate should be oriented perpendicular to the skin, allowing one distal corner of the plate to enter the wound first.

Once the correct position of the locking plate is confirmed, we will use provisional K-wires through the plate to keep it in an optimal position during the drilling and screw application. Subsequently, screws will be further inserted into the bone. Due to the smaller incision, it is recommended to place the retractors on the same side of the wound (Figure 6). Typically, within the surgical field, only the screw hole to be inserted and its immediate vicinity are visible. As long as this mobile window approach is employed, inserting distal screws should not pose any difficulty. When inserting screws near the proximal end, as mentioned earlier, it is important to maximize wrist flexion to ensure visibility of the proximal screw hole. Generally, we use six locking screws in the distal fragment and one cortical screw and one locking screw in the diaphysis.

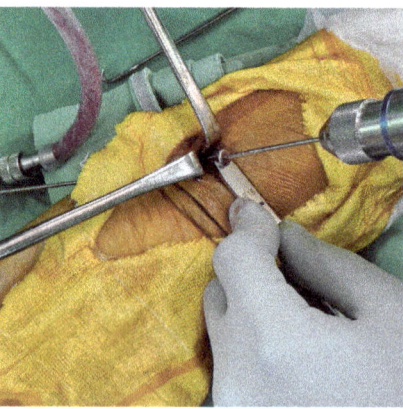

Figure 6. During drilling and screw insertion, it is recommended to place the retractors on the same side of the wound.

When all the screws were in place, we proceeded to suture the pronator quadratus using a 2-0 Vicryl suture with a 5/8 circle needle. Due to the limited visibility, we first retracted the side where the needle was to be inserted and then retracted the other side to suture the muscle on that side (Figure 7). In cases of significant displacement of the fracture, the pronator quadratus is often partially injured. Therefore, under normal circumstances, we were able to suture more than 2/3 of the dissected muscle, but suturing the most distal portion of the muscle was more challenging. The wound is finally closed with subcutaneous sutures using 3-0 Vicryl followed by 4-0 Vicryl in sequence (Figure 8). After the surgery, we instruct patients to wear a splint for two weeks for protection. After the two-week period, patients are no longer required to wear the splint, and we encourage them to start gentle wrist exercises.

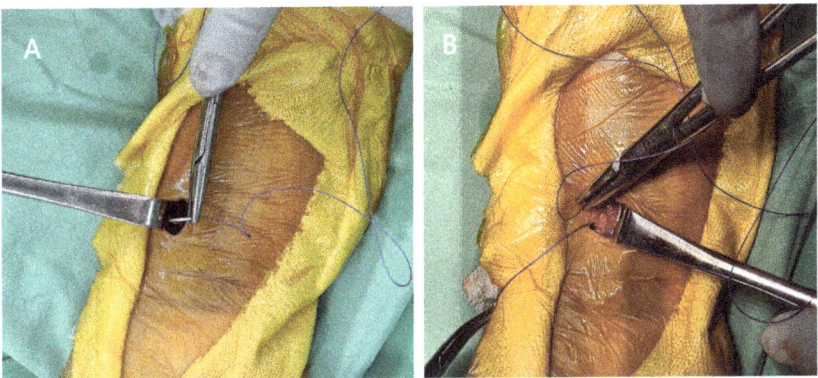

Figure 7. Pronator quadratus repair. (**A**) Retract the radial side where the needle was to be inserted first. (**B**) Retract the other side to suture the muscle on that side.

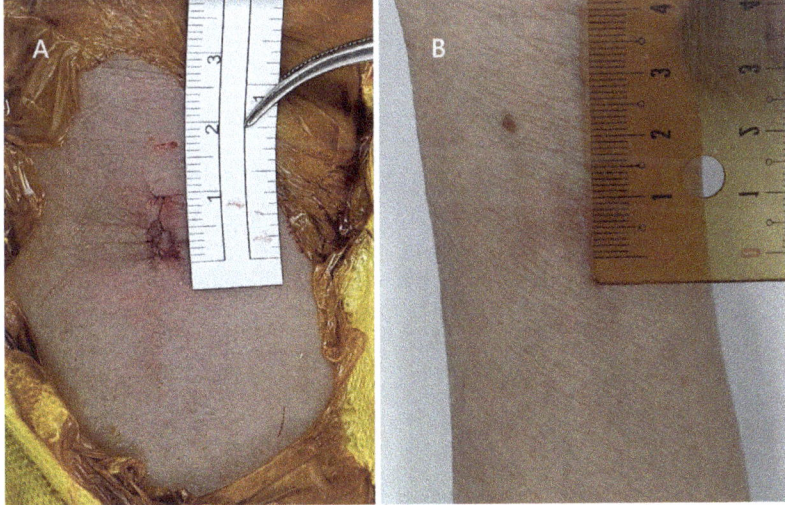

Figure 8. After wound closure. (**A**) Intraoperative photo. (**B**) An example of an 8 mm wound after wound healing.

2.3. Surgical Techniques of Conventional Incision Surgery

A pneumatic tourniquet is used at a pressure of 250 mmHg. A vertical incision between 30 and 50 mm is made at the radial border of the FCR. The distal end of the incision is about 15 mm proximal to the distal wrist crease. The subcutaneous tissue and the superficial tendon sheath were incised using scissors. After retracting the FCR tendon ulnarly, the deep tendon sheath was incised in the same manner. The pronator quadratus was incised vertically, preserving approximately 3 mm of the muscle on the radial side to facilitate subsequent repair. After the displaced fracture is reduced by manipulation and/or the Kapandji technique, a K-wire is often used through the radial styloid to temporarily stabilize it. A locking plate is then applied, and we check the plate position with an image intensifier. Screws are inserted for the final fixation of the fracture. The pronator quadratus is repaired using 2-0 Vicryl. The wound is finally closed with subcutaneous sutures using 3-0 Vicryl followed by 4-0 Vicryl in sequence. After the surgery, we instruct patients to wear a splint for two weeks for protection. After the two-week period, patients are no longer required to wear the splint, and we encourage them to start gentle wrist exercises.

2.4. Outcome Evaluations

The radiographic outcome, which included measurements of the volar tilt angle, radial inclination angle, ulna variance, and Soong grade [19] of the plate position, was assessed based on immediate post-operative plain films to determine the extent of fracture reduction. After the surgery, we conducted the same monthly X-ray imaging examination for the first three months post-surgery and approximately the sixth month to determine if there was any subsequent displacement. Taking into account measurement errors, we defined an angle change greater than 3 degrees and a distance measurement greater than 3 mm as indicative of subsequent displacement. All radiographic parameters were measured by CYH and THT in a blinded manner. Both observers measured the parameters twice, and the intervals between each time were >4 weeks.

We assessed patients' clinical outcomes in Oct 2023 using the visual analog scale (VAS) for pain intensity and patient-reported outcome measures, including the quick disabilities of the arm, shoulder, and hand (Q-DASH) score and patient-rated wrist evaluation (PRWE) [20]. Patient wound satisfaction was evaluated using a numerical rating scale (NRS), where patients provided a subjective score corresponding to their level of satisfaction, with 0 indicating the highest satisfaction and 10 indicating the lowest satisfaction. We also analyzed the complications in both groups, including those documented in the medical records and subsequent displacement of the fractures.

2.5. Statistical Analysis

All statistical analyses were performed using Real Statistics Resource Pack software (release 8.0) on a Microsoft Windows-based computer. The chi-square test was used to determine if two categorical variables between two groups are independent or if they are, in fact, related to one another. The Mann–Whitney U test was employed to compare the difference of continuous data between the two groups. Statistical significance was set at a p-value of <0.05. The interobserver and intraobserver reliabilities of the radiographic parameters were assessed using the intraclass correlation coefficient (ICC; model: two-way random; type: absolute agreement, single measures).

3. Results

3.1. Patient Characteristics

The characteristics of the patients are listed in Table 1. There were no significant differences among patients in terms of age, gender, BMI, injured side, and fracture classification. All cases in which an ultimate incision was intended result in an ultimate incision.

Table 1. Patient characteristics.

	Conventional	Ultimate Incision	p-Value
Number of patients	40	46	
Age, mean ± standard deviation (SD)	63.4 ± 16.0	60.7 ± 15.2	0.530
Sex (male/female)	12/28	8/38	0.167

Table 1. Cont.

	Conventional	Ultimate Incision	p-Value
Body mass index (BMI)	27.6 ± 2.1	26.5 ± 2.3	0.684
Laterality (right/left)	19/21	19/27	0.564
AO/OTA classification (A/B3/C1)	27/4/9	38/1/7	0.099

3.2. Radiographic Outcome

Regarding immediate post-operative radiographic outcome, there were no differences in the quality of fracture reduction in various parameters such as volar tilt angle, radial inclination angle, and ulna variance (Table 2). The mean time to union was 2.82 ± 0.4 months in the ultimate group and 2.68 ± 0.4 months in the conventional group ($p = 0.784$). The interobserver reliability (95% confidence interval of ICC: pre-operative volar tilt: 0.90–0.94, 0.89–0.93; radial inclination: 0.91–0.96, 0.90–0.95; ulna variance: 0.91–0.96, 0.88–0.94. Post-operative volar tilt: 0.90–0.94, 0.90–0.96; radial inclination: 0.89–0.94, 0.91–0.96; ulna variance: 0.88–0.94, 0.91–0.95 for each repeat) and intraobserver reliability (95% confidence interval of ICC: pre-operative volar tilt: 0.92–0.96, 0.90–0.94; radial inclination: 0.89–0.94, 0.91–0.96; ulna variance: 0.92–0.96, 0.90–0.95. Post-operative volar tilt: 0.91–0.96, 0.89–0.94; radial inclination: 0.89–0.96, 0.90–0.94; ulna variance: 0.88–0.95, 0.90–0.95 for each observer) were all high.

Table 2. Radiographic outcome.

	Conventional	Ultimate Incision	p-Value
Pre-operative parameter (mean ± SD)			
Volar tilt angle (°)	−13.1 ± 16.3	−14.6 ± 18.6	0.652
Radial inclination angle (°)	13.8 ± 9.8	15.0 ± 9.6	0.774
Ulna variance (mm)	3.1 ± 1.3	2.9 ± 1.5	0.446
Immediate post-operative parameter (mean ± SD)			
Volar tilt angle (°)	9.6 ± 5.0	9.0 ± 5.2	0.762
Radial inclination angle (°)	21.7 ± 4.2	21.9 ± 2.9	0.986
Ulna variance (mm)	0.5 ± 1.2	0.9 ± 1.2	0.166
Soong grade (grade 0/1/2)	20/18/2	29/14/3	0.378

3.3. Clinical Outcome

As for the clinical outcomes, both groups exhibited comparable results in the VAS, Q-Dash score, and PRWE. However, the ultimate mini-incision group displayed a significant increase in patient satisfaction with the wound, and this group also demonstrated a significantly shorter surgical duration compared to the other group (Table 3). The difference in surgical duration in minutes was 19.5 min.

Table 3. Clinical outcome.

Parameters (Mean ± SD)	Conventional	Ultimate Incision	p-Value
Pain VAS	0.7 ± 0.8	0.6 ± 0.7	0.684
Q-DASH	9.26 ± 10.6	5.42 ± 7.67	0.080
PRWE	12.2 ± 4.3	10.3 ± 4.1	0.134
Cosmetic NRS	1.93 ± 1.57	0.68 ± 0.87	<0.001
Surgical duration (min)	76.3 ± 22.4	59.8 ± 12.6	<0.001

The surgical duration is defined as the time from the first incision to the last suture.

3.4. Complications

In the ultimate mini-incision group, two cases experienced fracture re-displacement, while in the other group, one patient had an extensor pollicis longus rupture, and two had fracture re-displacement. Since all five patients were unwilling to undergo surgery again, conservative treatment was applied for these complications.

4. Discussion

The primary contribution of this study lies in confirming that, with the appropriate surgical indications, utilizing incisions smaller than one centimeter can yield clinical results and reduction quality comparable to conventional minimally invasive techniques. Moreover, there is a significant enhancement in patient satisfaction regarding the incision. Furthermore, the use of globally accessible locking plates in the surgery, as opposed to specially designed plates, provides surgeons reading this article with increased confidence in adopting this minimally invasive surgical approach by following our outlined procedural steps. The pearls and pitfalls of the technique are listed in Table 4.

Table 4. Pearls and pitfalls.

	Pearls	Pitfalls
Fracture type	Metaphysis and/or simple articular fractures	Avoid comminuted articular fractures.
Fracture reduction	1. Finger manipulation for fractures with volar cortices in contact; 2. Kapandji technique for large dorsal tilt; 3. Use of a bone levator, with the fracture site as the pivot point, to reduce the distal fragment;	Difficult to insert traditional reduction forceps into the ultimate incision.
Plate insertion	1. The plate is perpendicular to the skin, allowing one distal corner of the plate to enter the wound first; 2. Ensure that the pronator quadratus is not beneath the plate;	Avoid using retractors when inserting the plate.
Screw insertion	1. Mobile window approach; 2. Wrist flexion for proximal screws.	Avoid forceful wound retraction.

Many studies have explored the reduction of surgical incisions in the treatment of distal radius fractures. For example, Asmar et al. achieved open reduction and internal fixation of distal radius fractures through a 32 mm incision using a newly designed ultra-short plate, resulting in favorable clinical outcomes within a short surgical duration [21]. Other research endeavors have focused on further minimizing incision sizes. Lebailly et al., for instance, successfully utilized a volar plate (Step One®, Newclip Technics™, Haute-Goulaine, France) through a 15 mm incision, demonstrating its feasibility [21]. Subsequent investigations took a step further in reducing incision sizes. Ribeiro et al. reduced the incision to 1.2 cm, albeit necessitating two transverse incisions and the use of a specially designed plate [14]. Naito et al. reported a case series confirming that a 1 cm incision enables satisfactory functional recovery in patients [18], though the absence of a control group raises uncertainty about whether such small incisions might compromise clinical function and reduction quality. The present study builds upon these encouraging findings, aiming to extend the application of treating distal radius fractures with incisions smaller than or equal to one centimeter, utilizing a non-specially designed locking plate. We demonstrate that comparable quality of reduction and clinical outcomes can be achieved compared to larger incisions. Our results also indicate that the ultimate incisions significantly enhance patient satisfaction with the wound appearance. In our experience, patients are often surprised and impressed by the placement of the plate through such small incisions, boosting confidence in the surgeon's skill, which may be reflected in their satisfaction with the wound. Another unexpected finding is a significant reduction in surgical time. We attribute this to the smaller incisions and decreased soft tissue dissection, leading to a shorter duration for wound closure. Another potential contributing factor is the difference in surgeons; the diverse experiences and procedural rhythms among the surgical practitioners in the two groups may inevitably vary, possibly leading to the observed outcome.

Given that the pronator quadratus functions as a secondary forearm pronator and dynamically stabilizes the distal radioulnar joint, and an intact pronator quadratus can serve as a biological barrier for the flexor tendons, the question of whether the integrity or repair of the pronator quadratus contributes to clinical outcomes is a frequently debated topic [22–24]. Despite diverse perspectives in the literature [25–28], current high-level evidence suggests that the integrity or repair of the pronator quadratus does not definitively impact clinical results [22–24,29]. In our clinical practice, displaced fractures of the distal radius often coincide with a partial tear of the pronator quadratus. Attempting to preserve the pronator quadratus during surgery may also result in muscle injury, leading us to partially release the muscle during the procedure. Although there is no conclusive evidence mandating pronator quadratus repair, we have been using a mobile surgical window approach to repair the majority of the released muscle during surgery. Current follow-up results indicate no issues with flexor tendons, and patients demonstrate satisfactory functional scores. Another potential factor contributing to flexor tendon issues is the positioning of the locking plate. The reported rate of flexor tendon rupture after volar plates is around 0.57% [30–33], and some studies indicate that volar locking plate prominence is a risk factor for flexor tendon rupture, especially in Soong grade 2 cases [34]. Therefore, we made an effort during surgery to avoid unnecessarily placing the locking plate in Soong grade 2 conditions. This may be one of the reasons why there are currently no issues with flexor tendons, but long-term follow-up is necessary to confirm this.

In the "ultimate incision" group, there were two instances of post-operative re-displacement observed. We attribute this to the suboptimal placement of the locking plate. Taking one patient with a re-displaced fracture as an example, the plate was positioned too proximally, resulting in insufficient fixation strength of the distal screw on the distal bone fragment and subsequent re-displacement (Figure 9). Due to the constrained visibility in small incisions, there is a tendency for the plate to be situated in less-than-ideal positions, leading to fracture re-displacement. As a precautionary measure, we recommend placing the plate and inserting the initial 2–3 screws, followed by reassessing the plate position using an image intensifier. Once the position is confirmed to be satisfactory, the remaining screws can then be inserted to minimize the risk of fracture re-displacement.

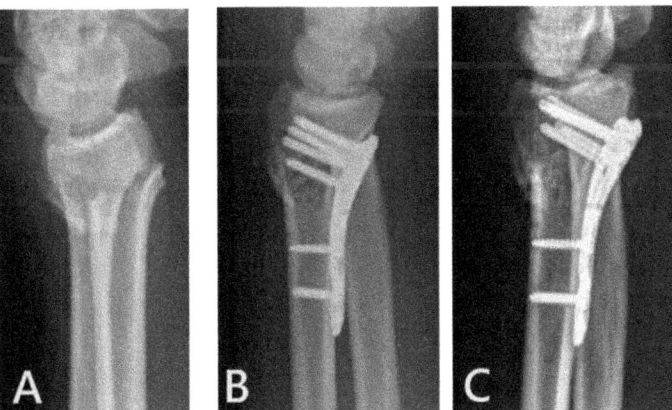

Figure 9. Re-displacement of fracture. (**A**) Pre-operative X-ray. (**B**) Immediate post-operative X-ray. (**C**) Follow-up X-ray.

This study has several limitations. Firstly, the patient follow-up duration is not extensive, with the shortest follow-up period being nine months. However, this duration is sufficient to assess reduction quality and alignment after the union of distal radius fractures.

Both patient groups underwent surgery during the same period, making the comparison of clinical outcomes between them representative, although long-term follow-up remains essential. Secondly, in our view, the "ultimate incision" approach may not be suitable for cases with comminuted joint surfaces. For joint fractures, we only included fractures with a C1 fracture pattern, as they usually behave like extraarticular fractures and can be well-managed even with the "ultimate incision" approach. Therefore, when using this surgical method, selecting appropriate surgical indications is crucial. Thirdly, as this is a retrospective study, there is still a possibility of selection bias in the fracture patterns of the patients. Future prospective studies are warranted to obtain a more thorough comparison in this aspect. Fourthly, because this study is a retrospective investigation and the number of patients is limited, although no serious complications occurred among these patients, it is not possible to confirm the potential for severe complications through this study. This needs to be verified through future larger-scale studies. Lastly, the ultimate incision group was all operated on by THT. Prior to performing surgery on this group of patients, the surgeon dedicated two years to surgeries on approximately 30 patients. During this period, the incision size progressed from 2 cm to 1.5 cm and was further reduced to 1 cm. Therefore, this surgical procedure entails a learning curve. The hope is that sharing insights from this study will help minimize the learning curve for other surgeons.

5. Conclusions

This study confirmed that treating distal radius fractures with wounds smaller than 10 mm using a non-specialized locking plate is a viable therapeutic approach. With regard to short-term outcomes, it does not compromise the quality of fracture reduction or functional scores and significantly improves wound satisfaction.

Author Contributions: C.-Y.H., C.-C.L., C.-W.C., M.-H.H., K.-W.W., T.-M.W., J.-H.W. and T.-H.T. contributed to the study's conception and design. Data collection and analysis were performed by C.-Y.H. and T.-H.T. The first draft of the manuscript was written by C.-Y.H. and T.-H.T. C.-Y.H., C.-C.L., C.-W.C., M.-H.H., K.-W.W., T.-M.W., J.-H.W. and T.-H.T. commented on previous versions of the manuscript. All authors have read and agreed to the published version of the manuscript.

Funding: This research received no external funding.

Institutional Review Board Statement: The study was conducted in accordance with the Declaration of Helsinki and approved by the Ethics Committee of the hospital (approval number: 202308080RIND) for studies involving humans.

Informed Consent Statement: Patient consent was waived because this is a retrospective study.

Data Availability Statement: The data that support the findings of this study are available from the corresponding author upon reasonable request.

Acknowledgments: We thank the nurse practitioners and resident surgeons of the National Taiwan University Hospital for their assistance during surgery.

Conflicts of Interest: The authors declare no conflict of interest.

References

1. Patel, D.; Kamal, R. Enhanced Approaches to the Treatment of Distal Radius Fractures. *Hand Clin.* **2023**, *39*, 515–521. [CrossRef] [PubMed]
2. van Delft, E.A.K.; van Bruggen, S.G.J.; van Stralen, K.J.; Bloemers, F.W.; Sosef, N.L.; Schep, N.W.L.; Vermeulen, J. Four weeks versus six weeks of immobilization in a cast following closed reduction for displaced distal radial fractures in adult patients: A multicentre randomized controlled trial. *Bone Jt. J.* **2023**, *105*, 993–999. [CrossRef] [PubMed]
3. Yang, Q.; Cai, G.; Liu, J.; Wang, X.; Zhu, D. Efficacy of cast immobilization versus surgical treatment for distal radius fractures in adults: A systematic review and meta-analysis. *Osteoporos. Int.* **2023**, *34*, 659–669. [CrossRef] [PubMed]
4. Chen, C.T.; Chou, S.H.; Huang, H.T.; Fu, Y.C.; Jupiter, J.B.; Liu, W.C. Comparison of distal radius fracture plating surgery under wide-awake local anesthesia no tourniquet technique and balanced anesthesia: A retrospective cohort study. *J. Orthop. Surg. Res.* **2023**, *18*, 746. [CrossRef] [PubMed]

5. Joo, P.Y.; Halperin, S.J.; Dhodapkar, M.M.; Adeclat, G.J.; Elaydi, A.; Wilhelm, C.; Grauer, J.N. Racial Disparities in Surgical Versus Nonsurgical Management of Distal Radius Fractures in a Medicare Population. *Hand* **2023**, 15589447231198267. [CrossRef] [PubMed]
6. Doering, T.A.; Mauck, B.M.; Calandruccio, J.H. Hot Topics in Hand and Wrist Surgery. *Orthop. Clin. N. Am.* **2021**, *52*, 149–155. [CrossRef] [PubMed]
7. Ensrud, K.E. Epidemiology of fracture risk with advancing age. *J. Gerontol. A Biol. Sci. Med. Sci.* **2013**, *68*, 1236–1242. [CrossRef] [PubMed]
8. Dempster, D.W. Osteoporosis and the burden of osteoporosis-related fractures. *Am. J. Manag. Care* **2011**, *17* (Suppl. S6), S164–S169.
9. Nellans, K.W.; Kowalski, E.; Chung, K.C. The epidemiology of distal radius fractures. *Hand Clin.* **2012**, *28*, 113–125. [CrossRef]
10. Oldrini, L.M.; Feltri, P.; Albanese, J.; Lucchina, S.; Filardo, G.; Candrian, C. Volar locking plate vs cast immobilization for distal radius fractures: A systematic review and meta-analysis. *EFORT Open Rev.* **2022**, *7*, 644–652. [CrossRef]
11. Nana, A.D.; Joshi, A.; Lichtman, D.M. Plating of the distal radius. *J. Am. Acad. Orthop. Surg.* **2005**, *13*, 159–171. [CrossRef] [PubMed]
12. Chaudhry, H.; Kleinlugtenbelt, Y.V.; Mundi, R.; Ristevski, B.; Goslings, J.C.; Bhandari, M. Are Volar Locking Plates Superior to Percutaneous K-wires for Distal Radius Fractures? A Meta-analysis. *Clin. Orthop. Relat. Res.* **2015**, *473*, 3017–3027. [CrossRef] [PubMed]
13. Zong, S.L.; Kan, S.L.; Su, L.X.; Wang, B. Meta-analysis for dorsally displaced distal radius fracture fixation: Volar locking plate versus percutaneous Kirschner wires. *J. Orthop. Surg. Res.* **2015**, *10*, 108. [CrossRef] [PubMed]
14. Ribeiro, E.; Campanholi, G.; Acherboim, M.; Ruggiero, G.M. Mini-Invasive Surgery for Distal Radius Fractures: A Double Incision under 12 mm. *J. Wrist Surg.* **2021**, *10*, 136–143. [CrossRef] [PubMed]
15. Lebailly, F.; Zemirline, A.; Facca, S.; Gouzou, S.; Liverneaux, P. Distal radius fixation through a mini-invasive approach of 15 mm. PART 1: A series of 144 cases. *Eur. J. Orthop. Surg. Traumatol.* **2014**, *24*, 877–890. [CrossRef] [PubMed]
16. Zemirline, A.; Naito, K.; Lebailly, F.; Facca, S.; Liverneaux, P. Distal radius fixation through a mini-invasive approach of 15 mm. Part 1: Feasibility study. *Eur. J. Orthop. Surg. Traumatol.* **2014**, *24*, 1031–1037. [CrossRef] [PubMed]
17. Zemirline, A.; Taleb, C.; Facca, S.; Liverneaux, P. Minimally invasive surgery of distal radius fractures: A series of 20 cases using a 15 mm anterior approach and arthroscopy. *Chir. Main* **2014**, *33*, 263–271. [CrossRef]
18. Naito, K.; Zemirline, A.; Sugiyama, Y.; Obata, H.; Liverneaux, P.; Kaneko, K. Possibility of Fixation of a Distal Radius Fracture With a Volar Locking Plate Through a 10 mm Approach. *Tech. Hand Up. Extrem. Surg.* **2016**, *20*, 71–76. [CrossRef]
19. Soong, M.; Earp, B.E.; Bishop, G.; Leung, A.; Blazar, P. Volar locking plate implant prominence and flexor tendon rupture. *J. Bone Jt. Surg. Am.* **2011**, *93*, 328–335. [CrossRef]
20. Kleinlugtenbelt, Y.V.; Krol, R.G.; Bhandari, M.; Goslings, J.C.; Poolman, R.W.; Scholtes, V.A.B. Are the patient-rated wrist evaluation (PRWE) and the disabilities of the arm, shoulder and hand (DASH) questionnaire used in distal radial fractures truly valid and reliable? *Bone Jt. Res.* **2018**, *7*, 36–45. [CrossRef]
21. Asmar, G.; Bellity, J.; Falcone, M.O. Surgical comfort and clinical outcomes of MIPO with an extra-short plate designed for distal radius fractures. *Eur. J. Orthop. Surg. Traumatol.* **2021**, *31*, 481–490. [CrossRef] [PubMed]
22. Zhang, D.; Meyer, M.A.; Earp, B.E.; Blazar, P. Role of Pronator Quadratus Repair in Volar Locking Plate Treatment of Distal Radius Fractures. *J. Am. Acad. Orthop. Surg.* **2022**, *30*, 696–702. [CrossRef] [PubMed]
23. Shi, F.; Ren, L. Is pronator quadratus repair necessary to improve outcomes after volar plate fixation of distal radius fractures? A systematic review and meta-analysis. *Orthop. Traumatol. Surg. Res.* **2020**, *106*, 1627–1635. [CrossRef] [PubMed]
24. Mulders, M.A.M.; Walenkamp, M.M.J.; Bos, F.; Schep, N.W.L.; Goslings, J.C. Repair of the pronator quadratus after volar plate fixation in distal radius fractures: A systematic review. *Strategies Trauma Limb Reconstr.* **2017**, *12*, 181–188. [PubMed]
25. Husain, T.M.; Jabbour, J.I.; Sudduth, J.D.; Lessard, A.S.; Patete, C.L.; Panthaki, Z.J.; Salloum, G.E. Pronator Quadratus Muscle Flap for Prevention of Flexor Tendon Rupture after Distal Radius Volar Plating. *Plast. Reconstr. Surg. Glob. Open* **2023**, *11*, e5227. [CrossRef] [PubMed]
26. Falk, S.S.I.; Maksimow, A.; Mittlmeier, T.; Gradl, G. Does access through the pronator quadratus influence pronation strength in palmar plate fixation of distal radius fractures in elderly patients? *Arch. Orthop. Trauma Surg.* **2023**, *143*, 5445–5454. [CrossRef]
27. Thalhammer, G.; Hruby, L.A.; Dangl, T.; Liebe, J.; Erhart, J.; Haider, T. Does the pronator-sparing approach improve functional outcome, compared to a standard volar approach, in volar plating of distal radius fractures? A prospective, randomized controlled trial. *J. Orthop. Traumatol.* **2023**, *24*, 16. [CrossRef]
28. Maniglio, M.; Truong, V.; Zumstein, M.; Bolliger, L.; McGarry, M.H.; Lee, T.Q. Should We Repair the Pronator Quadratus in a Distal Radius Fracture with an Ulnar Styloid Base Fracture? A Biomechanical Study. *J. Wrist Surg.* **2021**, *10*, 407–412. [CrossRef]
29. Turley, L.P.; Hurley, E.T.; White-Gibson, A.; Clesham, K.; Lyons, F. Pronator quadratus repair after volar plating for distal radius fractures: A systematic review and meta-analysis of randomized controlled trials. *Acta Orthop. Traumatol. Turc.* **2023**, *57*, 176–182. [CrossRef]
30. Lee, J.H.; Lee, J.K.; Park, J.S.; Kim, D.H.; Baek, J.H.; Kim, Y.J.; Yoon, K.T.; Song, S.H.; Gwak, H.G.; Ha, C.; et al. Complications associated with volar locking plate fixation for distal radius fractures in 1955 cases: A multicentre retrospective study. *Int. Orthop.* **2020**, *44*, 2057–2067. [CrossRef]
31. Azzi, A.J.; Aldekhayel, S.; Boehm, K.S.; Zadeh, T. Tendon Rupture and Tenosynovitis following Internal Fixation of Distal Radius Fractures: A Systematic Review. *Plast. Reconstr. Surg.* **2017**, *139*, 717e–724e. [CrossRef] [PubMed]

32. Sato, K.; Murakami, K.; Mimata, Y.; Doita, M. Incidence of tendon rupture following volar plate fixation of distal radius fractures: A survey of 2787 cases. *J. Orthop.* **2018**, *15*, 236–238. [CrossRef] [PubMed]
33. Thorninger, R.; Madsen, M.L.; Wæver, D.; Borris, L.C.; Duedal Rölfing, J.H. Complications of volar locking plating of distal radius fractures in 576 patients with 3.2 years follow-up. *Injury* **2017**, *48*, 1104–1109. [CrossRef] [PubMed]
34. Vasara, H.; Tarkiainen, P.; Stenroos, A.; Kosola, J.; Anttila, T.; Aavikko, A.; Nordback, P.H.; Aspinen, S. Higher Soong grade predicts flexor tendon issues after volar plating of distal radius fractures—A retrospective cohort study. *BMC Musculoskelet. Disord.* **2023**, *24*, 271. [CrossRef]

Disclaimer/Publisher's Note: The statements, opinions and data contained in all publications are solely those of the individual author(s) and contributor(s) and not of MDPI and/or the editor(s). MDPI and/or the editor(s) disclaim responsibility for any injury to people or property resulting from any ideas, methods, instructions or products referred to in the content.

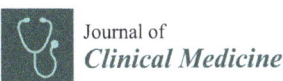

Systematic Review

Surgical Treatment in Post-Stroke Spastic Hands: A Systematic Review

Patricia Hurtado-Olmo [1], Ángela González-Santos [2,3,*], Javier Pérez de Rojas [4], Nicolás Francisco Fernández-Martínez [5,6,7], Laura del Olmo [8] and Pedro Hernández-Cortés [1,6,9]

1. Upper Limb Surgery Unit, Orthopedic Surgery Department, San Cecilio University Hospital of Granada, 18016 Granada, Spain
2. BIO 277 Group, Department of Physical Therapy, Faculty of Health Science, University of Granada, 18012 Granada, Spain
3. A02-Cuídate, Instituto de Investigación Biosanitaria, 18012 Granada, Spain
4. Department of Preventive Medicine and Public Health, San Cecilio University Hospital of Granada, 18016 Granada, Spain; jperezderojas@correo.ugr.es
5. Escuela Andaluza de Salud Pública (EASP), 18011 Granada, Spain
6. Instituto de Investigación Biosanitaria ibs, 18012 Granada, Spain
7. CIBER of Epidemiology and Public Health (CIBERESP), 28029 Madrid, Spain
8. Rehabilitation Department, San Cecilio University Hospital of Granada, 18016 Granada, Spain
9. Surgery Department, School of Medicine, Granada University, 18012 Granada, Spain
* Correspondence: angelagonzalez@ugr.es

Abstract: Background: For more than two decades, the surgical treatment of post-stroke spastic hands has been displaced by botulinum toxin therapy and is currently underutilized. **Objectives**: This article aimed to assess the potential of surgery for treating a post-stroke spastic upper extremity through a systematic review of the literature on surgical approaches that are adopted in different profiles of patients and on their outcomes and complications. **Methods**: Medline PubMed, Web of Science, SCOPUS, and Cochrane Library databases were searched for observational and experimental studies published in English up to November 2022. The quality of evidence was assessed using the Grading of Recommendations Assessment, Development and Evaluations (GRADE) system. **Results**: The search retrieved 501 abstracts, and 22 articles were finally selected. The GRADE-assessed quality of evidence was low or very low. The results of the reviewed studies suggest that surgery is a useful, safe, and enduring treatment for post-stroke spastic upper extremities, although most studied patients were candidates for hygienic improvements alone. Patients usually require an individualized combination of techniques. Over the past ten years, interest has grown in procedures that act on the peripheral nerve. **Conclusions**: Despite the lack of comparative studies on the effectiveness, safety, and cost of the treatments, botulinum toxin has displaced surgery for these patients. Studies to date have found surgery to be an effective and safe approach, but their weak design yields only poor-quality evidence, and clinical trials are warranted to compare these treatment options.

Keywords: stroke; muscle spasticity; upper extremity; hand; operative; surgical procedures; systematic review

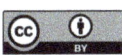

1. Introduction

Stroke is the principal cause of permanent disability among adults [1]. More than one-third of stroke patients develop spasticity that requires lifelong medical treatment and increases their dependence on others for daily living activities [2,3]. Upper extremity spasticity frequently results from upper motor neuron damage that is caused by stroke, traumatic brain injury, multiple sclerosis, spinal cord injury, or cerebral palsy [3]. The spastic upper extremity loses the functional position of the hand in space. Patients often have a deformity with internal rotation and shoulder adduction, elbow flexion, forearm pronation, wrist flexion, thumb adduction in palm, and/or flexion of triphalangeal fingers.

The deformity can have functional, cosmetic, and/or hygienic repercussions, depending on its intensity [4].

Currently, the first-choice treatment for localized spasticity is the intramuscular injection of botulinum toxin A [5–7], although this approach has some drawbacks. Thus, the injection can produce discomfort, the result persists for a maximum of only 3–4 months [8], and it is not useful for muscle or soft tissue contractures [9]. Around 30 years ago, patients with upper extremity spasticity after a first motor neuron injury were treated by surgery, but this option is now rarely considered in spasticity management protocols [7,10] and has been replaced by botulinum toxin therapy. However, no studies have compared the outcomes of these treatment modalities.

Various surgical procedures can be used to optimize function, reduce pain, and improve hygiene and esthetics in spastic upper extremities [11]. For instance, deformities can be corrected with single-event multilevel surgery, combining releases and elongations of soft tissues, tendon transfers, and joint stabilization procedures [12], or by centering on the nerve as the vehicle of spasticity. In this regard, different authors have proposed hyponeurotization, hyperselective neurectomy [13], and even rhizotomy of the C7 root of the affected extremity, followed by contralateral C7 nerve root transfer [14–16], to release the spasticity of the flexor musculature and strengthen weak extensor muscles.

Despite evidence of the long-term effectiveness of surgery in improving the function and hygiene of spastic upper extremities [12,17,18], it is now little used for this purpose [10], hampering evaluation of its true therapeutic potential and the risk of complications. We undertook a systematic review of the literature on surgical approaches that have been adopted in different profiles of patients and on their outcomes and complications, evaluating the quality of the published evidence. The aim was to guide clinical practice and to summarize available evidence for post-stroke patients with a spastic upper extremity who are interested in treatments other than botulinum toxin.

2. Material and Methods

This systemic review and its reporting followed the 2020 Preferred Reporting Items for Systematic reviews and Meta-Analyses (PRISMA) guidelines [19] (Table 1). The review protocol was prospectively registered in PROSPERO with ID CRD42022366686 (www.crd.york.ac.uk/PROSPERO, accessed on 15 November 2022).

Table 1. PICO format.

PICO for the research question: Which surgical approaches to adult patients with post-stroke spasticity of the upper extremity are effective in terms of improving their function, care, and quality of life?	
Patient	Adult patients with post-stroke spasticity of upper extremity.
Intervention	Surgical treatment of spastic upper extremity
Comparator	Untreated patients and/or (when available) patients treated with botulin toxin.
Results	• Improvement in function; • Improvement in pain; • Improvement in care; • Improvement in quality of life; • Complications.

3. Data Sources and Searches

The Medline PubMed, Web of Science, SCOPUS, and Cochrane Library databases were searched for studies up to November 2022 in accordance with the above protocol, using the following search strategy equation: (hand OR wrist OR thumb) AND (paralysis OR spastic* OR deformity* OR palsy) AND (transfer* OR surgery OR surgical OR neurectomy) AND (stroke OR cerebrovascular OR CVA). The reference lists of selected studies were also examined for relevant articles in a reverse search. Rayyan Systematic Review Screening

Software (https://www.rayyan.ai/, accessed on 16 May 2022) was employed to identify and eliminate duplicates.

4. Study Selection

The titles and abstracts of retrieved articles were independently screened by two reviewers (AGS, PHO) to select publications meeting the review's eligibility criteria. A third researcher (PHC) was consulted to resolve cases of disagreement. Inclusion criteria were as follows: observational or experimental design, from case series to clinical trials; evaluation of surgical treatment of post-stroke spastic upper extremity in patients of any age; and publication in English, regardless of the country of origin. Exclusion criteria were review articles, expert opinions, single case reports, exclusive focus on shoulder, cadaver research, qualitative research, and non-availability of whole text.

5. Data Extraction and Quality Assessment

The full texts of articles that were selected in the initial screening were reviewed independently by AGS and PHO to decide on their suitability for inclusion and to carry out data extraction and quality assessment procedures. PHC was consulted in cases of disagreement. Articles traced in the reverse search underwent the same process. Data were extracted on the author(s), year of publication, geographic origin, study type, sample size, baseline patient profile and diagnosis, surgical procedure, sample distribution, method of evaluation, efficacy and safety outcomes, and follow-up period.

The Grading of Recommendations Assessment, Development, and Evaluations (GRADE) was used to evaluate the quality of the evidence as high, moderate, low, or very low [20], and the Cochrane Collaboration tool served to assess the risk of bias. It was not possible to perform a meta-analysis due to the heterogeneity of patient samples, procedures, and outcomes.

6. Results

The search initially retrieved 501 abstracts (after removal of duplicates), 34 of which met the eligibility criteria. After reading the full texts of the studies, 19 were excluded, but 7 studies were added from the reverse search, leaving a total of 22 studies in the systematic review. Table 2 provides summarized information on the selected studies. Figure 1 depicts a flowchart of the review process.

Table 2. Summary of articles included in the review.

1st Author (Year)	Study Design	Sample Size: Patients Hands	Etiology of Spasticity	Groups (Surgical Procedure)	Gender	Age (Years)	Geographical Area	Time Since Diagnosis (Months)	Measurement Tools	Results	Complications	Follow-Up (Months)
Braun et al., 1974 [21]	Case series	23 / 24	CVA (21) TBI (3)	G1: STPTT	12M 12F	49 (23–63)	USA	36 (3–84)	Deformity correction Pain Hygiene	21 satisfactory results (87.5%) 3 unsatisfactory (12.5%)	3 recurrences of deformity (12.5%)	28 (12–30)
Keenan et al., 1987 [22]	Case series	27 / 27	CVA (6) TBI (20) Anoxia (1)	G1: FLFF	20M 7F	44 (5–62)	USA	45 (7–240)	- A 6-point functional scale for functional hands - Deformity correction for nonfunctional hands	- Functional hands: Improvement in 91%, deterioration in 9% - Nonfunctional hands: 100% improvement	Weak grip by overlengthening (9%) Unmasked intrinsic spasticity (30%)	33 (13–87)
Pinzur, 1991 [23]	Case series	18 / 18	CVA (13) CP (5)	G1: FOR and other selective tendon lengthening	NR	NR	USA	NR	Pinzur Functional scale [23]	Progression to assistive or independent function: 100%	NR	35 (24–64)
Pomerance y Keenan, 1996 [17]	Case series	14 / 15	TBI (9) CVA (5)	G1 STPTT + wrist arthrodesis	5M 9F	46 (26–81)	USA	NR	Hygiene Deformity correction	- Hygiene problem resolution: 100% - Mild under-correction: 26.67% - Mild over-correction: 33.33%	5 complications (33.3%): 2 arthrodesis nonunion and plate mobilization (13.3%) 1 postoperative edema 2 respiratory complications	12 (8–18)
Rayan y Young, 1999 [24]	Case series	9 / 11	CP (6) CVA (2) BTI (1)	G1: Wrist arthrodesis + 6 associated tendon release with hygienic goals	5M 4F	22	USA	NR	Subjective: - Satisfaction - Care burden Scale improvement Objective: - Union - Deformity correction - 17 tasks—hand function questionnaire	Subjective - Satisfaction: 8 total and 1 partial - Care burden scale: 9 improved Objective: - Union: 9 bone union - Deformity correction: mean of 85% - Secondary functional improvement: face washing, wheelchair propelling, and picking up objects: 90%	No complications reported	32 (12–62)

Table 2. Cont.

1st Author (Year)	Study Design	Sample Size: Patients Hands	Etiology of Spasticity	Groups (Surgical Procedure)	Gender	Age (Years)	Geographical Area	Time Since Diagnosis (Months)	Measurement Tools	Results	Complications	Follow-Up (Months)
Heijnen, 2008 [18]	Case series	6 / 6	CVA	G1: STPTT	6F	54 (36–73)	The Netherlands	60 (48–98)	- Inspection of skin condition - PROM: goniometry (shoulder, elbow, forearm, wrist, and metacarpophalangeal joints) - Muscle tone: Ashworth scale (shoulder, elbow, forearm, wrist, fingers, and thumb) - Hygiene: VAS - Pain: VAS	- Hygiene scored as very good (VAS:8.9) - Full passive opening of all hands - Resting position with flexion in MCP joints (20–60°) and extension of interphalangeal joints - Muscle tone: elbow, wrist and digit flexors improvement of 1–2 on Ashworth scale. Pain disappeared in 2 of 3 painful hands. All patients were satisfied.	No complications reported	19 (7–32)
Pappas, et al., 2010 [25]	Retrospective cohorts	23 / 23	CVA (16) TBI (6) Anoxia (1)	Surgery: STPTT + Ulnar motor branch neurectomy + wrist arthrodesis G1 (n = 11) Surgery without neurectomy of median nerve recurrent Branch G2 (n = 12) Surgery with neurectomy of median nerve	Group 1: 3M/8F Group 2: 5M/7F	48.35 (16–66) Group 1: 52.2 ± 15.7 Group 2: 44.8 ± 14.6	USA	NR	Postoperative intrinsic spastic TIP deformity development	Group 1: 5 of 11 patients developed intrinsic TIP deformity. Group 2: 2 of 12 patients developed intrinsic TIP deformity	No infection No sensation loss	16.1 (6–32)
Shin et al., 2010 [26]	Case series	14 / 14	CVA (5) CP (5) TBI (3) MS (1)	G1: Selective peripheral neurotomy (musculocutaneous)	10M 4F	37.29 (19–63)	Korea	-	MAS Satisfaction (VAS)	Patients' mean preoperative MAS score of 3.28 ± 0.12 was improved to 1.71 ± 0.12, 1.78 ± 0.18, 1.92 ± 0.16, and 1.78 ± 0.18 at 3, 6, and 12 months post-surgery and last follow-up. 65% satisfaction.	1 infection 1 transient paresthesia	30.71 (14–54)

Table 2. *Cont.*

1st Author (Year)	Study Design	Sample Size: Patients Hands	Etiology of Spasticity	Groups (Surgical Procedure)	Gender	Age (Years)	Geographical Area	Time Since Diagnosis (Months)	Measurement Tools	Results	Complications	Follow-Up (Months)
Facca et al., 2010 [27]	Case series	15 / 19	CVA (12) Lewy body disease (1) CP (1) Encephalitis (1)	G1: STPTT + complementary surgical procedures: arthrodesis, tendon surgery, peripheral neurotomy	11M 4F	55 (25–86)	France	116.8 (24–510)	MHS (6–20)	Mean MHS of 13.87 out of 20 pre-surgery vs. 9.67/20 post-surgery. Several imperfect results	2 incomplete thumb openings 2 unmasked intrinsic spasticity 1 wrist hyperextensions	6.13 (3–13)
Kwak et al., 2011 [28]	Case series	22 / 22	CVA (7) TBI (7) CP (7) MS (1)	G1: selective peripheral neurotomy (median nerve)	15M 7F	39.68 (19–63)	Korea	101 (19–367)	MAS Pain (VAS) Satisfaction (VAS)	Mean MAS score of 3.27 ± 0.46 pre-surgery vs. 1.82 ± 0.5, 1.73 ± 0.7, and 1.77 ± 0.81 at 3, 6, and 12 months post-surgery. Pain improved from 5.85 to 2.28. Satisfaction was 64.09 (30–90)	No recurrences 2 wound infections 1 paresthesia 1 dysesthesia	39.64 (14–93)
Anakwenze et al., 2013 [29]	Case series	42 / 42	CVA (30) TBI (11) CP (1)	G1: Fractional elbow flexor lengthening	26M 16F	50.9 (21–78)	USA	79.2	Passive and active motion. MAS	Active extension significantly improved (42° to 20°). Active arc of motion increased from 77 to 113°. Significant improvement in MAS recorded post-surgery (2.7 to 1.9).	2 wound infections	14
Thevenin-Lemoine et al., 2013 [30]	Case series	50 / 54	TBI (25) CP (10) CVA (11) Anoxia (2) Meningoencephalitis (2)	G1: Flexor-origin slide	35M 15F	32 ± 14 (15–65)	France	NR	Resting position of the wrist Zancolli and House Classifications	Wrist extension improved from −19 ± 35° pre-surgery to 21 ± 50° post-surgery. Significant improvement of 39°. Significant ($p < 0.01$) improvement in Zancolli and House scores. Ten nonfunctional hands became functional.	12 partial deformity recurrences 7 unmasked intrinsic spasticity	26 ± 21 (3–124)
Neuhaus et al., 2015 [31]	Case series	11 / 11	CVA (5) TBI (4) CP (2)	G1: Dorsal plate wrist arthrodesis	10M 1F	49 (19–78)	USA	240 (48–516)	Radiographic evaluation Deformity correction House score	Radiographic union 9/11 All patients improved appearance. Mean preoperative 66° of flexion changed to 4° of extension position. Mean House score of 2.8 pre-surgery vs. 4.8 post-surgery	2 edema and blisters 3 aggravated thumbs in palm deformity 1 Swan neck finger deformity	14 (3–42)

Table 2. Cont.

1st Author (Year)	Study Design	Sample Size: Patients Hands	Etiology of Spasticity	Groups (Surgical Procedure)	Gender	Age (Years)	Geographical Area	Time Since Diagnosis (Months)	Measurement Tools	Results	Complications	Follow-Up (Months)
Zheng et al., 2017 [16]	Randomized controlled trial	36 / 36	CP (13) TBI (12) CVA (9) Encephalitis (2)	G1: Contralateral C7 transfer + rehabilitation G2: Rehabilitation	36M	Group 1: 27 ± 9 Group 2: 26 ± 8	China	180 ± 108	UEFM MAS (assessment of five points, each scored from 0 to 5, with higher scores indicating more spasticity) Neurophysiological and fMRI assessment	Mean increase in Fugl-Meyer score for the paralyzed arm of 17.7 in surgery group vs. 2.6 in control group ($p < 0.001$). The smallest between-group difference in spasticity. Improvement in the thumb, with a 2-unit improvement in 6 patients in the surgery group, a 1-unit improvement in 9, and no change in 3. Transcranial magnetic stimulation and fMRI showed connectivity between ipsilateral hemisphere and paralyzed arm.	Paralyzed side: Shoulder or limb pain G1:13/18; G2: 8/18 Fatigue 15/18, hand numbness 16/18, elbow weakness 15/18, wrist extension weakness 16/18, sensory attenuation 16/18 No significant differences in sensorimotor functions assessed by neurologic examination between baseline and 12 months post-surgery in nonparalyzed limb.	12
Gatin et al., 2017 [32]	Case series	63 / 70	CVA (35) TBI (16) Neurodegenerative (6) Anoxia (4) PC (2)	G1: soft tissue surgery Interosseous tenotomy suture-less z plasty of flexor tendon Opening of first web space	40M 23F	51.3 ± 16.2 (24–87)	France	NR	Goal attainment scaling (GAS) transformed into a T score	Mean GAS score increased by 1.3 for hygiene, 1.1 for pain, and 1.0 for appearance	24 complications 7 postoperative edema 6 wound dehiscence 9 hypertonic deformity 1 cardiac failure 1 hardware intolerance	6.2 (1–30)
Peraut et al., 2018 [33]	Case series	26 / 26	CVA (22) TBI (3) Tumor (1)	G1: STPTT	17M 9F	57 (36–79)	France	NR	Deformity correction by Keenan classification Hygiene scale Pain (VAS) House score	All hands were type V before surgery. Postoperatively, 10 patients had type I and 12 patients had type II hands. Mean House score of all patients increased from 0 to 0.88, functional improvement was observed in seven patients, and hygienic care improvement in 25/26 hands.	10/26 (38.46%) intrinsic deformity 6/26 (23.07%) Swan neck deformity	47.7 (6.6–142.3)

Table 2. Cont.

1st Author (Year)	Study Design	Sample Size: Patients Hands	Etiology of Spasticity	Groups (Surgical Procedure)	Gender	Age (Years)	Geographical Area	Time Since Diagnosis (Months)	Measurement Tools	Results	Complications	Follow-Up (Months)
Gschwind, 2019 [12]	Case series	38 / 45	CVA (12) CP (10) TBI (7) Neurodegenerative (5) Anoxia (3) Encephalitis (1)	G1: Single-event multilevel surgery: tendon, neurectomy, and wrist stabilization	17M 21F	44 (17–83)	Australia	>24	Carer Burden Score	In all cases, the preoperative Carer Burden Score (mean 2.25, range 1.00–3.50) was significantly improved at 3 months post-surgery.	1 death unrelated to surgery 1 pressure sore in elbow 1 wound infection	6 (3–38)
AlHakeem et al., 2020 [34]	Prospective observational study	3 / 3	CVA (2) CP (1)	G1: FCR and ulnar nerve and carpal tunnel release	1M 2F	48.33 (20–73)	USA	42 (24–60)	Three-dimensional gait analysis before and 3, 6, and 12 months after surgery (Vicon Motion Capturing System)	Gait analysis demonstrated overall improvements in spatiotemporal parameters (cadence and walking speed) and in lower limb kinematics.	No complications reported	12
Bergfeldt, et al., 2020 [35]	Prospective observational study	30 / 30	CVA (13) Spinal cord injury (9) TBI (5) CP (2) Degenerative CNS disease (1)	G1: Tendon lengthening and muscle release.	23M 7F	57 (28–85)	Sweden	96 (12–288)	MAS Resting position and passive and active range of motion Pain (VAS) COPM	Significant improvements in all outcome measures: decreases in spasticity by 1.4 points and VAS by 1.3 points with increases in COPM (performance by 3.4 and satisfaction by 3.6) and in most measures of joint position and mobility	Increased spasticity and pain in 2 patients and hand weakness in 6 patients at 6 months post-surgery	12
Leclercq et al., 2021 [36]	Prospective observational study	42 (13 children) / 42	CVA (19) CP (16) Cord injury (3) TBI (2) Tumor (1) Degenerative CNS disease (1)	G1: Selective peripheral neurotomy	27M 15F	14.4 (6.4–17.9) for children 47.2 (20.8–74.2) for adults	France	216 in CP 93. 6 in the other etiologies	Rest position and active and passive range of motion. Ashworth and Tardieu spasticity scale House scores Goal attainment and VAS satisfaction	Effective reduction in spastic tone with no decrease in muscle strength. Comparison between 6 and 31 months showed persistence of improvements. The goal of surgery was reached in 93% of patients at the last follow-up. Mean satisfaction of 8.3/10	No complications	31

Table 2. Cont.

1st Author (Year)	Study Design	Sample Size: Patients Hands	Etiology of Spasticity	Groups (Surgical Procedure)	Gender	Age (Years)	Geographical Area	Time Since Diagnosis (Months)	Measurement Tools	Results	Complications	Follow-Up (Months)
Yang et al., 2021 [37]	Case series	2 / 2	CVA	G1: Contralateral C7 to C7 cross nerve transfer. For the lower limb, contralateral L5 to S1 cross nerve transfer	1M 1F	50 (36–64)	China	252	MAS UEFM MRC grade Barthel Index Hua Shan Grading	At 10 months post-surgery: reduction in MAS score to 1.5; increases in wrist and hand movements, with MRC 3 of 52 post-surgery vs. 28 pre-surgery and Fugl-Mayer score of 62 post-surgery to 51 pre-surgery	Mild soreness and discomfort on the unaffected side that disappeared at 3 months. No long-term complications	10
Feng et al., 2021 [38]	Retrospective multicenter cohort study. China and South Korea	425 / 425	G1: CVA (102); TBI (27); CP (32); Encephalitis (7) G2: CVA (209); CP (24); TBI (24); Encephalitis (1)	G1: Surgically treated (n = 168) CC7 cross transfer surgery G2: Rehabilitation alone (n = 257)	Group 1: 142M, 26F Group 2: 214M, 43F	Group 1: 35.8 ± 14.8 Group 2: 39.6 ± 14.5	China	Group 1: 85.2 ± 85.2 Group 2: 76.8 ± 79.2	UEFM. MAS Participant reported quality of life questionnaire	Significantly higher change in UEFM score between baseline and 2-year follow-up in the surgery group, which showed significant improvements at all joints	No severe complications or disabling sequelae. The most frequent complication was pain in shoulder, back, or limb in the first month post-surgery (58%) that generally disappeared within 6 months. A total of 194 instances involving the intact hand were reported within 1 month, but all disappeared within 6 months. A total of 244 instances of changes in muscle strength on the intact side	24

NR: not recorded. M: male, F: female; CP: cerebral palsy. TBI: traumatic brain injury. CVA: cerebrovascular accident. CNS: central nervous system. MS: multiple sclerosis; G1: Group 1. G2: Group 2; STPTT: Superficialis-to-Profundus Tendon Transfer; FLFF: fractional lengthening of finger flexors. FOR: Flexor-Origin Release; TIP deformity: Thumb in the palm deformity; MAS: Modified Ashworth Scale; VAS: visual analog scale. PROM: passive range of motion. MHS: Mini Hand Score (Facca et al., 2010) [27] fMRI: functional magnetic resonance imaging. COPM: Canadian Occupational Performance Measure. MRC: Medical Research Council Grade for motor function. UEFM: Upper-Extremity Fugl-Meyer Scale.

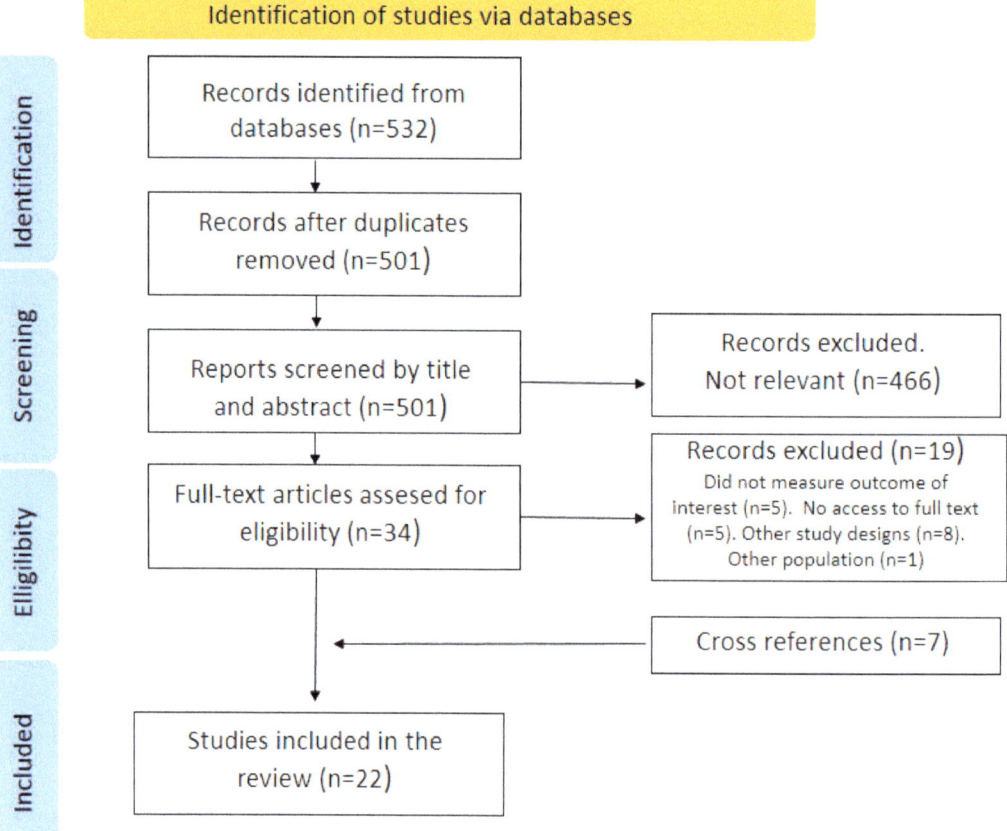

Figure 1. Preferred Reporting Items for Systematic Reviews and Meta-Analyses (PRISMA) flow chart of search results.

6.1. Quality of Evidence

Among the 22 reviewed studies, 19 (86.36%) provided level III evidence, and 21 (95.45%) obtained a low or very low score on the GRADE scale (Table 3) [39,40] (Figure 2).

Table 3. Quality of evidence and grade of recommendation for studies in the systematic review.

Study	Level of Evidence *	Source of Bias	Quality of Evidence **	Grade of Recommendation ***
Braun et al., 1973 [21]	3	No control; small sample; heterogeneous etiology; partly subjective evaluation method.	Very low	D
Keenan et al., 1987 [22]	3	No control; small sample; highly heterogeneous in etiology, age, and sex; partly subjective evaluation method.	Very low	D
Pinzur, 1991 [23]	3	Selection criteria unreported; no control; small sample; heterogeneous etiology; partly subjective evaluation method.	Very low	D

Table 3. Cont.

Study	Level of Evidence *	Source of Bias	Quality of Evidence **	Grade of Recommendation ***
Pomerance y Keenan, 1996 [17]	3	Selection criteria unreported; no control; small and heterogeneous sample; partly subjective evaluation method; short follow-up.	Very low	D
Rayan y Young, 1999 [24]	3	Selection criteria unreported; no control, very small and heterogeneous sample; partly subjective evaluation method.	Very low	D
Heijnen, 2008 [18]	3	No control; very small sample; partly subjective evaluation method.	Very low	D
Pappas et al., 2010 [25]	2+	Small sample; wide confidence interval; partly subjective evaluation method.	Low	C
Shin et al., 2010 [26]	3	Small sample; heterogeneous etiology; partly subjective evaluation method.	Very low	D
Facca et al., 2010 [27]	3	Selection criteria unreported; very small sample; heterogeneous etiology; partly subjective evaluation method.	Very low	D
Kwak et al., 2011 [28]	3	Small and heterogeneous sample; partly subjective evaluation method.	Very low	D
Anakwenze et al., 2013 [29]	3	Retrospective design; heterogeneous etiology.	Very low	D
Thevenin-Lemoine et al., 2013 [30]	3	Heterogeneous sample in etiology and sex; partly subjective evaluation method; highly heterogeneous follow-up.	Very low	D
Neuhaus et al., 2015 [31]	3	Very small and heterogeneous sample; partly subjective evaluation method; short and heterogeneous follow-up.	Very low	D
Zheng et al., 2017 [16]	1+	Small and heterogeneous sample; short follow-up; males only.	High	B
Gatin et al., 2017 [32]	3	Heterogeneous sample in etiology and sex; very short and heterogeneous follow-up.	Very low	D
Peraut et al., 2018 [33]	3	Small sample; heterogeneous etiology; highly heterogeneous follow-up.	Very low	D
Gschwind, 2019 [12]	3	Small sample; heterogeneous etiology; partly subjective evaluation method; highly heterogeneous follow-up	Very low	D
AlHakeem et al., 2020 [34]	3	Very short and heterogeneous sample.	Low	D
Bergfeldt et al., 2020 [35]	3	Small sample, heterogeneous etiology; partly subjective evaluation method.	Low	D
Leclercq et al., 2021 [36]	3	Heterogeneous etiology; mixture of children and adults; short follow-up.	Low	D

Table 3. Cont.

Study	Level of Evidence *	Source of Bias	Quality of Evidence **	Grade of Recommendation ***
Yang et al., 2021 [37]	3	Very small sample; short follow-up.	Very low	D
Feng et al., 2021 [38]	2+	Retrospective design; heterogeneous etiology; asymmetric sample size and sex of study groups.	Low.	C

* Level of evidence according to the Scottish Intercollegiate Guidelines Network [SIGN]), ranging from 1++ for high-quality meta-analyses, systematic reviews of clinical trials, or high-quality clinical trials with very small risk of bias to 4 for expert opinions. ** GRADE scale for quality of evidence (Aguayo-Albasini et al., 2014) [39], ranging from High, for high confidence in the agreement between real and estimated effect to Very low, for little confidence in the estimated effect, which is highly likely to differ from the real effect. *** Grade of recommendation according to the Scottish Intercollegiate Guidelines Network (SIGN) [40], ranging from A for at least one meta-analysis or clinical trial classified as 1++ and directly applicable to guideline target populations to D for level 3 or 4 scientific evidence or evidence extrapolated from studies classified as 2+.

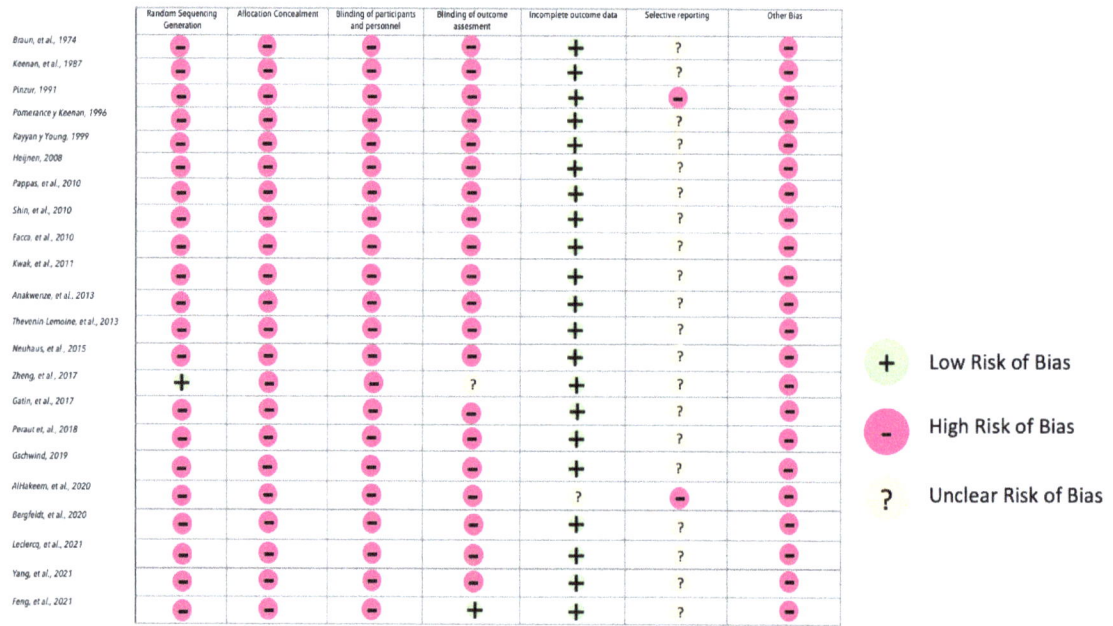

Figure 2. Summary of quality and risk of bias assessment using the Cochrane Collaboration tool [12,16–18,21–38].

Sixteen studies were retrospective case series [12,17,18,21–24,26–33,37], two were single-center [25] or multi-center [38] retrospective cohort studies, three were prospective case series [34–36], and one was a randomized controlled trial [16]. Only three studies included a comparative group, formed by patients who were treated with rehabilitation in two [16,38] and those undergoing a different surgical technique in the third [25]. No studies compared surgery and botulinum toxin treatment. The main sources of bias were a small sample size, a short follow-up period, the absence of a control group, a heterogeneous patient sample, and the partly subjective evaluation of outcomes (Table 3). The mean postoperative follow-up was 21.22 months (range, 6–47.7 months). The follow-up period was one year or shorter in eight (36.36%) of the studies.

6.2. Patient Profile

The studies reported on a total of 965 upper extremities in 939 patients. The patient samples were heterogenous in all except two studies [37,38], comprising not only patients with stroke but also those with other etiologies of upper extremity spasticity, including traumatic brain injury and cerebral palsy. Stroke sequelae in the upper extremity was observed in 355 (37.80%) of the patients. The goal of surgery was exclusively hygienic in ten studies [12,16–18,24,25,31–33], which included a total of 287 hands in 270 patients (i.e., 29.74% of hands in all reviewed studies and 28.75% of patients). Only two articles studied candidates for functional surgery [26,29], reporting on a total of 56 patients (5.96% of patients in reviewed studies). In the remaining studies, the patient sample was mixed, with functional and nonfunctional hands or hands of unspecified status [21,28,30,34–38,41]. None of the reviewed studies stratified their outcomes according to the etiology of the upper extremity spasticity or the patient profile. Overall, 690 males (73.48%) and 249 females (26.51%) were treated. Inadequate data are available to calculate the mean age of the global series, complicated by differences in the etiology of the patients' spasticity; however, the mean age was <50 years in 16 of the 22 studies. Figure 3 depicts the geographical origin of the reviewed articles.

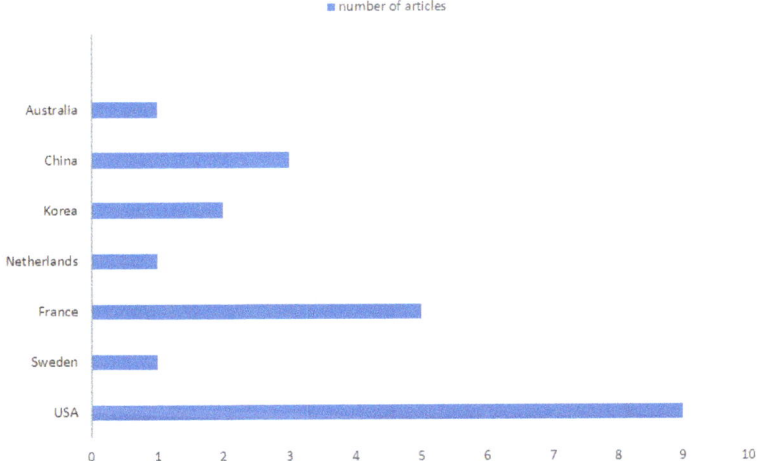

Figure 3. Distribution of the geographic origin of selected articles.

6.3. Types of Surgery

The most frequently reported surgical approaches (Table 4) were the transfer of *Superficialis*-to-*Profundus* (STP) flexors, muscle–tendon releases, wrist arthrodesis, and peripheral neurectomies. Contralateral C7 nerve root transfer was described in only three studies [16,37,38].

Table 4. Types of surgery and frequency of their application in the reviewed studies.

Type of Surgery	Number of Articles	Number of upper Extremities *	Percentage of Total **	Citations
Superficialis-to-Profundis tendon transfer	6	113	11.70%	Braun et al., 1974 [21]; Pomerance & Keenan, 1996 [17]; Heijnen, 2008 [18]; Pappas et al., 2010 [25]; Facca et al., 2010 [27]; Peraut et al., 2018 [33]

Table 4. Cont.

Type of Surgery	Number of Articles	Number of upper Extremities *	Percentage of Total **	Citations
Tendon and muscle lengthening or release	6	198	20.51%	Keenan et al., 1987 [22]; Pinzur, 1991 [23]; Rayyan & Young, 1999 [24]; Anakwenze et al., 2013 [29]; Gatin et al., 2017 [32]; Bergfeldt et al., 2020 [35]
Flexor origin release	3	75	7.77%	Pinzur, 1991 [23]; Thevenin-Lemoine et al., 2013 [30]; AlHakeem et al., 2020 [34]
Wrist Arthrodesis	6	124	12.84%	Pomerance y Keenan, 1996 [17]; Rayyan y Young, 1999 [24]; Pappas et al., 2010 [25]; Facca et al., 2010 [27]; Neuhaus et al., 2015 [31]; Gschwind, 2019 [12]
Selective peripheral neurectomy	6	165	17.09%	Pappas et al., 2010 [25]; Shin et al., 2010 [26]; Facca et al., 2010 [27]; Kwak et al., 2011 [28]; Gschwind, 2019 [12]; Leclercq et al., 2021 [36]
Contralateral C7 nerve transfer	3	206	21.34%	Zheng et al., 2017 [16]; Yang et al., 2021 [37]; Feng et al., 2021 [38]

Types of surgery performed in the reviewed studies. * Upper extremities treated in each study. ** Total = 710 upper extremities.

6.4. Effectiveness/Efficacy and Safety

Table 5 displays the different evaluations of outcomes, which can be classified as very good, especially for hygiene improvement and pain reduction, with patient satisfaction rates ranging between 65 [28] and 100% [18].

Table 5. Outcome evaluation methods used in the reviewed studies.

Evaluation Method		Citations
Resting position of the extremity; active and passive mobility		Braun et al., 1974 [21]; Pomerance and Keenan, 1996 [17]; Heijnen, 2008 [18]; Pappas et al., 2010 [25]; Anakwenze et al., 2013 [29]; Neuhaus et al., 2015 [31]; Peraut et al., 2018 [33]; Bergfeldt et al., 2020 [35]; Leclercq et al., 2021 [36].
Visual analog pain scale		Heijnen, 2008 [18]; Kwak et al., 2011 [28]; Peraut et al., 2018 [33]; Bergfeldt et al., 2020 [35].
Changes in hygiene and care capacities		Pomerance & Keenan, 1996 [17]; Rayyan & Young, 1999 [24]; Heijnen, 2008 [18]; Peraut et al., 2018 [33].
Modification of spasticity	Ashworth or Modified Ashworth Scale	Heijnen, 2008 [18]; Shin et al., 2010 [26]; Kwak et al., 2011 [28]; Anakwenze et al., 2013 [29]; Zheng et al., 2017 [16]; Bergfeldt et al., 2020 [35]; Yang et al., 2021 [37]; Feng et al., 2021 [38]; Leclercq et al., 2021 [36]
	Tardieu scale	Leclercq et al., 2021 [36]

Table 5. Cont.

Evaluation Method		Citations
Functional Scales	Pinzur 1985 functional scale	Pinzur, 1991 [23]
	17 tasks—hand function questionnaire	Rayyan & Young, 1999 [24]
	Mini Hand Score	Facca et al., 2010 [27]
	Zancolli classification	Thevenin-Lemoine et al., 2013 [30]
	House classification	Thevenin-Lemoine et al., 2013 [30]; Neuhaus et al., 2015 [31]; Peraut et al., 2018 [33]; Leclercq et al., 2021 [36]
	Fugl-Meyer Upper-Extremity Scale	Zheng et al., 2017 [16]; Yang et al., 2021 [37]; Feng et al., 2021 [38]
	Canadian Occupational Performance Measure	Bergfeldt et al., 2020 [35]
	Medical Research Council Grade	Yang et al., 2021 [37]
	Hua Shan Grading System	Yang et al., 2021 [37]
	Barthel Index	Yang et al., 2021 [37]
Goal Attainment Scale		Gatin et al., 2017 [32]; Leclercq et al., 2021 [36]
Modification of Care Burden	Care Burden Score	Gschwind, 2019 [12]
Modification of Gait		AlHakeem et al., 2020 [34]
Functional magnetic resonance and electrophysiology studies		Zheng et al., 2017 [16]
Patient evaluation of procedure using a visual analog satisfaction scale.		Shin et al., 2010 [26]; Kwak et al., 2011 [28]; Leclercq et al., 2021 [36]
Participant Reported Quality of Life Questionnaire		Feng et al., 2021 [38]

Hygiene improvement was reported in 87.5 [21]–100% of operated patients [17,18,22,24,33,42]. Kwak et al. [28] described a reduction in the visual analog scale (VAS) score for pain in a spastic upper extremity from 5.85 pre-surgery to 2.28 post-surgery. Gatin et al. [32] reported on 63 patients with a nonfunctional spastic hand who obtained post-surgical Goal Attainment Scaling (GAS) scores of 1.1 for analgesia, 1.0 for cosmetic appearance, and 1.3 for hygienic conditions, indicating that the outcomes were better or much better than expected. Gschwind et al. [12] studied 38 patients with severe spasticity and nonfunctional upper extremities and found a significant improvement in the Carer Burden Score at three months post-surgery.

Studies of postoperative functionality changes report statistically significant improvements in the Upper-Extremity Fugl-Meyer scale score (increases of 11–24 points vs. baseline or rehabilitation control group) [16,36–38] and in House Scale score [30,31,33] (increases of 0.88–2 points). Two research groups described an improvement in hands from nonfunctionality to a functionality of 18.51–100% [23,30]. Various studies have described a reduction in spasticity of between 0.8 and 2 points on the modified Ashworth scale [16,26,28,29,35–38], with a persistence of functional improvements and spasticity reduction for 12 to 31 months [28,36]. It was also reported by AlHakeem et al. [34] that gait was improved by spastic hand surgery in three patients.

No postoperative complications were reported by seven (31.81%) of the reviewed articles [18,24,25,34,36,38,41], and there have been no reports of surgery-related deaths. However, four studies [12,24,26,28] describe postoperative wound infections in between 2.63 [12] and 9.09% [28] of patients. The most frequently reported complications are incomplete correction [27] or deformity recurrence (12.50–27.27% of operated hands) [21,30,31], spasticity relapse (6.66–14.28%) [32,35], unmasking of intrinsic hand muscle spasticity with the emergence of new deformities such as swan neck fingers (9.09–38.46%) [27,30,31,33,42], and finally, prehension weakness due to excessive tendon elongation, observed in 9–20%

of patients undergoing tendon lengthening and muscle release [35,42]. Wrist arthrodesis nonunion has been described in between 0% [24,25,27] and 18.18% [31] of cases.

The only reported complications of peripheral nerve surgery have been mild, although two [25,36] of the seven studies did not provide any data on adverse effects. Paresthesia and dysesthesia were reported in less than 10% of peripheral neurectomies [26,28], and no severe or disabling sequelae were observed after crossed C7 nerve transfer, when the most common complication was pain in the shoulder, back, or extremity at one-month post-surgery (in 58%) that usually disappeared at six months [38]. In donor extremities, fatigue was reported in 41.66%, hand numbness in 44.44%, elbow weakness in 42.66%, wrist extension weakness in 44.44%, and sensory attenuation in 44.44% [16].

7. Discussion

We present the first systematic review of studies on post-stroke spastic upper extremities, based on a selection of 22 articles published up to 2022. Systematic reviews and meta-analyses have been performed on the efficacy of botulinum toxin type A in these patients [43–45] but not on the efficacy of surgery.

In 2021, Hashemi et al. published [46] a systematic review on the efficacy of surgery in treating spastic upper extremeties of different etiologies, and some study samples contained no patients with stroke (neither CVA nor Stroke was a search term). The larger number of items that were retrieved is attributable to their inclusion of publications in French or Farsi, review articles and updates, and series of patients whose shoulder alone was treated. Outcomes were analyzed as a function of anatomical site (i.e., shoulder, elbow, wrist, hand, or fingers) and main surgical procedure; however, no study included contralateral C7 root transfer, probably the most innovative surgical approach to date. The authors were unable to draw specific conclusions about the efficacy of surgery because of the differences among studies in patient samples and procedures. The same problem of heterogenous populations and the failure to stratify outcomes by the cause of spasticity also limited earlier systematic reviews on thumb-in-palm deformity by Smeulders et al. in 2005 [47] and on peripheral neurectomy by Yong et al. in 2018 [48]. All cases of upper extremity spastic paresis result from upper motor neuron syndrome, but treatment decisions must take account of the etiology and the age and profile of patients [49]. The surgical goal differs between patients whose hands have functional possibilities and those with more severe upper extremity spasticity and nonfunctional hands. Surgical endpoints for the latter group of patients are solely related to hygiene, esthetics, or comfort, and the same evaluation methods cannot be applied. In this regard, Feng et al. (2021) reduced the variability in assessment methods by focusing on quality-of-life changes and patient-reported outcomes [38]. The follow-up period varied among the studies but was generally too short (≤ 12 months) to confirm the longer-term efficacy of surgery.

7.1. Efficacy and Safety

7.1.1. Superficialis-to-Profundus Tendon (STP) Transfer

STP transfer was first proposed in 1974 by Braun et al. [21] to improve hand hygiene in patients with spastic clenched-fist deformities of the hand and no volitional control [50]. Although it impairs their prehension capacity, it is performed in patients with stroke sequelae with no expectation of a functional hand from surgery. It is associated with fewer complications in comparison to flexor-origin release, because it requires lesser dissection, and it is less laborious and faster than the selective elongation of all flexor tendons.

STP transfer must frequently be combined with wrist flexor elongation and arthrodesis [17,27] or peripheral neurectomies [25,27] to improve deformity correction.

Published outcomes have been very good, with an improvement in hygienic conditions in 100% of patients and satisfaction rates of 87 [39]–100% [17,18]. Pain relief was not always evaluated, but the intervention was described as having a beneficial effect against pain in most cases [18,33], and Peraut et al. [33] observed functional improvement on the House Scale in 7 out of 26 patients.

Published complications include over-correction, incomplete correction, deformity by the unmasking of intrinsic spasticity, and partial baseline deformity recurrence. No systemic complications have been reported. Some authors [18,25] observed no complications, while Peraut et al., 2018 [33], reported postoperative deformities through the "unmasking" of intrinsic spasticity in 38.46% and swan neck finger deformities in 23.07%. Recurrences of the deformity (in 12.5%) were only observed by Braun et al. [21].

7.1.2. Tendon and Muscle Release (Including Flexor-Origin Release)

A selective fractioned elongation of wrist and finger flexors or flexor-pronator-origin slide can be performed to improve function in patients with deformity due to extrinsic flexor spasticity who retain volitive control and sensitivity [50]. These procedures may be combined with tendon transfers to improve wrist extension, mainly from the *flexor carpi ulnaris* (FCU) to the *Extensor Carpi Radialis Longus* (ECRL), but only Gatin et al. [32] described this approach for stroke sequelae. Transfers for extension in infantile cerebral palsy involves a risk of reverse postoperative deformities and alteration of the post-prehension release phase [51], and this possibility should also be considered in post-stroke patients.

Very good outcomes have been reported for these techniques, including significant and consistent improvements in rest position, spasticity, pain, and function [32,35]. Function improvement was achieved in >90% of patients, with volitive control after either selective fractioned tendon elongation [42] or flexor-origin release [23].

Although AlHakeem et al. described an improvement in gait function in 2020 [34], it was only observed in three patients, and it would be due to the change in positioning of the upper extremity rather than to the surgical procedure per se.

The rate (<30%) and types of local complications [32] that are observed for flexor-origin release were similar to those reported for STP, including prehension weakness (9 [42]–20% [35]), over-correction, incomplete correction, deformity by "unmasking" of intrinsic spasticity (12 [30]–30% [42]), and partial recurrence of baseline deformity (22% [30]).

Some of these complications may be reduced with the application of surgery under WALANT (Wide-Awake Local Anesthesia No Tourniquet) versus general anesthesia, as recently proposed by Kumar and Ho [52], because it permits the active collaboration and mobility of patients and a more precise calibration, customizing each fractional tendon elongation in real time. The authors observed no under- or over-corrections when adopting this approach.

7.1.3. Wrist Arthrodesis

All reports on post-stroke wrist arthrodesis have involved patients with nonfunctional hands who were treated for hygiene improvement alone [12,17,24,25,27,31]. In spastic patients with no volitive hand control, wrist arthrodesis is more reproducible and long-lasting in comparison to isolated soft tissue procedures [24]. First-row carpectomy is often necessary to place the wrist in a neutral or slightly extended position [41], and other procedures are frequently associated, including STP, carpal tunnel release, thumb-long flexor elongation, and sometimes ulnar nerve motor branch neurectomy to treat intrinsic spasticity [17,52].

Again, published results are very good and report hygienic improvement [17,24,31,53], wrist flexion correction of between 66° [31] and 85° [24], and reduced carer burden [12] in virtually all patients. A screwed compression or neutralization plate with autograft was used as an internal fixation method by all authors except for Rayyan and Young (1999) [24], who employed a structural iliac graft.

Only local complications have been reported, although these affected one-third of the patients studied by Pomerance and Keenan (1996) [17]. The procedure-specific complication is non-consolidated pseudoarthrosis; however, although a nonunion rate of 13% was observed by Pomerance and Keenan in 1996 [17], more recent articles have not reported this complication. Once more, the procedure can be complicated by the unmasking of intrinsic spasticity and swan neck finger deformity [31,44].

7.1.4. Selective Peripheral Neurotomy

In 1913, partial or selective neurectomy of specific motor nerve fascicles was proposed by Stoffel [54] to improve function in patients with upper extremity spasticity, and the treatment gained in popularity after the publication of the study by Brunelli and Brunelli [55]. The authors initially resected 50% of nerve branches at their muscle insertion points; however, observations of spasticity recurrence due to the "adoption" phenomenon [55] led them to resect 80% of branches or carry out a second neurectomy some months after the first intervention. This procedure has recently been refined [13,56], and partial neurectomy is now performed at the insertion point of each muscle motor branch.

Neurectomy is most frequently performed in the ulnar nerve motor branch [12,25,27], median nerve recurrent branch [25,28], musculocutaneous nerve [26,36], and the nerves of *Pronator Teres* (PT), *Flexor carpi radialis* (FCR), and FCU [36]. A pre-surgical anesthetic block of peripheral nerves allows for differentiation between spasticity and contracture. The published neurectomy outcomes have been very good, obtaining a significant decrease in spasticity on the modified Ashworth scale, with mean patient satisfaction rates ranging between 64.09 [28] and 83% [36]. Virtually no complications are reported, except for some cases of surgical wound infection. There has been little research on "intrinsic minus" hand deformities, and only Facca et al. [27] described incomplete corrections, observed in around half of patients. Despite expectations related to the adoption phenomenon [55], authors observed no recurrences [28] or only a slight relapse in spasticity, and improvements remained statistically significant at the final follow-up evaluation [26,28,36].

7.1.5. Contralateral C7 Nerve Transfer

Cervical nerve root transfer from the contralateral side has been used to repair brachial plexus root avulsion since 1986 [57]. Variants of this technique include the interposition of a free nerve graft [57], passing the nerve graft through the retropharyngeal and prespinal space instead of the subcutaneous tunnel on the anterior surface of the neck and chest [58], or direct coaptation of the transfer without nerve graft interposition [59]. Different receptor nerves have been utilized in C7 transfer, and Xu et al. were the first to employ the C7 root of the affected side as receptor in a child with spastic paralysis [14]. In 2018, the first clinical trial of contralateral C7 transfer obtained significantly better results compared with rehabilitation [16] in the reduction in spasticity on the modified Ashworth scale and the improvement in function on the Fugl-Maier scale. Functional magnetic resonance imaging (f-MRI) was used to verify the activation of the ipsilateral brain hemisphere with mobility of the affected arm. In 2021, Feng et al. published the largest contralateral C7 transfer trial to date [38] in more than 400 patients, including 168 who underwent the intervention. There was a predominance of patients with stroke in both the surgery and rehabilitation groups, and contralateral C7 transfer achieved significant improvements in spasticity and function (Fugl-Maier scale). The published complications were all mild, including slight weakness, fatigue, soreness, and discomfort on the unaffected side, and they disappeared at 3–6 months post-surgery [16,37,38]. However, this research was conducted in the specific socio-cultural setting of Asia. It may not be so easy to convince patients in many Western settings to transfer nerve elements from the unaffected extremity, on which they may depend for a certain level of function and independence. For this reason, the proposal to transfer these elements from the affected extremity (as both receptor and donor) is of particular interest, avoiding any risk to the healthy arm.

Nerve transfer is an innovative surgical approach to upper extremity paralysis that is well documented in patients with brachial plexus sequelae and is under evaluation for tetraplegic patients; however, it has not yet been described for spastic upper extremities. Waxweiler et al. [60] and Jaloux et al. [61] combined neurectomy with nerve transfer, performing a partial nerve transfer from spastic muscles (elbow flexor, FCR, and PT) to "recipient" motor branches of weak wrist and finger extensor muscles (ECRL, *Extensor Carpi Radialis Brevis*). The aim was to reduce the spasticity of the former and simultaneously activate the latter.

In general, surgery has proved to be an effective treatment option that offers long-lasting results with a low rate of major complications. This raises questions about the status of botulinum toxin as a first-line treatment for regional post-stroke spasticity of the upper extremity [43], given the absence of comparative data on the effectiveness, safety, and economic cost of the two approaches. Beutel et al. [10] investigated upper extremity reconstructive surgery in patients with stroke or TBI in the USA National Inpatient Sample (NIS) database between 2001 and 2012. They reported that 80% of 730,000 new cases of stroke/year survived the acute episode, 76% of the survivors developed spasticity, and 50% of these spastic patients could benefit from surgery [62]. Nevertheless, only 2132 patients underwent surgery during the 12-year study period, i.e., less than 1% of the suitable candidates for surgery, indicating a marked underutilization of upper extremity reconstructive surgery in this patient population.

7.2. Other Therapies

The assessment of the therapeutic potential of surgery does not imply an opposition to treatment with toxin or other conservative therapies. The multiple nonsurgical options that are available for the rehabilitation of upper extremity spasticity should be integrated in a multidisciplinary approach to optimize function and prevent deformity in post-stroke patients. Thus, control of baseline muscle tone can be improved by medication, botulinum toxin injection, and chemodenervation, allowing therapists to maximize muscle strengthening, maintain joint integrity, and increase task-specific training [63]. Orthotics can reduce deformity and improve function [64], and radial extracorporeal shock wave therapy (RESWT) has also been proposed for spasticity reduction [65]. Megna et al. studied post-stroke patients with spastic upper extremities and observed a greater spasticity reduction (modified Asworth scale) in patients who were treated with a combination of physical therapy, botulinum toxin injection, and RESWT than in those receiving physiotherapy and botulinum toxin alone [66]. Promisingly, new technologies are developing novel tools for rehabilitation of the spastic hand, notably robotic therapy [67], virtual reality [68], transcranial magnetic stimulation [69], and brain–computer interface systems [70].

7.3. Strengths and Limitations of the Review

The main limitation of this review is the poor quality of the scientific evidence that is offered by the studies, largely due to their design and the heterogeneity of patient samples. Furthermore, inadequate information is provided to enable the stratification of types of patients and procedures for comparison, and studies differ in their outcome evaluation methods, which are sometimes highly subjective. Finally, follow-up periods have been too short to evaluate outcomes and complications over the longer term. It was not feasible to search the gray literature, which might possibly have caused some publication bias, and it was not possible to perform a meta-analysis due to the heterogeneity of patient profiles and evaluated outcomes. Strengths of our systematic review include its compliance with the rigorous PRISMA guidelines and its synthesis of the scant available information on an issue of major clinical relevance.

8. Conclusions

The results of this review suggest that surgery is a useful, safe, and durable treatment option for post-stroke spastic upper extremities, although most studied patients were only candidates for hygienic improvement. Patients often require an individualized combination of techniques, and there has been renewed interest over the past ten years in procedures that act on the nerve. However, the reviewed studies provide only weak evidence due to their design and heterogeneous patient populations. There is a need for clinical trials to compare surgery and botulinum toxin in the treatment of these patients. The aim is not to exclude one of these approaches but rather to explore how their potential and indications might be integrated within a multidisciplinary treatment protocol in a complementary manner.

Author Contributions: Conceptualization: P.H.-C., Á.G.-S. and P.H.-O.; Methodology: Á.G.-S., J.P.d.R. and N.F.F.-M.; Software: Á.G.-S. and P.H.-O.; Validation: J.P.d.R. and N.F.F.-M.; Formal Analysis: P.H.-O., Á.G.-S. and P.H.-C.; Investigation: P.H.-O., Á.G.-S., L.d.O. and P.H.-C.; Data Curation: P.H.-O., Á.G.-S., L.d.O. and P.H.-C.; Writing—original draft preparation: P.H.-O., Á.G.-S., L.d.O. and P.H.-C.; Writing—review and editing: J.P.d.R. and N.F.F.-M.; Visualization: All authors; Supervision: P.H.-C., J.P.d.R. and N.F.F.-M.; Project Administration and Funding Acquisition: P.H.-C. All authors have read and agreed to the published version of the manuscript.

Funding: Project "PI20/01574", funded by Instituto de Salud Carlos III (ISCIII) and co-funded by the European Union. This research forms part of the doctoral thesis of Patricia Hurtado-Olmo, developed under the Doctoral Program in Clinical Medicine and Public Health at the University of Granada (Spain).

Data Availability Statement: Data are contained within the article.

Acknowledgments: Richard Davies M.A. for language review of the manuscript.

Conflicts of Interest: The authors declare no conflicts of interest.

References

1. GBD 2019 Stroke Collaborators. Global, regional, and national burden of stroke and its risk factors, 1990–2019: A systematic analysis for the Global Burden of Disease Study 2019. *Lancet Neurol.* **2021**, *20*, 795–820. [CrossRef]
2. Kjellström, T.; Norrving, B.; Shatchkute, A. Helsingborg Declaration 2006 on European stroke strategies. *Cerebrovasc. Dis.* **2007**, *23*, 231–241. [CrossRef]
3. Angulo-Parker, F.J.; Adkinson, J.M. Common Etiologies of Upper Extremity Spasticity. *Hand Clin.* **2018**, *34*, 437–443. [CrossRef]
4. Seruya, M. The Future of Upper Extremity Spasticity Management. *Hand Clin.* **2018**, *34*, 593–599. [CrossRef]
5. Winter, T.; Wissel, J. Treatment of spasticity after stroke. *Neurol. Rehabil.* **2013**, *19*, 285–309.
6. Schnitzler, A.; Ruet, A.; Baron, S.; Buzzi, J.C.; Genet, F. Botulinum toxin A for treating spasticity in adults: Costly for French hospitals? *Ann. Phys. Rehabil. Med.* **2015**, *58*, 265–268. [CrossRef]
7. Morone, G.; Baricich, A.; Paolucci, S.; Bentivoglio, A.R.; De Blasiis, P.; Carlucci, M.; Violi, F.; Levato, G.; Pani, M.; Carpagnano, L.F.; et al. Long-Term Spasticity Management in Post-Stroke Patients: Issues and Possible Actions—A Systematic Review with an Italian Expert Opinion. *Healthcare* **2023**, *11*, 783. [CrossRef]
8. Bakheit, A.M. The pharmacological management of post-stroke muscle spasticity. *Drugs Aging* **2012**, *29*, 941–947. [CrossRef] [PubMed]
9. Ward, A.B. A literature review of the pathophysiology and onset of post-stroke spasticity. *Eur. J. Neurol.* **2012**, *19*, 21–27. [CrossRef] [PubMed]
10. Beutel, B.G.; Marascalchi, B.J.; Melamed, E. Trends in Utilization of Upper Extremity Reconstructive Surgery Following Traumatic Brain Injury and Stroke. *Hand* **2020**, *15*, 35–40. [CrossRef] [PubMed]
11. Rhee, P.C. Surgical Management of Upper Extremity Deformities in Patients with Upper Motor Neuron Syndrome. *J. Hand Surg. Am.* **2019**, *44*, 223–235. [CrossRef]
12. Gschwind, C.R.; Yeomans, J.L.; Smith, B.J. Upper limb surgery for severe spasticity after acquired brain injury improves ease of care. *J. Hand Surg. Eur. Vol.* **2019**, *44*, 898–904. [CrossRef]
13. Leclercq, C. Selective Neurectomy for the Spastic Upper Extremity. *Hand Clin.* **2018**, *34*, 537–545. [CrossRef]
14. Xu, W.-D.; Hua, X.-Y.; Zheng, M.-X.; Xu, J.-G.; Gu, Y.-D. Contralateral C7 nerve root transfer in treatment of cerebral palsy in a child: Case report. *Microsurgery* **2011**, *31*, 404–408. [CrossRef]
15. Hua, X.Y.; Qiu, Y.Q.; Li, T.; Zheng, M.X.; Shen, Y.D.; Jiang, S.; Xu, J.G.; Gu, Y.D.; Xu, W.D. Contralateral peripheral neurotization for hemiplegic upper extremity after central neurologic injury. *Neurosurgery* **2015**, *76*, 187–195. [CrossRef]
16. Zheng, M.X.; Hua, X.Y.; Feng, J.T.; Li, T.; Lu, Y.C.; Shen, Y.D.; Cao, X.H.; Zhao, N.Q.; Lyu, J.Y.; Xu, J.G.; et al. Trial of Contralateral Seventh Cervical Nerve Transfer for Spastic Arm Paralysis. *N. Engl. J. Med.* **2018**, *378*, 22–34. [CrossRef]
17. Pomerance, J.F.; Keenan, M.A. Correction of severe spastic flexion contractures in the nonfunctional hand. *J. Hand Surg. Am.* **1996**, *21*, 828–833. [CrossRef] [PubMed]
18. Heijnen, I.C.; Franken, R.J.; Bevaart, B.J.; Meijer, J.W. Long-term outcome of superficialis-to-profundus tendon transfer in patients with clenched fist due to spastic hemiplegia. *Disabil. Rehabil.* **2008**, *30*, 675–678. [CrossRef] [PubMed]
19. Page, M.J.; McKenzie, J.E.; Bossuyt, P.M.; Boutron, I.; Hoffmann, T.C.; Mulrow, C.D.; Shamseer, L.; Tetzlaff, J.M.; Akl, E.A.; Brennan, S.E.; et al. The PRISMA 2020 statement: An updated guideline for reporting systematic reviews. *BMJ* **2021**, *372*, n71. [CrossRef] [PubMed]
20. Guyatt, G.H.; Oxman, A.D.; Vist, G.E.; Kunz, R.; Falck-Ytter, Y.; Alonso-Coello, P.; Schünemann, H.J.; GRADE Working Group. GRADE: An emerging consensus on rating quality of evidence and strength of recommendations. *BMJ* **2008**, *336*, 924–926. [CrossRef] [PubMed]
21. Braun, R.M.; Vise, G.T.; Roper, B. Preliminary experience with superficialis-to-profundus tendon transfer in the hemiplegic upper extremity. *J. Bone Jt. Surg. Am.* **1974**, *56*, 466–472. [CrossRef]

22. Keenan, M.A.; Korchek, J.I.; Botte, M.J.; Smith, C.W.; Garland, D.E. Results of transfer of the flexor digitorum superficialis tendons to the flexor digitorum profundus tendons in adults with acquired spasticity of the hand. *J. Bone Jt. Surg. Am.* **1987**, *69*, 1127–1132. [CrossRef]
23. Pinzur, M.S. Flexor origin release and functional prehension in adult spastic hand deformity. *J. Hand Surg. Br.* **1991**, *16*, 133–136. [CrossRef]
24. Rayan, G.M.; Young, B.T. Arthrodesis of the spastic wrist. *J. Hand Surg. Am.* **1999**, *24*, 944–952. [CrossRef]
25. Pappas, N.; Baldwin, K.; Keenan, M.A. Efficacy of median nerve recurrent branch neurectomy as an adjunct to ulnar motor nerve neurectomy and wrist arthrodesis at the time of superficialis to profundus transfer in prevention of intrinsic spastic thumb-in-palm deformity. *J. Hand Surg. Am.* **2010**, *35*, 1310–1316. [CrossRef]
26. Shin, D.K.; Jung, Y.J.; Hong, J.C.; Kim, M.S.; Kim, S.H. Selective musculocutaneous neurotomy for spastic elbow. *J. Korean Neurosurg. Soc.* **2010**, *48*, 236–239. [CrossRef] [PubMed]
27. Facca, S.; Louis, P.; Isner, M.E.; Gault, D.; Allieu, Y.; Liverneaux, P. Braun's flexor tendons transfer in disabled hands by central nervous system lesions. *Orthop. Traumatol. Surg. Res.* **2010**, *96*, 656–661. [CrossRef] [PubMed]
28. Kwak, K.W.; Kim, M.S.; Chang, C.H.; Kim, S.W.; Kim, S.H. Surgical results of selective median neurotomy for wrist and finger spasticity. *J. Korean Neurosurg. Soc.* **2011**, *50*, 95–98. [CrossRef] [PubMed]
29. Anakwenze, O.A.; Namdari, S.; Hsu, J.E.; Benham, J.; Keenan, M.A. Myotendinous lengthening of the elbow flexor muscles to improve active motion in patients with elbow spasticity following brain injury. *J. Shoulder Elbow Surg.* **2013**, *22*, 318–322. [CrossRef]
30. Thevenin-Lemoine, C.; Denormandie, P.; Schnitzler, A.; Lautridou, C.; Allieu, Y.; Genêt, F. Flexor origin slide for contracture of spastic finger flexor muscles: A retrospective study. *J. Bone Jt. Surg. Am.* **2013**, *95*, 446–453. [CrossRef] [PubMed]
31. Neuhaus, V.; Kadzielski, J.J.; Mudgal, C.S. The role of arthrodesis of the wrist in spastic disorders. *J. Hand Surg. Eur. Vol.* **2015**, *40*, 512–517. [CrossRef]
32. Gatin, L.; Schnitzler, A.; Calé, F.; Genêt, G.; Denormandie, P.; Genêt, F. Soft Tissue Surgery for Adults with Nonfunctional, Spastic Hands Following Central Nervous System Lesions: A Retrospective Study. *J. Hand Surg. Am.* **2017**, *42*, 1035.e1–1035.e7. [CrossRef]
33. Peraut, E.; Taïeb, L.; Jourdan, C.; Coroian, F.; Laffont, I.; Chammas, M.; Coulet, B. Results and complications of superficialis-to-profundus tendon transfer in brain-damaged patients, a series of 26 patients. *Orthop. Traumatol. Surg. Res.* **2018**, *104*, 121–126. [CrossRef] [PubMed]
34. AlHakeem, N.; Ouellette, E.A.; Travascio, F.; Asfour, S. Surgical Intervention for Spastic Upper Extremity Improves Lower Extremity Kinematics in Spastic Adults: A Collection of Case Studies. *Front. Bioeng. Biotechnol.* **2020**, *8*, 116. [CrossRef] [PubMed]
35. Bergfeldt, U.; Strömberg, J.; Ramström, T.; Kulbacka-Ortiz, K.; Reinholdt, C. Functional outcomes of spasticity-reducing surgery and rehabilitation at 1-year follow-up in 30 patients. *J. Hand Surg. Eur. Vol.* **2020**, *45*, 807–812. [CrossRef] [PubMed]
36. Leclercq, C.; Perruisseau-Carrier, A.; Gras, M.; Panciera, P.; Fulchignoni, C.; Fulchignoni, M. Hyperselective neurectomy for the treatment of upper limb spasticity in adults and children: A prospective study. *J. Hand Surg. Eur. Vol.* **2021**, *46*, 708–716. [CrossRef] [PubMed]
37. Yang, F.; Chen, L.; Wang, H.; Zhang, J.; Shen, Y.; Qiu, Y.; Qu, Z.; Li, J.; Xu, W. Combined contralateral C7 to C7 and L5 to S1 cross nerve transfer for treating limb hemiplegia after stroke. *Br. J. Neurosurg.* **2021**, *10*, 1–4. [CrossRef] [PubMed]
38. Feng, J.; Li, T.; Lv, M.; Kim, S.; Shin, J.H.; Zhao, N.; Chen, Q.; Gong, Y.; Sun, Y.; Zhao, Z.; et al. Reconstruction of paralyzed arm function in patients with hemiplegia through contralateral seventh cervical nerve cross transfer: A multicenter study and real-world practice guidance. *EClinicalMedicine* **2022**, *43*, 101258. [CrossRef]
39. Aguayo-Albasini, J.L.; Flores-Pastor, B.; Soria-Aledo, V. Sistema GRADE: Clasificación de la calidad de la evidencia y graduación de la fuerza de la recomendación [GRADE system: Classification of quality of evidence and strength of recommendation]. *Cirugía Española* **2014**, *92*, 82–88. [CrossRef] [PubMed]
40. Scottish Intercollegiate Guidelines Network (SIGN). *SIGN 50: A Guideline Developers' Handbook*; SIGN Publication No. 50; SIGN: Edinburgh, UK, 2011. Available online: https://www.sign.ac.uk/assets/sign50_2011.pdf (accessed on 17 October 2023).
41. Pinzur, M.S. Carpectomy and fusion in adult-acquired hand spasticity. *Orthopedics* **1996**, *19*, 675–677. [CrossRef]
42. Keenan, M.A.; Abrams, R.A.; Garland, D.E.; Waters, R.L. Results of fractional lengthening of the finger flexors in adults with upper extremity spasticity. *J. Hand Surg. Am.* **1987**, *12*, 575–581. [CrossRef] [PubMed]
43. Esquenazi, A.; Albanese, A.; Chancellor, M.B.; Elovic, E.; Segal, K.R.; Simpson, D.M.; Smith, C.P.; Ward, A.B. Evidence-based review and assessment of botulinum neurotoxin for the treatment of adult spasticity in the upper motor neuron syndrome. *Toxicon* **2013**, *67*, 115–128. [CrossRef] [PubMed]
44. Dong, Y.; Wu, T.; Hu, X.; Wang, T. Efficacy and safety of botulinum toxin type A for upper limb spasticity after stroke or traumatic brain injury: A systematic review with meta-analysis and trial sequential analysis. *Eur. J. Phys. Rehabil. Med.* **2017**, *53*, 256–267. [CrossRef]
45. Hara, T.; Momosaki, R.; Niimi, M.; Yamada, N.; Hara, H.; Abo, M. Botulinum Toxin Therapy Combined with Rehabilitation for Stroke: A Systematic Review of Effect on Motor Function. *Toxins* **2019**, *11*, 707. [CrossRef]
46. Hashemi, M.; Sturbois-Nachef, N.; Keenan, M.A.; Winston, P. Surgical Approaches to Upper Limb Spasticity in Adult Patients: A Literature Review. *Front. Rehabil. Sci.* **2021**, *2*, 709969. [CrossRef]
47. Smeulders, M.J.; Coester, A.; Kreulen, M. Surgical treatment for the thumb-in-palm deformity in patients with cerebral palsy. *Cochrane Database Syst. Rev.* **2005**, CD004093. [CrossRef] [PubMed]

48. Yong, L.Y.; Wong, C.H.L.; Gaston, M.; Lam, W.L. The Role of Selective Peripheral Neurectomy in the Treatment of Upper Limb Spasticity. *J. Hand Surg. Asian Pac. Vol.* **2018**, *23*, 181–191. [CrossRef]
49. Gart, M.S.; Adkinson, J.M. Considerations in the Management of Upper Extremity Spasticity. *Hand Clin.* **2018**, *34*, 465–471. [CrossRef]
50. Waljee, J.F.; Chung, K.C. Surgical Management of Spasticity of the Thumb and Fingers. *Hand Clin.* **2018**, *34*, 473–485. [CrossRef]
51. Patterson, J.M.; Wang, A.A.; Hutchinson, D.T. Late deformities following the transfer of the flexor carpi ulnaris to the extensor carpi radialis brevis in children with cerebral palsy. *J. Hand Surg. Am.* **2010**, *35*, 1774–1778. [CrossRef]
52. Kumar, A.; Ho, P.C. Novel Use of the Wide-Awake Local Anesthesia No Tourniquet Technique for Release of Spastic Upper Limbs. *J. Hand Surg. Glob. Online* **2022**, *4*, 442–447. [CrossRef] [PubMed]
53. Duquette, S.P.; Adkinson, J.M. Surgical Management of Spasticity of the Forearm and Wrist. *Hand Clin.* **2018**, *34*, 487–502. [CrossRef] [PubMed]
54. Stoffel, A. Treatment of spastic contractures. *Am. J. Orthop. Surg.* **1913**, *210*, 611.
55. Brunelli, G.; Brunelli, F. Partial selective denervation in spastic palsies (hyponeurotization). *Microsurgery* **1983**, *4*, 221–224. [CrossRef] [PubMed]
56. Leclercq, C.; Gras, M. Hyperselective neurectomy in the treatment of the spastic upper limb. *Phys. Med. Rehabil. Int.* **2016**, *3*, 1075.
57. Gu, Y.D.; Zhang, G.M.; Chen, D.S.; Yan, J.G.; Cheng, X.M.; Chen, L. Seventh cervical nerve root transfer from the contralateral healthy side for treatment of brachial plexus root avulsion. *J. Hand Surg. Br.* **1992**, *17*, 518–521. [CrossRef]
58. Mcguiness, C.N.; Kay, S.P.J. The prespinal route in contralateral C7 nerve root transfer for brachial plexus avulsion injuries. *J. Hand Surg. Am.* **2002**, *27B*, 159–160. [CrossRef]
59. Wang, S.; Yiu, H.-W.; Li, P.; Li, Y.; Wang, H.; Pan, Y. Contralateral C7 nerve root transfer to neurotize the upper trunk via a modified prespinal route in repair of brachial plexus avulsion injury. *Microsurgery* **2012**, *32*, 183–188. [CrossRef]
60. Waxweiler, C.; Remy, S.; Merlini, L.; Leclercq, C. Nerve transfer in the spastic upper limb: Anatomical feasibility study. *Surg. Radiol. Anat.* **2022**, *44*, 183–190. [CrossRef]
61. Jaloux, C.; Bini, N.; Leclercq, C. Nerve transfers in the forearm: Potential use in spastic conditions. *Surg. Radiol. Anat.* **2022**, *44*, 1091–1099. [CrossRef]
62. Tafti, M.A.; Cramer, S.C.; Gupta, R. Orthopaedic management of the upper extremity of stroke patients. *J. Am. Acad. Orthop. Surg.* **2008**, *16*, 462–470. [CrossRef] [PubMed]
63. Black, L.; Gaebler-Spira, D. Nonsurgical Treatment Options for Upper Limb Spasticity. *Hand Clin.* **2018**, *34*, 455–464. [CrossRef] [PubMed]
64. Kerr, L.; Jewell, V.D.; Jensen, L. Stretching and Splinting Interventions for Poststroke Spasticity, Hand Function, and Functional Tasks: A Systematic Review. *Am. J. Occup. Ther.* **2020**, *74*, 7405205050p1–7405205050p15. [CrossRef] [PubMed]
65. Gjerakaroska Savevska, C.; Nikolikj Dimitrova, E.; Gocevska, M. Effects of radial extracorporeal shock wave therapy on hand spasticity in poststroke patient. *Hippokratia* **2016**, *20*, 309–312. [PubMed]
66. Megna, M.; Marvulli, R.; Farì, G.; Gallo, G.; Dicuonzo, F.; Fiore, P.; Ianieri, G. Pain and Muscles Properties Modifications After Botulinum Toxin Type A (BTX-A) and Radial Extracorporeal Shock Wave (rESWT) Combined Treatment. *Endocr. Metab. Immune Disord. Drug Targets* **2019**, *19*, 1127–1133. [PubMed]
67. Zhang, C.; Li-Tsang, C.W.; Au, R.K. Robotic approaches for the rehabilitation of upper limb recovery after stroke: A systematic review and meta-analysis. *Int. J. Rehabil. Res.* **2017**, *40*, 19–28. [CrossRef]
68. Chen, J.; Or, C.K.; Chen, T. Effectiveness of Using Virtual Reality-Supported Exercise Therapy for Upper Extremity Motor Rehabilitation in Patients with Stroke: Systematic Review and Meta-analysis of Randomized Controlled Trials. *J. Med. Internet Res.* **2022**, *24*, e24111. [CrossRef]
69. Lüdemann-Podubecká, J.; Bösl, K.; Nowak, D.A. Repetitive transcranial magnetic stimulation for motor recovery of the upper limb after stroke. *Prog. Brain Res.* **2015**, *218*, 281–311.
70. Monge-Pereira, E.; Ibañez-Pereda, J.; Alguacil-Diego, I.M.; Serrano, J.I.; Spottorno-Rubio, M.P.; Molina-Rueda, F. Use of Electroencephalography Brain-Computer Interface Systems as a Rehabilitative Approach for Upper Limb Function After a Stroke: A Systematic Review. *PMR* **2017**, *9*, 918–932. [CrossRef]

Disclaimer/Publisher's Note: The statements, opinions and data contained in all publications are solely those of the individual author(s) and contributor(s) and not of MDPI and/or the editor(s). MDPI and/or the editor(s) disclaim responsibility for any injury to people or property resulting from any ideas, methods, instructions or products referred to in the content.

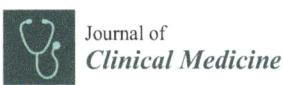 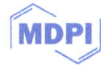

Article

Hydrotherapy after Rotator Cuff Repair Improves Short-Term Functional Results Compared with Land-Based Rehabilitation When the Immobilization Period Is Longer

Alexandre Lädermann [1,2,3], Alec Cikes [4,5], Jeanni Zbinden [1], Tiago Martinho [1], Anthony Pernoud [6,*] and Hugo Bothorel [6]

1. Division of Orthopaedics and Trauma Surgery, La Tour Hospital, 1217 Meyrin, Switzerland
2. Faculty of Medicine, University of Geneva, 1205 Geneva, Switzerland
3. Division of Orthopaedics and Trauma Surgery, Department of Surgery, Geneva University Hospitals, 1205 Geneva, Switzerland
4. Division of Orthopaedics and Trauma Surgery, Genolier Clinic, 1272 Genolier, Switzerland
5. Synergy Medical Centre, Medbase Group, 1007 Lausanne, Switzerland
6. Research Department, La Tour Hospital, 1217 Meyrin, Switzerland
* Correspondence: anthony.pernoud@latour.ch; Tel.: +41-22-719-78-74

Abstract: Background: The evidence of hydrotherapy after rotator cuff repair (RCR) is limited as most studies either used it as an adjuvant to standard land-based therapy, or have different initiation timing. This study aimed to compare hydrotherapy and land-based therapy with varying immobilization time. **Methods:** Patients who underwent RCR with a 10-days or 1-month immobilization duration (early or late rehabilitation) were prospectively randomized. **Results:** Constant scores significantly differed at three months only, with the best score exhibited by the late hydrotherapy group (70.3 ± 8.2) followed by late land-based (61.0 ± 5.7), early hydrotherapy (55.4 ± 12.8) and early land-based (54.6 ± 13.3) groups ($p < 0.001$). There was a significant interaction between rehabilitation type and immobilization duration ($p = 0.004$). The effect of hydrotherapy compared to land-based therapy was large at three months when initiated lately only (Cohen's d, 1.3; 95%CI, 0.9–1.7). However, the relative risk (RR) of postoperative frozen shoulder or retear occurrence for late hydrotherapy was higher compared to early hydrotherapy (RR, 3.9; 95%CI, 0.5–30.0). **Conclusions:** Hydrotherapy was more efficient compared to land-based therapy at three months only and if initiated lately. Even though initiating hydrotherapy later brought greater constant scores at three months, it might increase the risk of frozen shoulders or retear compared to early hydrotherapy.

Keywords: arthroscopic rotator cuff repair; immobilization duration; rehabilitation; hydrotherapy; land-based therapy; constant score

Citation: Lädermann, A.; Cikes, A.; Zbinden, J.; Martinho, T.; Pernoud, A.; Bothorel, H. Hydrotherapy after Rotator Cuff Repair Improves Short-Term Functional Results Compared with Land-Based Rehabilitation When the Immobilization Period Is Longer. *J. Clin. Med.* **2024**, *13*, 954. https://doi.org/10.3390/jcm13040954

Academic Editor: Christian Ehrnthaller

Received: 19 December 2023
Revised: 31 January 2024
Accepted: 3 February 2024
Published: 7 February 2024

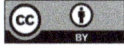

Copyright: © 2024 by the authors. Licensee MDPI, Basel, Switzerland. This article is an open access article distributed under the terms and conditions of the Creative Commons Attribution (CC BY) license (https://creativecommons.org/licenses/by/4.0/).

1. Introduction

Shoulder pain constitutes a highly prevalent complaint, with estimates suggesting s lifetime prevalence as high as 67% [1]. Among the numerous causes of this discomfort, rotator cuff tears (RCT) stand out, accounting for approximately one-third of reported shoulder complaints [2]. This particular pathology is among the most frequently encountered musculo-tendinous injuries seen and treated by orthopedic surgery. RCTs may emerge either due to the degeneration of tendons comprising the rotator cuff or as a consequence of trauma [3]. In degenerative rotator cuff diseases, several risk factors have been identified, with age playing a significant role in its development [4]. Consequently, this condition is notably prevalent among adults age over 50 years old and within the elderly population, with an anticipated increase in prevalence as the population continues to age [5–9]. The essential role of the rotator cuff in shoulder function renders addressing this pathology critical. RCTs contribute to shoulder pain, increased stiffness, and decreased strength, considerably hindering individuals in performing daily activities, even as basic as combing hair [10,11]. Moreover, this condition incurs considerable societal and economic burdens due to productivity losses and functional decline [12].

Conservative treatment has been primarily indicated for degenerative RCT, demonstrating satisfactory outcomes, particularly in addressing rotator cuff-related shoulder pain [13] or improving active forward range of motion [14]. A delayed surgical intervention, however, can increase the risk of anatomical deterioration including muscle atrophy, fatty infiltration and an increase in tear size [15]. Consequently, surgical intervention for RCT has been increasingly performed [5], either as first-line treatment or following unsuccessful conservative approaches, with improved long-term outcomes [16]. Surgical procedures encompass open interventions, mini-open approaches or arthroscopy techniques, each bearing distinct advantages and disadvantages. Although historically, open procedures prevailed [17], technological and surgical advancements led to the adoption of arthroscopic methods. Arthroscopy has become the gold standard for rotator cuff repair (RCR) as it is a minimally invasive approach reducing complications, pain, and stiffness compared to open procedure [18]. While arthroscopic RCR grants satisfactory outcomes for most patients [19], stiffness remains a common post-operative complication contributing to functional disability, pain and frustration [20]. This emphasizes the importance of post-operative rehabilitation since it helps, when supervised by physiotherapists, at reducing the occurrence of such complications and alleviate patient symptoms [21].

There are numerous rehabilitation modalities after arthroscopic RCR. The main modality that can be considered is the timing of initial mobilizations post-surgery, which can be early, delayed, or strict (no mobilization). Despite the importance of post-operative rehabilitation, there is a lack of high-quality evidence-based studies to guide clinicians, and no consensus regarding the most appropriate protocol [22–24]. Delayed mobilization might minimize strain at the repair site as the tendon begins to heal, potentially leading to improved healing rates [25]. Delayed range of motion, however, could maximize tendon adhesions and stiffness. On the other hand, early rehabilitation helps prevent joint stiffness, facilitating a quicker return to functionality and daily activities [23,26–28]. However, long-term outcomes might remain comparable to those obtained after a delayed rehabilitation, which advocates for a longer immobilization time [27,28]. Furthermore, early rehabilitation needs to be performed progressively and cautiously as it could entail a higher risk of re-rupture due to excessive load with regard to the tendon's healing state [29]. Therefore, hydrotherapy has been introduced during early rehabilitation to diminish joint stress, aiding in shoulder mobilization for patients experiencing pain, anxiety, or dysfunctional muscular activation [30].

Hydrotherapy reduces strain, allowing patients to engage in active range of motion. This activity is essential for tissue healing from a physiological standpoint [31]. Additionally, it holds neurophysiological importance as it enhances proprioception and replicates physiological activation patterns without compromising tendon repair [30]. Despite these advantages, the evidence of hydrotherapy benefits after RCR remains limited. Most of the studies either employed it as an adjuvant therapy to standard land-based rehabilitation [30] or restricted its application to selected patients only [32,33]. Recently, two randomised clinical trials have reported contradictory findings concerning the effects of hydrotherapy compared to land-based therapy [21,34], though they differed in terms of tear size studied (small-medium vs. small-large) and immobilization duration before rehabilitation initiation (10 days or 1 month). The authors of the present study therefore aimed to investigate if, on a comparable group of patients, the benefits of hydrotherapy over land-based therapy depend on immobilization time after RCR. We hypothesized that hydrotherapy's effects would be more pronounced if rehabilitation initiation occurs later.

2. Materials and Methods

The data utilized in this study originate from two clinical studies conducted by Dufournet et al. [34] and Cikes et al. [21]. Thus, patients who underwent primary arthroscopic

RCR at La Tour Hospital or Bois-Cerf Clinic between 2012 and 2019 were eligible. Inclusion criteria were (1) small to medium sized symptomatic supraspinatus and/or infraspinatus tendon tears [35], (2) grade 1 to 2 tendon retraction according to Patte [36], (3) fatty infiltration stage ≤ 2 [37], and failure of conservative treatment during a minimum of six months in case of degererative lesions. Rotator cuff tears in this study were either traumatic or degenerative. Degenerative lesions were failure of conservative treatment, which involved standard land-based physiotherapy over a 6-month period. Additionally, cortisone injections were administered during this timeframe. A mandatory period of at least 3 months post-injection, was observed before the surgical intervention. Since the study performed by Dufournet et al. [34] included lesions of all sizes, 24 patients (26.1%) were not included in the present study due to the presence of large lesions. Exclusion criteria were (1) patients unable to follow the study protocol, (2) other types of rotator cuff lesion (bony rotator cuff (A), medial tendinous disruption (B2), tendon-to-tendon adhesion 'Fosbury flop tear' (B3), and musculotendinous junction lesion (C type)) [35], (3) patients with subscapularis tendon lesions, (4) associated superior labrum anterior posterior (SLAP) lesion, or (5) frozen shoulder [38]. In both studies, patients were randomized between the rehabilitation protocols and provided their written informed consent. Furthermore, ethical approval was granted by the local ethics committee for both (CER–VD-481/15, 13 January 2016; CCER–2016-02242, 27 July 2017), and the studies registered at ClinicalTrials.gov (NCT05106842) and our National Clinical Trials Portal (SNCTP No. 000002244).

2.1. Pre- and Post-Operative Clinical Assessment

Data were collected through independent assessors at baseline before the surgical intervention and at 3, 6, and 24 months post-operatively. Patients characteristics included age, sex, and dominant side. Functional status was assessed by the Constant score, a validated questionnaire ranging from a score of 0 (indicating the worst functional status) to 100 (indicating the best functional status) [39].

2.2. Surgical Procedure

The surgery was performed under general anesthesia and with ultrasound (US)-guided interscalene brachial plexus block with the patients placed in a beach-chair position. Adjuvant acromioplasty was performed only in patients who had radiographic signs of dynamic impingement [40], and resection of the distal part of the clavicle was performed when pain was elicited by palpation of the acromioclavicular joint. Biceps tenodesis or tenotomy was performed when the posterior wall of the bicipital groove was damaged. All repairs were carried out using two anchors, of which one was implanted at the bone–cartilage junction, and one was implanted at the lateral part of the greater tuberosity [41]. At the end of the intervention, all repairs were complete and "watertight", with adequate restoration of the tendons to their footprints. Post-operative care included regular wound dressing twice per week with removal of skin closure sutures 10 days after surgery.

2.3. Rehabilitation Protocol

Patients had to wear a sling for four weeks, ensuring the positioning of the shoulder in an internally rotated stance. During the immobilization phase, patients were advised to engage in gentle self-passive motion exercises. The immobilization duration varied between two groups: patients operated and rehabilitated at La Tour hospital had a 10-day immobilization period (Early rehabilitation group), whereas patients operated and rehabilitated at Bois-Cerf Clinic underwent a 30-day immobilization (Late rehabilitation group). The early rehabilitation group started supervised physiotherapy at 10 days, after skin closure removal. The exercises consisted in progressive passive motion for three weeks, followed by active motion until the third postoperative month [42]. At three months, patients then began strengthening exercises. The Late rehabilitation group started supervised physiotherapy at one month post-operatively with progressive passive and active motion for two weeks, two to three times a week, before proceeding to strengthening exercises. In both the Early and Late groups, patients were allocated to receive either standard land-based therapy or hydrotherapy. Consequently, our final study cohort comprised four distinct groups: (1) Early rehabilitation with Hydrotherapy (Early–Hydrotherapy), (2) Late rehabilitation with Hydrotherapy (Late–Hydrotherapy), (3) Early rehabilitation with Land-based therapy (Early–Land-based), (4) Late rehabilitation with Land-based therapy (Late–Land-based). Hydrotherapy sessions were performed in a swimming pool with a depth ranging between 125 and 140 cm depth. Patients were instructed to kneel or sit to submerge their shoulders during exercises, performed in water heated to a temperature ranging between 28 to 34 °C.

2.4. Statistical Analyses

The sample size was determined *a priori* for both studies. In Dufournet et al. study [34], it was calculated in order to ensure the detection of a minimal clinically important difference (MCID) of 20° in active forward flexion between patients undergoing aquatic therapy and standard land-based therapy. The sample size in Cikes et al. study [21] was performed to detect a minimal clinically important difference in Constant score, corresponding to a 10.4 points change [43]. In this study, the sample size was calculated to detect at least a medium effect (f = 0.253, partial eta square = 0.06) of a physiotherapy type (aquatic vs. land-based) in postoperative Constant scores while considering the differences in therapy onset times (early vs. late). Parameters for the sample size calculation were estimated according to a 'worst-case scenario' approach, with low correlation among repeated measures (r = 0.2) and nonsphericity correction (ε = 0.5). To achieve a power of 0.8 in those circumstances, a minimum total sample size of 96 patients was required (24 per group).

Descriptive statistical methods were used to summarize the data. Continuous variables were reported as the mean along with the standard deviation (mean ± SD), additionally displaying the range from the minimum to the maximum values (min-max). Categorical data were reported as counts (n) and proportions. The normality of the distributions for continuous variable was assessed using the Shapiro–Wilk test and the normality of the residuals was visually assessed on a Q–Q plot. Two-way mixed ANOVA tests were conducted at each follow-up point to evaluate the effect of rehabilitation type (hydro- vs. land-based therapy) and the commencement timing of rehabilitation (Early vs. Late) on post-operative Constant scores. Effect sizes calculated with this ANOVA analysis were expressed in generalized eta squared (η^2_G) and interpreted as follows: small (0.01 to 0.05), medium (0.06 to 0.13) and large ($\geq$0.14). Post-hoc analyses comparing groups of patients at each time point were conducted using Wilcoxon rank sum tests or unpaired Student t-tests. Analyses comparing patient data at different follow-up time points were performed with Wilcoxon signed rank tests or paired Student t-tests. Tests were adjusted for multiple comparisons using the Bonferroni correction. Categorical variables were compared using Chi-squared tests or Fischer tests. To evaluate and compare the effect of hydrotherapy versus land-based therapy for the two different immobilization durations at different follow-ups, Cohen effect sizes were computed and interpreted as follows: negligeable (0.00 to 0.19), small (0.20 to 0.49), medium (0.50 to 0.79) and large ($\geq$0.80). The analyses were performed using R (version 4.1.3, R Foundation for Statistical Computing, Vienna, Austria), following the intention to treat analysis method, and with *p*-values less than 0.05 considered as significant.

3. Results

A total of 191 patients were eligible and six patients declined to participate to the study (3.1%). The study enrolled a cohort of 185 patients, among whom 92 patients were allocated to land-based therapy, comprising 29 (16%) patients who commenced physiotherapy early, and 63 (34%) who initiated it at a later phase. Conversely, 93 patients underwent hydrotherapy, with 33 (18%) in the early rehabilitation group, and 60 (32%) in the late rehabilitation group (Figure 1).

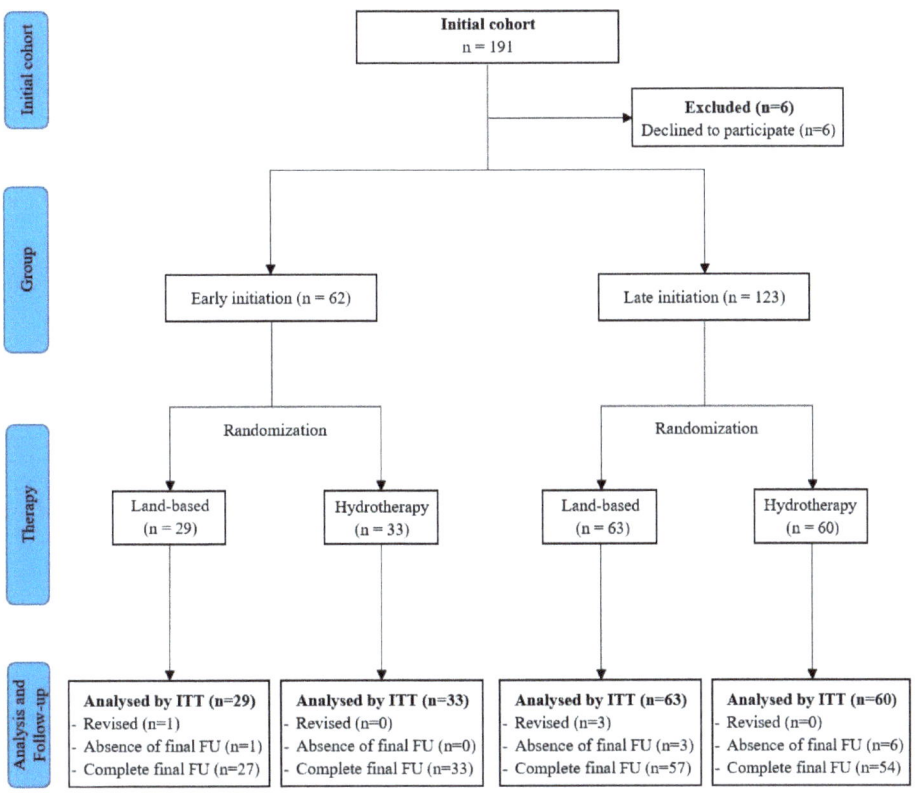

Figure 1. Flow diagram of patients' selection.

There was no statistical difference among the four groups concerning patient age ($p = 0.121$), dominancy of the affected side ($p = 0.114$) or gender distribution ($p = 0.992$) (Table 1). However, it is worth mentioning that patients allocated to the early hydrotherapy group had a slightly greater pre-operative Constant score (58.0 ± 16.7) compared with those in the late hydrotherapy group (50.6 ± 3.2) ($p = 0.009$) (Figure 2).

Table 1. Demographic and pre-operative data.

	Land-Based Therapy (n = 92)					Hydrotherapy (n = 93)					p-Value LB vs. H	
	Early (n = 29)		Late (n = 63)			Early (n = 33)		Late (n = 60)				
	Mean ± SD	(Min–Max)	Mean ± SD	(Min–Max)	p-Value	Mean ± SD	(Min–Max)	Mean ± SD	(Min–Max)	p-Value	Early	Late
	n (%)		n (%)			n (%)		n (%)				
Male gender	16 (55%)		36 (57%)		1.000	19 (58%)		33 (55%)		0.983	1.000	0.954
Dominant side	20 (69%)		33 (52%)		0.205	25 (76%)		35 (58%)		0.146	0.754	0.630
Age at surgery	56.0 ± 7.5	(45.0–75.0)	56.8 ± 5.4	(47.0–67.0)	0.624	52.8 ± 9.5	(37.0–69.0)	56.2 ± 5.2	(46.0–67.0)	0.063	0.146	0.811
Score Constant	55.9 ± 15.9	(21.0–88.0)	50.4 ± 3.3	(44.0–57.0)	0.125	58.0 ± 16.7	(30.0–87.5)	50.6 ± 3.2	(44.0–57.0)	**0.009**	1.000	1.000

H, Hydrotherapy; LB, Land-based; Max, Maximum; Min, Minimum; n, Number of patients; SD, Standard deviation. Bold and underlined p-values indicate statistically significant differences.

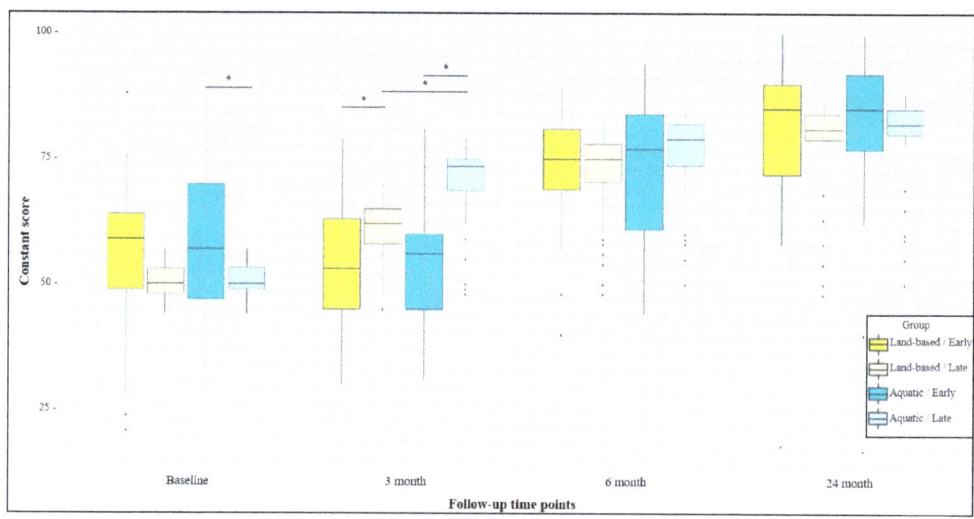

Figure 2. Pre-operative and post-operative Constant score depending on type of rehabilitation (Land-based therapy vs. Hydrotherapy) and the physiotherapy beginning (Early vs. Late). Black dots indicate outliers. Black stars indicate statistically significant difference between the groups at a given follow-up.

Post-Operative Outcomes

Patients who initiated physiotherapy early had no improvements at three months from baseline scores, regardless of rehabilitation protocol. Patients who started physiotherapy lately, on the other hand, had an improvement at three months both for the land-based rehabilitation (mean improvement of 10.6 points, $p < 0.001$) and the Hydrotherapy (mean improvement of 19.7 points, $p < 0.001$). At three months post-operatively, patients who initiated land-based physiotherapy later showed a significantly higher Constant score than those who initiated it early (mean difference of 6.4 points, $p = 0.042$), though this difference was not clinically relevant. At the same time-point, patients who initiated lately hydrotherapy had a statistically significant higher Constant score than those who initiated it early (mean difference of 14.9 points, $p < 0.001$), with this difference being clinically relevant. From three to six post-operative months, all groups statistically improved, exceeding a difference that seems to be clinically relevant, except for the Late–Hydrotherapy group. No statistically significant difference was observed neither between the land-based therapy and aquatic therapy groups when physiotherapy was initiated early (mean difference of 1.1 point, $p = 1.000$) or at a later phase (mean difference of 3.3 points, $p = 0.478$). At 6 months, all groups plateaued and no clinically relevant improvement was observed at 24 months. Only the Late-Land-based group had a statistical improvement (mean improvement of 6.6 points, $p = 0.003$). No differences were observed at 24 postoperative months, neither between patients who initiated early and lately land-based therapy (mean difference 1.0 point, $p = 1.000$), nor between patients who initiated early and lately aquatic therapy (mean difference of 0.4 point, $p = 1.000$). Likewise, initiating physiotherapy early after surgery was not statistically superior at 24 months in the land-based group (mean difference of 0.0 point, $p = 1.000$) and hydrotherapy group (1.5 point, $p = 1.000$) (Table 2).

Table 2. Comparison of post-operative scores between the rehabilitation type (Land-based vs. Hydrotherapy) and the beginning of therapy (Early vs. Late).

| | Land-Based Therapy (n = 92) | | | | | Hydrotherapy (n = 93) | | | | | p-Value LB vs. H | |
| | Early (n = 29) | | Late (n = 63) | | | Early (n = 33) | | Late (n = 60) | | | | |
	Mean ± SD	(Min–Max)	Mean ± SD	(Min–Max)	p-Value	Mean ± SD	(Min–Max)	Mean ± SD	(Min–Max)	p-Value	Early	Late
Constant												
3 months	54.6 ± 13.3	(30.0–79.0)	61.0 ± 5.7	(45.0–70.0) *	**0.042**	55.4 ± 12.8	(31.0–81.0)	70.3 ± 8.2	(48.0–79.0) *	**≤0.001**	1.000	**≤0.001**
6 months	72.6 ± 12.3	(40.0–90.0) *	72.2 ± 8.6	(48.0–82.0) *	1.000	73.7 ± 13.7	(44.0–94.0) *	75.5 ± 9.5	(50.0–86.0) *	1.000	1.000	0.478
24 months	79.8 ± 16.2	(18.0–100.0)	78.8 ± 9.0	(48.0–87.0) *	1.000	79.8 ± 18.0	(17.0–100.0)	80.3 ± 8.6	(50.0–88.0)	1.000	1.000	1.000

H, Hydrotherapy; LB, Land-based; Max, Maximum; Min, Minimum; SD, Standard deviation; * indicates significant difference with previous follow-up (Wilcoxon signed rank test with Bonferroni correction). Bold and underlined p-values indicate statistically significant differences.

The two-way ANOVA revealed an effect of the rehabilitation type ($p = 0.001$), and the immobilization duration ($p < 0.001$), with an interaction between those two factors ($p = 0.004$) at a three-month follow-up solely (Table 3).

Table 3. Two-way mixed ANOVA (type III tests) for Constant score at the different follow-up.

Follow-Up	Effect	DFn	DFd	F	p-Value	Ges
3 month	Rehabilitation	1	181	11.786	**0.001**	0.061
	Immobilization	1	181	52.562	**<0.001**	0.225
	Rehabilitation × Immobilization	1	181	8.372	**0.004**	0.044
6 month	Rehabilitation	1	181	1.808	0.180	0.010
	Immobilization	1	181	0.2	0.655	0.001
	Rehabilitation × Immobilization	1	181	0.471	0.493	0.003
24 month	Rehabilitation	1	181	0.158	0.692	0.001
	Immobilization	1	181	0.017	0.895	0.000
	Rehabilitation × Immobilization	1	181	0.16	0.690	0.001

DF, Degrees of Freedom; F, F-Statistic; Ges, Generalized eta squared. Bold and underlined p-values indicate statistically significant associations.

Cohen effect sizes showed that, at a three-month follow-up, hydrotherapy had a large effect compared to land-based therapy when initiated later only (Cohen's d, 1.34; 95%CI, 0.95–1.73). A tendency was also observed at 6 months post-operatively in favor of the late hydrotherapy protocol (Cohen's d, 0.35; 95%CI, −0.01–0.70) (Figure 3).

The rate of complications was higher for patients who initiated their rehabilitation lately for both the land-based and aquatic rehabilitation groups. Patients who initiated physiotherapy lately had more revisions (2.4% vs. 1.6%) and more complications (19.5% vs. 6.5%) for those allocated to the hydrotherapy ($p = 0.033$), and we observed a tendency also for those who underwent conventional land-based therapy ($p = 0.071$).

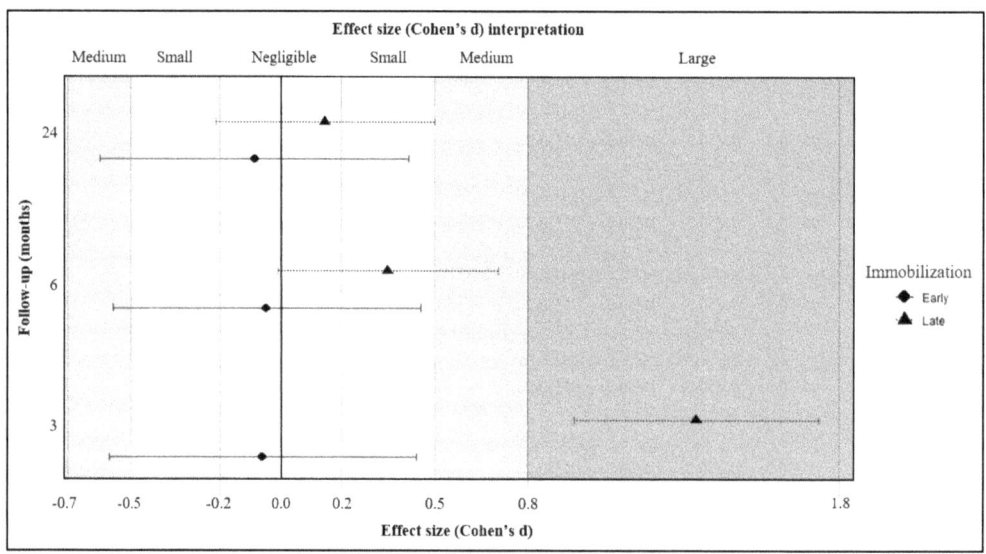

Figure 3. Effect size of early and late hydrotherapy (compared to land-based rehabilitation) at each follow-up time point.

4. Discussion

Hydrotherapy is an interesting modality in rehabilitation due to its capacity to facilitate shoulder mobilization while exerting lesser strain on muscles and tendons. However, evidence concerning the effects of hydrotherapy remains relatively sparse. Recent investigations by Cikes et al. [21] and Dufournet et al. [34] explored this thematic, albeit yielding contradictory outcomes. Nevertheless, there was an important methodological difference between the two studies, as the post-operative immobilization duration differed greatly, with patients included in the Dufournet et al. study having a 10-day immobilization period, while patients included in the Cikes et al. study had a 30-day immobilization period. The objective of this study was therefore to assess the potential interaction between rehabilitation type (Land-based therapy vs. Hydrotherapy) and the duration of immobilization (Early vs. Late). The main finding of this study was that hydrotherapy had a large effect at three months in improving the functional patient status (compared to land-based rehabilitation) only for those who were immobilized for longer period, confirming the interaction between the rehabilitation type and the immobilization duration.

Previous studies have shown that shoulder recovery can be accelerated using hydrotherapy rather than land-based therapy [21,32]. Aquatic therapy facilitates passive or active range of motion exercises with reduced strain on the musculo-tendinous structures. This reduced stress on muscles and tendons allows for earlier engagement of the affected shoulder, potentially enhancing improving the healing process without compromising long-term tendon integrity [32,44]. Despite the increasing interest in hydrotherapy, the current literature remains limited with studies based on small sample sizes [32,33], or where hydrotherapy is combined with standard therapy [32], thereby complicating the assessment of aquatic therapy's independent effect. In this study, however, we identified that hydrotherapy had a particular efficient role for patients who were first immobilized for a longer period (Cohen's d: 1.34, 95%CI [0.95–1.73], who may have stiffer shoulders [45]. Among the patients undergoing hydrotherapy, thaose who started therapy lately demonstrated a significantly higher score of 15 points at a three-month follow-up compared to those who started immediately after surgery ($p < 0.001$), exceeding the minimal clinically important difference. Likewise, Sekome et al. found beneficial short-term effects of hydrotherapy for patients experiencing knee stiffness [46]. Conversely, we found that hydrotherapy had a negligible short-term effect when initiated promptly, as patients may be less likely to develop stiffness due to rapid mobilization (Cohen's d: −0.06 [−0.57–0.44]). Consistently, akin to the preceding studies, there was no effect of hydrotherapy at 6 months ($p = 1.000$) and at 24 months post-operatively ($p = 1.000$).

The disparities between early and delayed rehabilitation initiation have been largely reported for the traditional land-based therapy. The results, however, differ according to the studies, with some reporting an improved range of motion, function and pain up to six months [23], while others reported no differences [27,28,47]. Most of these differences are transient stiffness, and results are equivalent at a 1-year follow-up [23,25,27,48,49]. In our study, we found that traditional land-based therapy provided higher Constant score at three post-operative months when started later ($p = 0.042$). Nevertheless, this difference didn't reach a clinical importance (mean improvement 6.4) [43]. As found in the aforementioned studies, this difference had vanished at later follow-ups ($p = 1.000$). The immobilization duration also had an effect on the two-year complication rate with patients who initiated physiotherapy lately having more complications (20% vs. 7%) and revisions (4% vs. 2%). Patients undergoing hydrotherapy early had less complications (3% vs. 12%) and less revisions (0% vs. 3%). Thus, rehabilitation protocol modalities should be guided by the desire to have good results quickly or to privilege the absence of complications in the longer term. Therefore, all patients should not necessarily be allocated to an aquatic-based therapy since the results are heterogeneous depending on the immobilization duration, and the burden (financial, temporal, etc.) that this therapy can add on the patient. However, caution is required in inferring the figures as the design of our study does not provide the necessary power to assess complication rates and revision rates. Further studies are needed to compare the long-term repair integrity associated with the rehabilitation modalities.

Limitations

Related to the different modalities, neither clinicians nor patients were blinded to their rehabilitation. The surgical interventions were carried out by two distinct experienced surgeons operating in two different centers. However, to mitigate this potential bias, effect sizes regarding the impact rehabilitation type were computed by comparing groups within the same center. Moreover, only the Constant score was used whereas other PROMs would have been of interest such as the pain measured on a visual analog scale or the American Shoulder and Elbow Surgeons score. Additionally, these patient-reported scores are inherently subjective as they rely on patient responses and their initial health condition. Consequently, patients exposed to a longer period of immobilization might start physiotherapy in a relatively worse condition, potentially influencing their perception of improvement, thereby rating their progress more positively. Therefore, complementing these findings with more objective measures such as range of motions would indeed be beneficial and informative.

5. Conclusions

Hydrotherapy is a modality that provides superior results at a short-term follow-up in patients who initiated physiotherapy later compared to land-based therapy. At long-term follow-up, however, there was no difference in Constant score between the groups. This absence of discrepancy persisted irrespective of the type of rehabilitation employed or the duration of immobilization.

Author Contributions: Conceptualization, A.L., A.C., J.Z. and T.M.; methodology, A.L., A.P. and H.B.; validation, A.L., A.C., J.Z. and T.M.; formal analysis, A.P. and H.B.; investigation, A.L. and A.C.; resources, A.L. and A.C.; writing—original draft preparation, A.P.; writing—review and editing, A.L., A.C., J.Z., H.B. and T.M.; visualization, A.P. and H.B.; supervision, A.L. and H.B.; project administration, A.L. and H.B. All authors have read and agreed to the published version of the manuscript.

Funding: This research received no external funding.

Institutional Review Board Statement: This investigation was based on the data of two published studies that were conducted in accordance with the Declaration of Helsinki, and were both approved by local ethic committees (CER-VD-481/15, 13 January 2016; CCER-2016-02242, 27 July 2017).

Informed Consent Statement: Informed consent was obtained from all subjects involved in the study.

Data Availability Statement: The data presented in this study are available from the corresponding author upon reasonable request.

Conflicts of Interest: A.L. receives royalties from Stryker and Medacta, is a paid consultant for Arthrex, Stryker, Medacta, and Enovis, and is a board member of the French Arthroscopic Society. Other authors declare no conflict of interest.

References

1. Luime, J.J.; Koes, B.W.; Hendriksen, I.J.; Burdorf, A.; Verhagen, A.P.; Miedema, H.S.; Verhaar, J.A. Prevalence and incidence of shoulder pain in the general population; a systematic review. *Scand. J. Rheumatol.* **2004**, *33*, 73–81. [CrossRef]
2. Bunker, T. Rotator cuff disease. *Curr. Orthop.* **2002**, *3*, 223–233. [CrossRef]
3. Hashimoto, T.; Nobuhara, K.; Hamada, T. Pathologic evidence of degeneration as a primary cause of rotator cuff tear. *Clin. Orthop. Relat. Res.* **2003**, *415*, 111–120. [CrossRef] [PubMed]
4. Codding, J.L.; Keener, J.D. Natural History of Degenerative Rotator Cuff Tears. *Curr. Rev. Musculoskelet. Med.* **2018**, *11*, 77–85. [CrossRef] [PubMed]
5. Karjalainen, T.V.; Jain, N.B.; Heikkinen, J.; Johnston, R.V.; Page, C.M.; Buchbinder, R. Surgery for rotator cuff tears. *Cochrane Database Syst. Rev.* **2019**, *12*, CD013502. [CrossRef] [PubMed]
6. Teunis, T.; Lubberts, B.; Reilly, B.T.; Ring, D. A systematic review and pooled analysis of the prevalence of rotator cuff disease with increasing age. *J. Shoulder Elb. Surg.* **2014**, *23*, 1913–1921. [CrossRef] [PubMed]
7. Vidal, C.; Lira, M.J.; de Marinis, R.; Liendo, R.; Contreras, J.J. Increasing incidence of rotator cuff surgery: A nationwide registry study in Chile. *BMC Musculoskelet. Disord.* **2021**, *22*, 1052. [CrossRef] [PubMed]
8. Yanik, E.L.; Chamberlain, A.M.; Keener, J.D. Trends in rotator cuff repair rates and comorbidity burden among commercially insured patients younger than the age of 65 years, United States 2007–2016. *JSES Rev. Rep. Tech.* **2021**, *1*, 309–316. [CrossRef]
9. Paloneva, J.; Lepola, V.; Aarimaa, V.; Joukainen, A.; Ylinen, J.; Mattila, V.M. Increasing incidence of rotator cuff repairs—A nationwide registry study in Finland. *BMC Musculoskelet. Disord.* **2015**, *16*, 189. [CrossRef]
10. Littlewood, C.M.S.; Walters, S. Epidemiology of Rotator Cuff Tendinopathy: A Systematic Review. *Shoulder Elb.* **2013**, *5*, 256–265. [CrossRef]
11. McCabe, R.A.; Nicholas, S.J.; Montgomery, K.D.; Finneran, J.J.; McHugh, M.P. The effect of rotator cuff tear size on shoulder strength and range of motion. *J. Orthop. Sports Phys. Ther.* **2005**, *35*, 130–135. [CrossRef]
12. Parikh, N.; Martinez, D.J.; Winer, I.; Costa, L.; Dua, D.; Trueman, P. Direct and indirect economic burden associated with rotator cuff tears and repairs in the US. *Curr. Med. Res. Opin.* **2021**, *37*, 1199–1211. [CrossRef]
13. Paraskevopoulos, E.; Plakoutsis, G.; Chronopoulos, E.; Maria, P. Effectiveness of Combined Program of Manual Therapy and Exercise Vs Exercise Only in Patients With Rotator Cuff-related Shoulder Pain: A Systematic Review and Meta-analysis. *Sports Health* **2023**, *15*, 727–735. [CrossRef]
14. Longo, U.G.; Rizzello, G.; Petrillo, S.; Loppini, M.; Maffulli, N.; Denaro, V. Conservative Rehabilitation Provides Superior Clinical Results Compared to Early Aggressive Rehabilitation for Rotator Cuff Repair: A Retrospective Comparative Study. *Medicina* **2019**, *55*, 402. [CrossRef]
15. Moosmayer, S.; Gartner, A.V.; Tariq, R. The natural course of nonoperatively treated rotator cuff tears: An 8.8-year follow-up of tear anatomy and clinical outcome in 49 patients. *J. Shoulder Elb. Surg.* **2017**, *26*, 627–634. [CrossRef]
16. Chalmers, P.N.; Ross, H.; Granger, E.; Presson, A.P.; Zhang, C.; Tashjian, R.Z. The Effect of Rotator Cuff Repair on Natural History: A Systematic Review of Intermediate to Long-Term Outcomes. *JB JS Open Access* **2018**, *3*, e0043. [CrossRef]
17. Colvin, A.C.; Egorova, N.; Harrison, A.K.; Moskowitz, A.; Flatow, E.L. National trends in rotator cuff repair. *J. Bone Joint Surg. Am.* **2012**, *94*, 227–233. [CrossRef] [PubMed]
18. Tauro, J.C. Arthroscopic rotator cuff repair: Analysis of technique and results at 2- and 3-year follow-up. *Arthroscopy* **1998**, *14*, 45–51. [CrossRef] [PubMed]
19. Aleem, A.W.; Brophy, R.H. Outcomes of rotator cuff surgery: What does the evidence tell us? *Clin. Sports Med.* **2012**, *31*, 665–674. [CrossRef]
20. Namdari, S.; Green, A. Range of motion limitation after rotator cuff repair. *J. Shoulder Elb. Surg.* **2010**, *19*, 290–296. [CrossRef] [PubMed]
21. Cikes, A.; Kadri, F.; van Rooij, F.; Ladermann, A. Aquatic therapy following arthroscopic rotator cuff repair enables faster improvement of Constant score than land-based therapy or self-rehabilitation therapy. *J. Exp. Orthop.* **2023**, *10*, 2. [CrossRef]
22. Bouche, P.A.; Gaujac, N.; Descamps, J.; Conso, C. Assessment of several postoperative protocols after rotator cuff repair: A network meta-analysis. *Orthop. Traumatol. Surg. Res.* **2022**, *108*, 103418. [CrossRef]

23. Keener, J.D.; Galatz, L.M.; Stobbs-Cucchi, G.; Patton, R.; Yamaguchi, K. Rehabilitation following arthroscopic rotator cuff repair: A prospective randomized trial of immobilization compared with early motion. *J. Bone Joint Surg. Am.* **2014**, *96*, 11–19. [CrossRef]
24. Nabergoj, M.; Bagheri, N.; Bonnevialle, N.; Gallinet, D.; Barth, J.; Labattut, L.; Metais, P.; Godeneche, A.; Garret, J.; Clavert, P.; et al. Arthroscopic rotator cuff repair: Is healing enough? *Orthop. Traumatol. Surg. Res.* **2021**, *107*, 103100. [CrossRef]
25. Cuff, D.J.; Pupello, D.R. Prospective randomized study of arthroscopic rotator cuff repair using an early versus delayed postoperative physical therapy protocol. *J. Shoulder Elb. Surg.* **2012**, *21*, 1450–1455. [CrossRef]
26. Gallagher, B.P.; Bishop, M.E.; Tjoumakaris, F.P.; Freedman, K.B. Early versus delayed rehabilitation following arthroscopic rotator cuff repair: A systematic review. *Phys. Sportsmed.* **2015**, *43*, 178–187. [CrossRef]
27. Mazuquin, B.; Moffatt, M.; Gill, P.; Selfe, J.; Rees, J.; Drew, S.; Littlewood, C. Effectiveness of early versus delayed rehabilitation following rotator cuff repair: Systematic review and meta-analyses. *PLoS ONE* **2021**, *16*, e0252137. [CrossRef] [PubMed]
28. Sheps, D.M.; Silveira, A.; Beaupre, L.; Styles-Tripp, F.; Balyk, R.; Lalani, A.; Glasgow, R.; Bergman, J.; Bouliane, M.; Shoulder; et al. Early Active Motion Versus Sling Immobilization After Arthroscopic Rotator Cuff Repair: A Randomized Controlled Trial. *Arthroscopy* **2019**, *35*, 749–760.e742. [CrossRef] [PubMed]
29. Houck, D.A.; Kraeutler, M.J.; Schuette, H.B.; McCarty, E.C.; Bravman, J.T. Early Versus Delayed Motion After Rotator Cuff Repair: A Systematic Review of Overlapping Meta-analyses. *Am. J. Sports Med.* **2017**, *45*, 2911–2915. [CrossRef] [PubMed]
30. Speer, K.P.; Cavanaugh, J.T.; Warren, R.F.; Day, L.; Wickiewicz, T.L. A role for hydrotherapy in shoulder rehabilitation. *Am. J. Sports Med.* **1993**, *21*, 850–853. [CrossRef] [PubMed]
31. Levin, S. Early Mobilization Speeds Recovery. *Phys. Sportsmed.* **1993**, *21*, 70–74. [CrossRef] [PubMed]
32. Brady, B.; Redfern, J.; MacDougal, G.; Williams, J. The addition of aquatic therapy to rehabilitation following surgical rotator cuff repair: A feasibility study. *Physiother. Res. Int.* **2008**, *13*, 153–161. [CrossRef] [PubMed]
33. Burmaster, C.; Eckenrode, B.J.; Stiebel, M. Early Incorporation of an Evidence-Based Aquatic-Assisted Approach to Arthroscopic Rotator Cuff Repair Rehabilitation: Prospective Case Study. *Phys. Ther.* **2016**, *96*, 53–61. [CrossRef] [PubMed]
34. Dufournet, A.; Chong, X.L.; Schwitzguebel, A.; Bernimoulin, C.; Carvalho, M.; Bothorel, H.; Ladermann, A. Aquatic Therapy versus Standard Rehabilitation after Surgical Rotator Cuff Repair: A Randomized Prospective Study. *Biology* **2022**, *11*, 610. [CrossRef] [PubMed]
35. Ladermann, A.; Burkhart, S.S.; Hoffmeyer, P.; Neyton, L.; Collin, P.; Yates, E.; Denard, P.J. Classification of full-thickness rotator cuff lesions: A review. *EFORT Open Rev.* **2016**, *1*, 420–430. [CrossRef] [PubMed]
36. Patte, D. Classification of rotator cuff lesions. *Clin. Orthop. Relat. Res.* **1990**, *254*, 81–86. [CrossRef]
37. Goutallier, D.; Postel, J.M.; Bernageau, J.; Lavau, L.; Voisin, M.C. Fatty muscle degeneration in cuff ruptures. Pre- and postoperative evaluation by CT scan. *Clin. Orthop. Relat. Res.* **1994**, *304*, 78–83. [CrossRef]
38. Abrassart, S.; Kolo, F.; Piotton, S.; Chih-Hao Chiu, J.; Stirling, P.; Hoffmeyer, P.; Ladermann, A. 'Frozen shoulder' is ill-defined. How can it be described better? *EFORT Open Rev.* **2020**, *5*, 273–279. [CrossRef]
39. Constant, C.R.; Murley, A.H. A clinical method of functional assessment of the shoulder. *Clin. Orthop. Relat. Res.* **1987**, *214*, 160–164. [CrossRef]
40. Ladermann, A.; Chague, S.; Preissmann, D.; Kolo, F.C.; Zbinden, O.; Kevelham, B.; Bothorel, H.; Charbonnier, C. Acromioplasty during repair of rotator cuff tears removes only half of the impinging acromial bone. *JSES Int.* **2020**, *4*, 592–600. [CrossRef]
41. Collin, P.; McCoubrey, G.; Ladermann, A. Posterosuperior rotator cuff repair by an independent double-row technique. Technical note and radiological and clinical results. *Orthop. Traumatol. Surg. Res.* **2016**, *102*, 405–408. [CrossRef]
42. Barth, J.; Andrieu, K.; Fotiadis, E.; Hannink, G.; Barthelemy, R.; Saffarini, M. Critical period and risk factors for retear following arthroscopic repair of the rotator cuff. *Knee Surg. Sports Traumatol. Arthrosc.* **2017**, *25*, 2196–2204. [CrossRef] [PubMed]
43. Kukkonen, J.; Kauko, T.; Vahlberg, T.; Joukainen, A.; Aarimaa, V. Investigating minimal clinically important difference for Constant score in patients undergoing rotator cuff surgery. *J. Shoulder Elb. Surg.* **2013**, *22*, 1650–1655. [CrossRef]
44. Killian, M.L.; Cavinatto, L.; Galatz, L.M.; Thomopoulos, S. The role of mechanobiology in tendon healing. *J. Shoulder Elb. Surg.* **2012**, *21*, 228–237. [CrossRef] [PubMed]
45. Sarver, J.J.; Peltz, C.D.; Dourte, L.; Reddy, S.; Williams, G.R.; Soslowsky, L.J. After rotator cuff repair, stiffness--but not the loss in range of motion--increased transiently for immobilized shoulders in a rat model. *J. Shoulder Elb. Surg.* **2008**, *17*, 108S–113S. [CrossRef] [PubMed]
46. Sekome, K.; Maddocks, S. The short-term effects of hydrotherapy on pain and self-perceived functional status in individuals living with osteoarthritis of the knee joint. *S. Afr. J. Physiother.* **2019**, *75*, 476. [CrossRef] [PubMed]
47. Kim, Y.S.; Chung, S.W.; Kim, J.Y.; Ok, J.H.; Park, I.; Oh, J.H. Is early passive motion exercise necessary after arthroscopic rotator cuff repair? *Am. J. Sports Med.* **2012**, *40*, 815–821. [CrossRef] [PubMed]
48. Thomson, S.; Jukes, C.; Lewis, J. Rehabilitation following surgical repair of the rotator cuff: A systematic review. *Physiotherapy* **2016**, *102*, 20–28. [CrossRef]
49. Yi, A.; Villacis, D.; Yalamanchili, R.; Hatch, G.F., 3rd. A Comparison of Rehabilitation Methods After Arthroscopic Rotator Cuff Repair: A Systematic Review. *Sports Health* **2015**, *7*, 326–334. [CrossRef]

Disclaimer/Publisher's Note: The statements, opinions and data contained in all publications are solely those of the individual author(s) and contributor(s) and not of MDPI and/or the editor(s). MDPI and/or the editor(s) disclaim responsibility for any injury to people or property resulting from any ideas, methods, instructions or products referred to in the content.

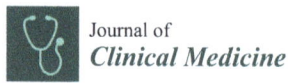 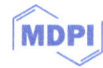

Article

The Influence of Temporary Epiphysiodesis of the Proximal End of the Tibia on the Shape of the Knee Joint in Children Treated for Leg Length Discrepancy

Grzegorz Starobrat [1], Anna Danielewicz [1,*], Tomasz Szponder [2], Magdalena Wójciak [3], Ireneusz Sowa [3], Monika Różańska-Boczula [4] and Michał Latalski [1]

[1] Department of Paediatric Orthopaedics, Medical University of Lublin, 20-093 Lublin, Poland; starobrat@o2.pl (G.S.); michallatalski@umlub.pl (M.L.)
[2] Department and Clinic of Animal Surgery, Faculty of Veterinary Medicine, University of Life Sciences, 20-612 Lublin, Poland; tomasz.szponder@up.lublin.pl
[3] Department of Analytical Chemistry, Medical University of Lublin, 20-093 Lublin, Poland; magdalena.wojciak@umlub.pl (M.W.); ireneusz.sowa@umlub.pl (I.S.)
[4] Department of Applied Mathematics and Computer Science, University of Life Sciences in Lublin, 20-033 Lublin, Poland; monika.boczula@up.lublin.pl
* Correspondence: anna.danielewicz@umlub.pl

Abstract: Background: Leg length discrepancy (LLD) is a common problem in the daily clinical practice of pediatric orthopedists. Surgical treatment using LLD temporary epiphysiodesis with eight-plate implants is a minimally invasive, safe, and well-tolerated procedure that provides good treatment effects with a relatively low percentage of complications. The main aim of this retrospective study was to determine the effect of epiphysiodesis on the shape of the proximal tibia. **Methods:** The retrospective study was based on medical records from 2010 to 2019. Radiographs taken before the epiphysiodesis and at 6-month intervals until the end of the treatment were investigated. A total of 60 patients treated for LLD were included in the study (24 girls, 36 boys). They were divided into three groups depending on the duration of the LLD treatment: group I (18 months), group II (30 months), and group III (42 months of treatment). Radiological parameters were assessed, including the roof angle (D), the slope angles (α and β), and the specific parameters of the tibial epiphysis, namely LTH (lateral tubercle height), MTH (medial tubercle height), and TW (tibial width). **Results:** The roof angle decreased in all the groups, which was accompanied by an increase in the β or α angle. LTH, MTH and TW also increased, and the differences before and after the treatment for the treated legs were statistically significant in all the studied groups. The greatest change in the shape of the articular surface of the proximal tibia occurred after 42 months of treatment. **Conclusions:** The study showed that epiphysiodesis affects the proximal tibial articular surface over prolonged treatment. Thus, there is a need for future long-term follow-up studies to elucidate the potential effects of LLD egalization.

Keywords: leg length discrepancy; temporary epiphysiodesis; eight-plate; growth plate; knee deformity

Citation: Starobrat, G.; Danielewicz, A.; Szponder, T.; Wójciak, M.; Sowa, I.; Różańska-Boczula, M.; Latalski, M. The Influence of Temporary Epiphysiodesis of the Proximal End of the Tibia on the Shape of the Knee Joint in Children Treated for Leg Length Discrepancy. *J. Clin. Med.* **2024**, *13*, 1458. https://doi.org/10.3390/jcm13051458

Academic Editor: Christian Ehrnthaller

Received: 15 December 2023
Revised: 26 February 2024
Accepted: 29 February 2024
Published: 2 March 2024

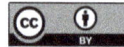

Copyright: © 2024 by the authors. Licensee MDPI, Basel, Switzerland. This article is an open access article distributed under the terms and conditions of the Creative Commons Attribution (CC BY) license (https://creativecommons.org/licenses/by/4.0/).

1. Introduction

Leg length discrepancy (LLD) of the lower limbs may result from structural deformations, i.e., real differences in the length of bones that make up a given limb segment [1–3]. Leg length discrepancy occurs in approximately two-thirds of the population of children. LLD up to approximately 5 mm occurs in approximately 10–12% of the population, and LLD above 10 mm occurs in approximately 4% of the population.

The modern Multiplier app and Paley Growth app include a number of features used in a variety of clinical contexts, including upper- and lower-limb LLD calculation, epiphysiodesis time, and limb growth charts. It also contains information on other growth disorders [4].

Epiphysiodesis is a method of treating LLD that involves surgically blocking the growth plate in order to inhibit the growth of the longer limb. The first procedures involved irreversible destruction of the bone growth region, and the following years brought the development of reversible methods enabling safer control of limb growth [5].

Epiphysiodesis with flexible plates in the shape of the figure "8" and two screws (Figure 1) was introduced in 2007 by Stevens (Orthofix; McKinney, TX, USA).

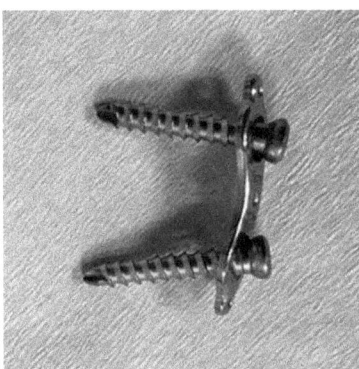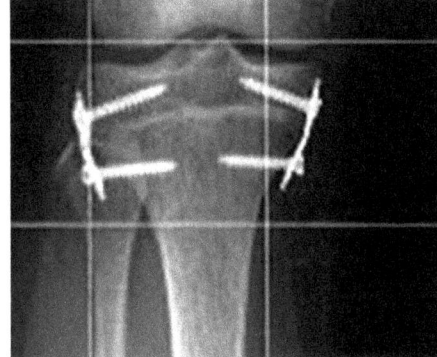

Figure 1. Eight-plate implant and X-ray image of the knee joint showing eight-plate implants used for the treatment of leg length discrepancy.

These implants were developed as a response to complications that occurred when using Blount staples. The strong compression with a stiff pin damaged the growth plate, which prevented it from functioning after the implant was removed. Other complications included damage or dislodgement during treatment [6].

There are no studies in the literature presenting the influence of temporal epiphysiodesis on the shape of the knee articular surface. Most of the available works on epiphysiodesis analyze the degree of its effectiveness—compensation of LLD—in various contexts. The impact of epiphysiodesis on the shape of the knee joint, the duration of treatment followed by joint deformation, and, consequently, biomechanics disorders has not been subjected to a broader analysis so far. Thus, the main aim of this study was to determine the effect of epiphysiodesis on the shape of the proximal tibia and establish a time frame for the safe use of this procedure. The following radiological parameters were assessed: the roof angle (D), the slope angles (α and β), and the specific parameters of the tibial epiphysis, namely LTH (lateral tubercle height), MTH (medial tubercle height), and TW (tibial width).

2. Materials and Methods

2.1. Selection of Participants

The study protocol and consent form were approved by the Bioethics Committee of the Medical University of Lublin (number KE-0254/81/2020, dated 30 April 2020). Our study was retrospective in nature. Medical records from 2010 to 2019, available in the archives of the Pediatric Orthopedic Clinic at the Medical University of Lublin, were analyzed. The inclusion criterion was idiopathic leg length discrepancy of lower limbs treated by temporary epiphysiodesis of the proximal tibia using eight-plate implants. The indication for the treatment was the presence of an active growth plate, indicating skeletal immaturity. The exclusion criteria included an etiology of shortening other than idiopathic and surgical procedures in the limb segment planned for treatment.

In the end, 60 cases were qualified for the study (24 girls, 36 boys). They were divided into 3 groups depending on the duration of the LLD treatment (group I (18 months), group II (30 months), and group III (42 months)). The characteristics of the groups are given in Table 1.

Table 1. Characteristics of participants.

Parameter	Group I	Group II	Group III
Duration of treatment (months)	18	30	42
Number/(boys/girls)	24/(12/12)	24/(18/6)	12/(6/6)
Age y.m average/(range)	13.2/(12.2–13.80)	10.11/(10.2–11.11)	9.0/(8.6–9.6)
Age y.m boys average/(range)	13.0/(12.2–13.11)	11.3/(10.7–11.11)	9.2/(9.0–9.6)
Age y.m girls average/(range)	13.3/(2.11–13.10)	10.6/(10.2–10.11)	8.11/(8.10–9.6)
LLD cm average/(range)	2.0/(1.5–2.8)	2.6/(1.4–3.6)	2.4/(1.6–3.6)
LLD cm boys average/(range)	2.1/(1.5–2.8)	2.6/(1.5–2.8)	2.5/(2.0–3.2)
LLD cm girls average/(range)	2.0/(1.5–2.6)	2.6/(1.4–3.6)	2.4/(1.6–3.6)

y.m—year.months; LLD—leg length discrepancy.

2.2. Study Design

Radiographs taken before the planned epiphysiodesis procedure and at intervals of +/− 6 months until the end of the treatment were assessed. A full-length standing AP radiograph of the lower limbs (body X-ray) was used to assess angular and linear parameters. A single radiographic exposure of both lower limbs was performed, with the radiation beam centered on the knees from a distance of approximately 180 cm and the patient standing upright with both patellas pointing directly forward. To illustrate changes in the tibial plate surface expressed in degrees, measurements of the angles of the triangle proposed by R. Sinha from the connection of the tibial articular line (the line connecting the external highest points of the tibial condyles—green line in Figure 2), the medial line of the tibial plate inclination (the line between the highest point in the projection of the medial intercondylar tubercle and the point defining the outermost upper end of the medial condyle—blue line in Figure 2) (angle α), and the lateral line of the tibial plate inclination (the line between the highest point in the projection of the lateral intercondylar tubercle and the point defining the outer highest upper end of the lateral condyle—orange line in Figure 2) (angle β) were performed [7].

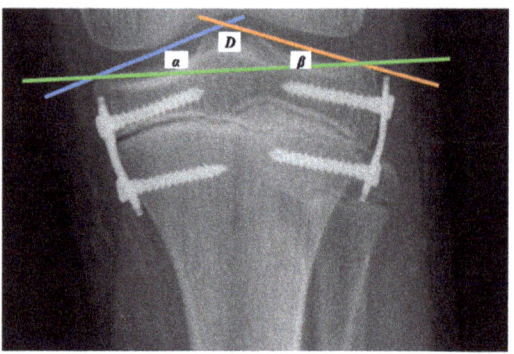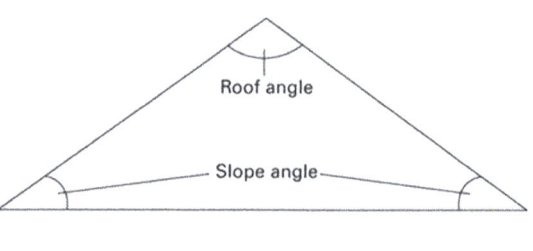

Figure 2. A graphic image of the tibial articular line (green line), the medial line of the tibial plate inclination (blue line), and the lateral tibial plate slope (orange line), as well as a graphical representation of the roof angle.

The "tibial roof" angle (D) is included between the medial and lateral lines of the tibial plate inclination, defined as the result of the difference in the acute angles of the triangle formed by the lines (the medial tibial plate inclination line, the lateral line of the tibial plate inclination, and the tibial articular line (180 minus α, minus β)) [7].

To illustrate changes in the tibial plate surface expressed in millimeters, the changes in the height of the intercondylar tubercles of the medial MLH (dimension measured from the tibial articular line to the highest point in the projection of the medial intercondylar tubercle;

blue arrow) (Figure 3) and lateral LTH (dimension measured from the tibial articular line to the highest point in the projection of the lateral intercondylar tubercle; orange arrow) (Figure 3) were assessed. Changes in the width of the distal tibial epiphysis were illustrated by the TW parameter (width of the tibial epiphysis measured between the widest points of the proximal tibial epiphysis, one located on the lateral and the other on the medial cortex; black arrow) (Figure 3).

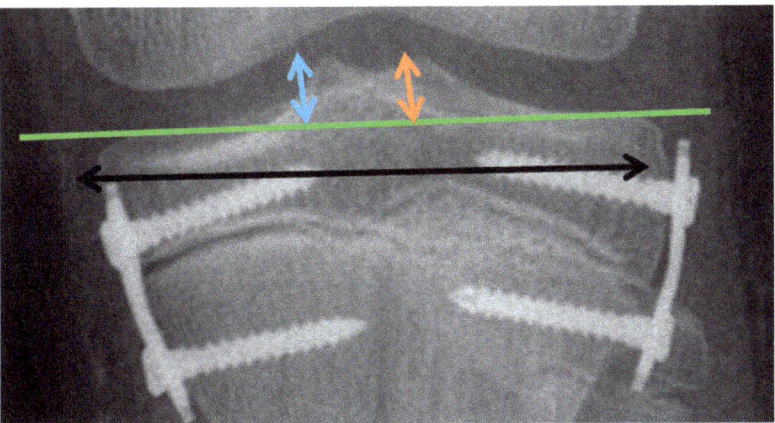

Figure 3. Graphical display of linear parameters. MLH (dimension measured from the tibial articular line to the highest point in the projection of the medial intercondylar tubercle) (blue arrow); LTH (dimension measured from the tibial articular line to the highest point in the projection of the lateral intercondylar tubercle) (orange arrow); and TW (width of the tibial epiphysis measured between the widest points of the proximal tibial epiphysis, one located on the lateral and the other on the medial cortex) (black arrow).

Data regarding the following characteristics (parameters) were collected for each person. For each feature, 4 measurements (group I), 6 measurements (group II), and 8 measurements (group III) were performed and repeated at equal time intervals (every 6 months). Observations were made for both the longer (treated) limb ("d") and the shorter (non-treated) limb ("k").

2.3. Statistical Analysis

Each measurement was performed three times. Statistical evaluation of the data was performed using Statistica ver. 13.1 software. The significance level of the tests was $\alpha = 0.05$. Since no normal distribution of the characteristics (Shapiro–Wilk test, $p < 0.05$) and no homogeneity of the relevant variances (Levene's test) were confirmed, non-parametric tests were used to assess the relationships. When comparing measurements between subsequent time points, the Friedman test (equivalent to one-way analysis of variance for repeated measurements) was used, and the Wilcoxon paired test was used to compare two dependent features. Box-and-whisker plots were made to illustrate the changes.

3. Results

In this study, changes in the tibial plate surface were assessed using measurements of the D, α, and β angles (degree value), as well as the parameters of the tibial epiphysis (in mm), both after the treatment and at various time periods.

A decrease in the D angle reflects the elevation of both tubercles of the tibial plate, an increase in the α angle illustrates the lowering of the medial part of the tibial plate, and an increase in the β angle reflects the lifting of the lateral part of the tibial plate. In turn, an increase in LTH and MTH indicates a change in the shape of the articular surface of the tibia to a more conical one due to the apparent hyperactivity of the middle part of the growth plate. This may result in the loosening of the ACL (anterior cruciate ligament) and the PCL (posterior cruciate ligament), consequently creating a sense of instability.

3.1. Changes in the Investigated Parameters Evaluated after the Completion of the Treatment

The results for all the investigated parameters expressed as the difference between the values obtained after and before the treatment and the statistical analysis of the significance of the differences between the values obtained at the beginning and after the treatment are summarized in Tables 2 and 3, respectively.

Table 2. Changes in the investigated parameters from the beginning to the end of the treatment period.

Parameter	Group I (0–18 Months)			Group II (0–30 Months)			Group III (0–42 Months)		
	Girls	Boys	Total	Girls	Boys	Total	Girls	Boys	Total
Δ D angle (degrees)	6–16 (av. 9.5)	1–15 (av. 8.9)	1–16 (av. 9.1)	8–9 (av. 8.3)	9–15 (av. 12.0)	8–15 (av. 10.2)	8–9 (av. 8.6)	6–14 (av. 10.3)	8–14 (av. 9.4)
Δ α angle (degrees)	1–8.9 (av. 4.9)	5.1–6.8 (av. 7.3)	1–8.9 (av. 5.1)	1.9–2.2 (av. 2.0)	6.3–9.6 (av. 8.3)	1.9–9.6 (av. 5.15)	2.8–7.4 (av. 4.3)	5.7–8.9 (av. 7.3)	2.8–7.4 (av. 5.8)
Δ β angle (degrees)	1.5–16 (av. 6.25)	0.5–2.7 (av. 1.9)	0.5–16 (av. 4)	3.2–3.6 (av. 3.4)	1–7.1 (av. 3)	1–7.1 (av. 3.2)	6.1–8.8 (av. 7.9)	3.9–6.1 (av. 5)	3.9–8.8 (av. 6.45)
Δ MTH (mm)	0.6–2.6 (av. 1.6)	0.7–1.9 (av. 1.4)	0.6–2.6 (av. 1.5)	1.5–2.2 (av. 1.9)	0.5–3.6 (av. 2.3)	0.5–3.6 (av. 2.1)	1.3–2.1 (av. 1.5)	1.2–2.5 (av. 1.9)	1.2–2.5 (av. 1.7)
Δ LTH (mm)	2.4–4.7 (av. 2.4)	0.7–1.7 (av. 1.2)	0.7–4.7 (av. 3.6)	2.6–3.8 (av. 3.4)	0.3–3.8 (av. 2.4)	0.3–3.8 (av. 2.9)	0.3–2.1 (av. 0.9)	2.1–3.6 (av. 2.8)	0.3–3.6 (av. 1.8)
Δ TW (mm)	0.3–17.7 (av. 6.6)	1.8–13.3 (av. 9.4)	0.3–17.7 (av. 8)	0.9–1.1 (av. 1.0)	1.4–5.7 (av. 1.8)	0.9–5.7 (av. 1.4)	1.6–9.9 (av. 4.3)	9.9–12.2 (av. 11)	1.6–12.2 (av. 7.6)

Δ—difference between the measurements at the beginning and after the treatment; D—angle between the medial and lateral lines of the tibial plate inclination; β—angle between the medial line of the tibial plate inclination and the joint line of the tibia; α—angle between the lateral line of the tibial plate inclination and the joint line of the tibia; MTH—dimension measured from the tibial articular line to the highest point in the projection of the medial intercondylar tubercle; LTH—dimension measured from the tibial articular line to the highest point in the projection of the lateral intercondylar tubercle; TW—width of the tibial epiphysis between the farthest points of the proximal tibial epiphysis located on the lateral and medial cortex.

Table 3. Statistical significance of the differences (p) in values obtained before and after the treatment.

Parameter	G I (0–18 Months)		G II (0–30 Months)		G III (0–42 Months)	
	Girls	Boys	Girls	Boys	Girls	Boys
D angle l	0.0007	0.0102	0.0002	0.0001	0.0039	0.0039
D angle k	0.0004	0.0555	0.2709	0.6358	0.0277	0.5706
α angle l	0.2615	0.4079	0.5492	0.0001	0.4407	0.7419
α angle k	0.0011	0.4936	0.0795	0.6269	0.0609	0.6226
β angle l	0.0117	0.0776	0.6586	0.0007	0.0041	0.0206
β angle k	0.0005	0.6823	0.1617	0.0001	0.1311	0.9943
MTH l	0.0001	0.0001	0.0001	0.0001	0.00001	0.00001
MTH k	0.0103	0.4677	0.0245	0.0001	0.02707	0.2056
LTH l	0.0001	0.0001	0.0001	0.0001	0.0001	0.0001
LTH k	0.7839	0.5299	0.0291	0.0001	0.0001	0.8245
TW l	0.0001	0.0001	0.01231	0.0001	0.0001	0.0001
TW k	0.0001	0.0001	0.0001	0.0001	0.0001	0.0001

l—longer leg; k—shorter leg.

In groups I, II, and III, the D angle decreased significantly during the treatment, which was accompanied by an increase in the β or α angle. The lateral tubercle (LT) and medial tubercle (MT) height and the tibial width (TW) increased, and the differences before and after the treatment for the treated legs were statistically significant in all the studied groups. TW also changed in a statistically significant manner in the non-treated legs. In turn, the lateral tubercle height in the non-treated legs only changed in the boys in groups II and III and in the girls in group II. No statistically significant differences were observed for MT in the boys.

3.2. Changes in the Investigated Parameters Evaluated Every Six Months during the Treatment

To track changes in the tibial plate surface over time, the parameters were assessed every six months. The results were expressed as the difference in measurements for the treated limb (longer—d) and the non-treated limb (shorter—k). The goal of this part was to verify whether the changes in parameter values at adjacent time points were the same for the non-treated limb (k) and the treated limb (d). For this purpose, a non-parametric Wilcoxon test was performed. The results for groups I, II, and III are shown in Tables 4–6, respectively.

Table 4. P probability values (longer leg vs. shorter leg) for the Wilcoxon test—comparison in different time periods for group I.

	Girls						Boys					
Period	D	α	β	MLH	LTH	TW	D	α	β	MLH	LTH	TW
0–6 m	0.0277	0.0281	0.9165	0.0125	0.0047	0.3078	0.4631	0.0022	0.0277	0.0022	0.0995	0.6379
6–12 m	0.0277	0.0121	0.6002	0.0229	0.0229	0.0229	0.2489	0.0022	0.3454	0.6949	0.0281	0.1579
12–18 m	0.0277	0.0121	0.4631	0.0022	0.0995	0.3078	0.0277	0.1579	0.6002	0.0229	0.0121	0.6379

D—decrease in Δ D angle; α—increase in Δ α angle; β—increase in Δ β angle; MLH—increase in medial tubercle height; LTH—increase in Δ medial tubercle height; TW—increase in Δ width of the tibial epiphysis.

Table 5. P probability values (longer leg vs. shorter leg) for the Wilcoxon test—comparison in different time periods for group II.

	Girls						Boys					
Period	D	α	β	MLH	LTH	TW	D	α	β	MLH	LTH	TW
0–6 m	0.0678	0.1159	0.0277	0.9165	0.9165	0.0277	0.0707	0.0011	0.0096	0.0479	0.0002	0.0011
6–12 m	0.0277	0.9265	0.0479	0.0277	0.0277	0.0277	0.0002	0.0096	0.0033	0.0018	0.7174	0.0151
12–18 m	0.0277	0.0277	0.9165	0.0277	0.1158	0.9165	0.0011	0.6791	0.4204	0.0311	0.0014	0.4379
18–24 m	0.0277	0.0277	0.1158	0.1797	0.0277	0.0277	0.2667	0.7771	0.0006	0.0049	0.0582	0.4459
24–30 m	0.4652	0.0277	0.4631	0.0277	0.0277	0.0277	0.4459	0.0096	0.0057	0.0386	0.0084	0.0311

D—decrease in Δ D angle; α—increase in Δ α angle; β—increase in Δ β angle; MLH—increase in medial tubercle height; LTH—increase in Δ medial tubercle height; TW—increase in Δ width of the tibial epiphysis.

Table 6. P probability values (longer leg vs. shorter leg) for the Wilcoxon test—comparison in different time periods for group III.

	Girls						Boys					
Period	D	α	β	MLH	LTH	TW	D	α	β	MLH	LTH	TW
0–6 m	0.1158	0.1158	0.0277	0.1158	0.0277	0.0277	0.1158	0.1158	0.9165	0.4631	0.4631	0.1158
6–12 m	0.0678	0.0277	0.9165	0.0277	0.0277	0.0277	0.0678	0.9165	0.9165	0.4631	0.0277	0.9158
12–18 m	0.0678	0.0277	0.0277	0.4631	0.9165	0.1158	0.0678	0.4631	0.0277	0.4631	0.4631	0.1158
18–24 m	0.4652	0.0277	0.0277	0.0277	0.0277	0.9165	0.0678	0.9165	0.9165	0.0277	0.0277	0.1158
24–30 m	0.0277	0.1158	0.0277	0.0277	0.0277	0.0277	0.1797	0.9165	0.9165	0.9165	0.4631	0.4631
30–36 m	0.9165	0.9165	0.0277	0.0277	0.0277	0.0277	0.0277	0.9165	0.0277	0.4631	0.4631	0.1158
36–42 m	0.1158	0.9165	0.0277	0.1158	0.1158	0.0277	0.1158	0.0277	0.9165	0.4652	0.1158	0.1277

D—decrease in Δ D angle; α—increase in Δ α angle; β—increase in Δ β angle; MLH—increase in medial tubercle height; LTH—increase in Δ medial tubercle height; TW—increase in Δ width of the tibial epiphysis.

Statistically significant differences in parameter D were demonstrated in all the groups ($p < 0.05$), but in group I of the boys, only in the period of 12–18 months (Table 4). In group II, statistically significant differences were observed in the period of 6–18 months (boys) and 6–24 months (girls) (Table 5). In group III, the changes were observed from 6 to 18 and from 24 to 30 months in the group of girls, and from 6 to 18 and from 30 to 42 months in the boys (Table 6). The α angle increased significantly during the treatment. In group I, changes occurred from 0 to 18 months (girls) and from 0 to 12 months (boys) (Table 4). In group II, visible changes were observed in the periods of 12–30 months (girls) and 0–12 and 24–30 months (boys) (Table 5). Statistically significant differences in the girls from group III were observed between 6 and 24 months, and differences in the group of boys were notable in the last stage of treatment, i.e., at 42–48 months (Table 6). The highest changes in the β angle were observed in the girls from group III (Table 6) and in the boys from group II (Table 5), where this parameter increased significantly during most of the treatment period. The highest differences in the lateral tubercle height and in the medial tubercle height in the different treatment periods were found in the groups of girls and in the boys from groups I and II (Tables 4 and 5, respectively). Statistically significant changes for TW were noted for the girls in groups II and III and for the boys in group II in almost all the investigated period ranges (Tables 5 and 6).

Box-and-whisker plots were created to illustrate the changes noted in the specific time periods. An example presenting the results obtained for group III is shown in Figure 4.

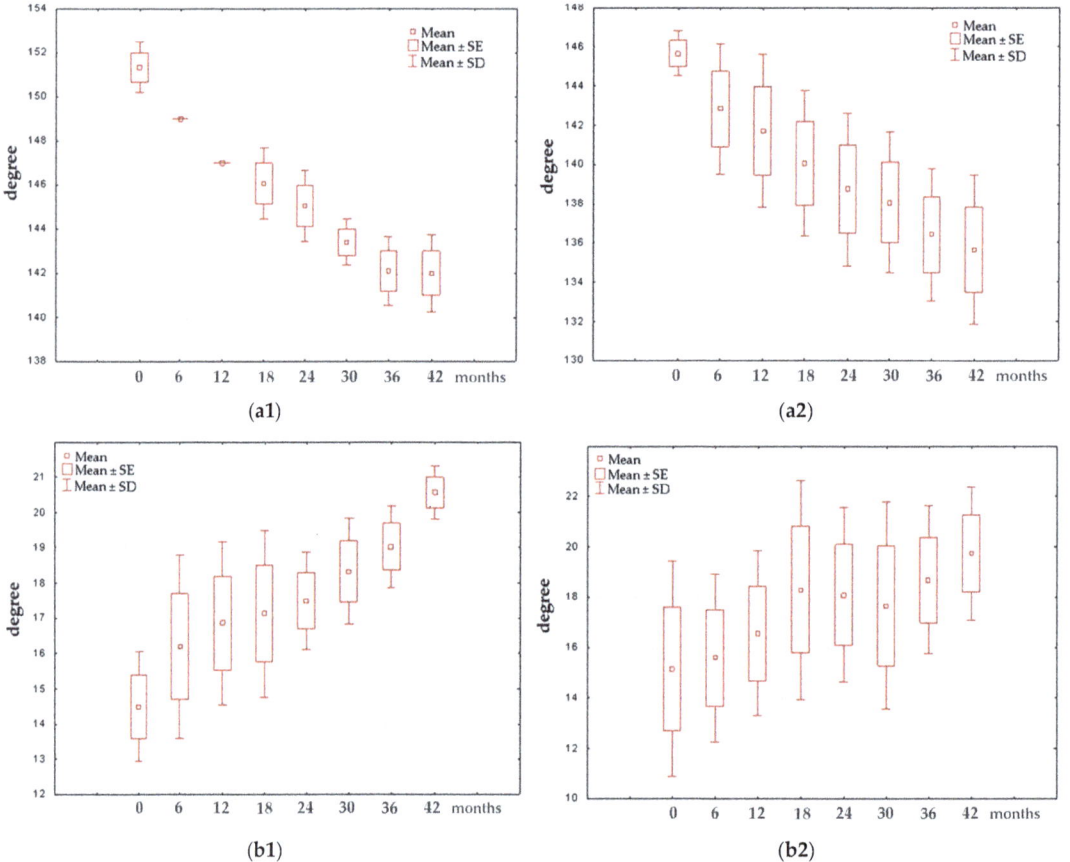

Figure 4. *Cont.*

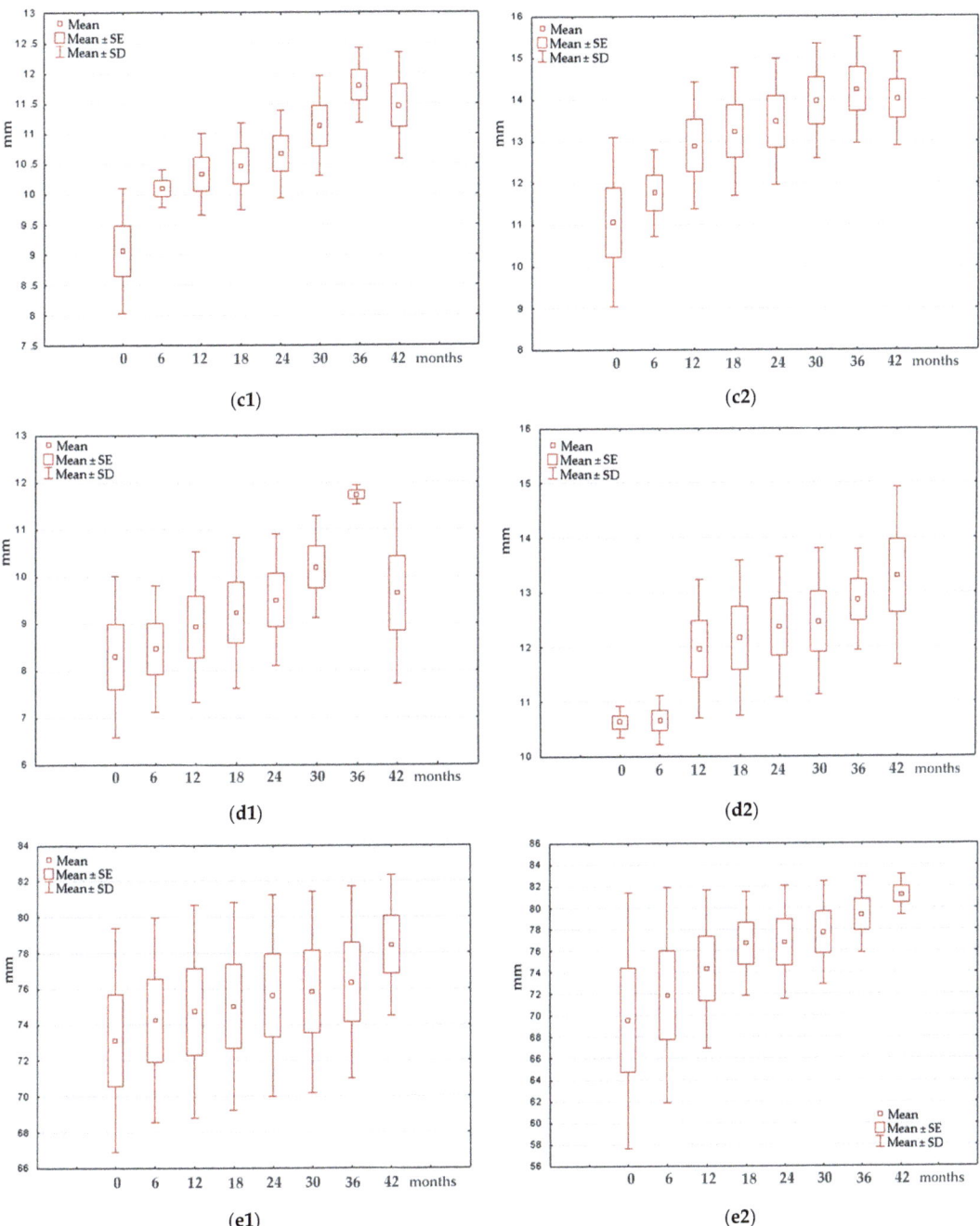

Figure 4. Example of box-and-whisker plots illustrating changes in the investigated parameters over the specific time periods for group III: (**a1**,**a2**)—roof angle (D) in the group of girls and boys, respectively; (**b1**,**b2**)—slope angle β in the group of girls and boys, respectively; (**c1**,**c2**)—lateral tubercle height (LTH) in the group of girls and boys, respectively; (**d1**,**d2**)—medial tubercle height (MTH) in the group of girls and boys, respectively; (**e1**,**e2**)—tibial width (TW) in the group of girls and boys, respectively.

4. Discussion

Epiphysiodesis using eight-plate implants is a minimally invasive method of correcting LLD. It is well tolerated and accepted by pediatric patients and their parents. It is offered to patients as an alternative to long surgical treatment requiring external fixators and burdened with a higher risk of complications, e.g., lengthening using the Ilizarov method. We have found several scientific papers in which, in addition to the effects of LLD treatment with temporary epiphysiodesis-egalization, complications are also described. These are mainly cases of implant damage—its rupture, dislodgement, or displacement. They also describe permanent damage to the growth plate; after the implant was removed, the plate did not resume its function, causing a disruption of the leg axis [8–15]. Due to the limited literature on the analysis of changes in the shape of the proximal tibial base treated with an eight-plate implant, in this discussion, we used reports of authors examining the results of LLD treatment also using other types of implants.

In 2007, P. Stevens began research on an implant intended to reduce the number of complications often observed during epiphysiodesis treatment of LLD using a Blount staple. In the same year, the researcher published an article in which he described the technique of asymmetrical temporary epiphysiodesis using a flexible plate in the shape of the figure "8" and two screws (Orthofix GmbH, Lewisville, TX, USA) [6]. This method was originally dedicated to the treatment of leg axis disorders [13,14,16,17]. The simple surgical technique of reducing the number of implants to one (in the case of staples, several were used) and the good results presented by other authors resulted in the extension of the indications, and this method was used for symmetrical epiphysiodesis in the treatment of LLD [18,19]. The introduction of these implants solved the main problem of temporary epiphysiodesis, i.e., permanent damage to the growth plate. The implant, which facilitates gradual inhibition of growth, does not damage the growth plate. The screws are not rigidly mounted in the plate, and the angle can be increased (up to a maximum of 60 degrees). Further mechanisms of gradual epiphysiodesis include the narrowing of the plate by half of its length and the flexibility of the material from which it is made. The plate begins to bend under the pressure of growth forces. This implant design also moves the point of support of the epiphysiodesis forces away by approximately 30 mm from its outer part, which increases the surface area of impact of these forces [6]. We had similar observations when analyzing the study groups. We did not observe any cases of permanent growth damage. Patients whose leg normalization occurred before the end of growth had their implants removed, and follow-up examinations confirmed further normal growth of the operated limb. We did not observe any damage to the implant itself, but deformations of the plate were visible, especially in the patients from group III.

According to the theory of the inventors of the implant, the use of eight-plate implants in symmetric epiphysiodesis causes different effects on the growth plate, depending on the distance from the implant. Columns of chondrocytes located closer to the implant are inhibited more strongly, and those closer to the center of the joint are less inhibited. This provides a graphic image of the triangle formed by the medial line of the tibial plate slope, the lateral line of the tibial plate slope, and the tibial articular line. In turn, the angle defined as the result of the difference between the acute angles of the triangle, i.e., the roof angle D, was described by R. Sinha et al. in 2018 as the main parameter determining possible disorders of the articular surface of the tibia [7]. This is the first work that, almost 10 years after the introduction of eight-plate implants for the treatment of LLD, describes changes in the articular surfaces of the knee. In his work, the researcher tried to graphically and mathematically present how the shape of the tibial epiphysis changes during LLD treatment with epiphysiodesis using eight-plate implants. In the material of 42 patients, the author proved that the shape of the joint changed in almost half of the examined patients (46%), and the roof angle decreased by an average of 5 degrees (from 1 to 18 degrees) during the treatment. Sinha's work, however, had limitations, namely, the size of the group of patients treated due to LLD (only 8 cases) and their combination with the group of patients treated due to KD axis disorder (34 cases). The average follow-up time was 1.8 years (from 0.5 to 5 years).

The results presented by R. Sinha confirm the observations reported by scientists who compared the results of temporary epiphysiodesis with the final one. They claim that temporary epiphysiodesis with eight-plate implants causes a change in the shape of the joint. This may be related to the design of the implant, i.e., the possibility of changing the angle of the screw in relation to the plate causes a delay in the process of epiphysiodesis [18,20].

In 2016, E. Gaumetou et al. assessed the effectiveness of LLD treatment using eight-plate implants on a group of 32 patients. The results were very unsatisfactory; in the case of the proximal tibial metaphysis, only 13 patients (42%) achieved the expected KD compensation. Eight patients (20%) reported pain up to 18 months after treatment, and five (12.5%) required revision of the implant position. The author also reported asymmetries in the shape of the tibial plate of the treated limb visible on radiographs [18].

In turn, in 2019, Borbasa presented the results of a comparison of irreversible epiphysiodesis with temporary epiphysiodesis (using eight-plate implants). The researcher compared the results of KD correction, which spoke in favor of irreversible epiphysiodesis (group of 21 patients). After a year, a reduction in LLD by an average of 8.4 mm was achieved in this group compared to the reversible one (group of 17 patients), where the average reduction in LLD was 5.7 mm. After a two-year observation period, these differences were even greater, i.e., by an average of 17.9 mm in the irreversible epiphysiodesis and an average of 12.2 mm in the reversible variant. The author also presented a high revision rate for reversible epiphysiodesis (17.6% to 4.8%), with the main reason being implant migration. He also commented negatively on temporal epiphysiodesis, highlighting its unpredictability for growth cartilage activity after implant removal and possible asymmetries in the shape of the knee joint [21]. All the above-mentioned works indicate that the LLD treatment method using eight-plate implants is not so perfect.

In our analysis, we assessed the impact of eight-plate implants on the width of the knee joint ("TW" parameter). This parameter has not been assessed so far in the available literature. During the treatment with the implants, the width of the tibial base increased compared to the other limb in groups II and III. This parameter increased from 0.9 mm to 5.7 mm (dia. 1.4 mm) in group II (30-month treatment) and from 1.6 mm to 12.2 mm (dia. 7.6 mm) in group III (42-month treatment). This can significantly change the congruence of the knee joint. These results give another argument to opponents of temporal epiphysiodesis who believe that the shorter limb, considered responsible for the occurrence of leg length asymmetry, should be treated for LLD. It is known that changing the surface of the knee joint may accelerate the development of knee arthrosis [22–24].

In the available literature, authors do not specify the time frame for the use of temporal epiphysiodesis. Most researchers suggest that the so-called safe duration of use of this method should not exceed 24 months. This belief is based on reports provided by the authors of the method, Blount and Clark, on the limitations of temporal epiphysiodesis. They reported that implants kept in the growth cartilage area for longer than 2 years may permanently damage it. However, they do not explain the mechanism by which this damage would occur [25]. These observations were confirmed by Phemister in frequent correspondence with the authors of temporal epiphysiodesis [26].

Our research shows changes in the shape of the joint and limb axis when the treatment period is substantially exceeded (24 months). The smallest changes were observed in group I (treatment for up to 18 months). The age of the patients is also important; this group comprised teenagers aged from 12 years and 2 months to 13 years and 10 months (on average, 13 years and 2 months). In other studies comparing epiphysiodeses, the average age of patients ranged from 10 to 14 years at the time of surgical treatment. In 2018, W. Lee presented the results of a comparison of temporal epiphysiodesis, depending on the type of implant used. The group included 19 patients aged from 10.0 to 13.8 years (mean 12.1) [27]. A similar average age of patients treated with epiphysiodesis, i.e., 13.3 years, was presented in 2017 by Bayhan et al. In their study, a larger group of patients was analyzed, i.e., 72 cases with LLD. In the temporal group, an average LLD correction of 12 mm was achieved (41%), and in the irreversible group, of 16 mm after 24 months of treatment [28]. The work covered a treatment period of 24 months, ending with the removal of the implants. In our study, the greatest changes occurred in group III (the youngest patients) and at the longest treatment duration of 48 months.

Limitations of the study: Our work is not without limitations. Firstly, it is a relatively small research group (60 patients), although it is still larger than those in the works of the above-mentioned authors. Moreover, we did not analyze lateral X-rays. This would facilitate the assessment of the shape of the knee joint in the sagittal plane. Despite the use of digital measurement tools, the measurements are not that precise. The use of CT and MRI would facilitate a more accurate assessment of the surface. However, these methods are not used to assess the progress of LLD treatment. It should also be mentioned that the skeletal maturity of the patients was not assessed.

This topic requires further research and the analysis of subsequent groups of patients. The effect of the eight-plate implant on sensitive growth cartilage is still not fully understood. We should look at our actions more broadly and be aware of the consequences they may cause. Thus, there is a need for future long-term follow-up studies to elucidate the potential effects of LLD treatment on the tibial surface.

Author Contributions: Conceptualization, G.S., A.D. and M.L.; methodology, G.S., A.D., T.S. and M.L.; software, G.S. and M.R.-B.; validation, G.S. and M.R.-B.; formal analysis, G.S. and A.D.; investigation, G.S., A.D. and M.L.; resources, G.S., A.D. and M.L.; data curation, G.S., A.D., T.S. and M.L.; writing—original draft preparation, G.S., A.D., M.W., I.S. and M.L.; writing—review and editing, G.S., A.D., M.W., I.S. and M.L.; visualization, G.S., A.D., M.W. and M.R.-B.; supervision, G.S., A.D., M.W., I.S. and M.L.; project administration, G.S., A.D., M.W. and M.L.; funding acquisition, M.L. All authors have read and agreed to the published version of the manuscript.

Funding: This research received no external funding.

Institutional Review Board Statement: This study was approved by the Bioethics Committee of the Medical University of Lublin (number KE-0254/81/2020).

Informed Consent Statement: Not applicable.

Data Availability Statement: The data presented in this study are available upon request from the corresponding author.

Conflicts of Interest: The authors declare no conflicts of interest.

References

1. Baylis, W.J.; Rzonca, E.C. Functional and Structural Limb Length Discrepancies: Evaluation and Treatment. *Clin. Podiatr. Med. Surg.* **1988**, *5*, 509–520. [CrossRef] [PubMed]
2. Danbert, R.J. Clinical Assessment and Treatment of Leg Length Inequalities. *J. Manip. Physiol. Ther.* **1988**, *11*, 290–295.
3. Walsh, M.; Connolly, P.; Jenkinson, A.; O'Brien, T. Leg Length Discrepancy—An Experimental Study of Compensatory Changes in Three Dimensions Using Gait Analysis. *Gait Posture* **2000**, *12*, 156–161. [CrossRef] [PubMed]
4. Paley, J.; Talor, J.; Levin, A.; Bhave, A.; Paley, D.; Herzenberg, J.E. The Multiplier Method for Prediction of Adult Height. *J. Pediatr. Orthop.* **2004**, *24*, 732–737. [CrossRef]
5. Birch, J.G.; Samchukov, M.L. Use of the Ilizarov Method to Correct Lower Limb Deformities in Children and Adolescents. *J. Am. Acad. Orthop. Surg.* **2004**, *12*, 144–154. [CrossRef]
6. Stevens, P.M. Guided Growth for Angular Correction: A Preliminary Series Using a Tension Band Plate. *J. Pediatr. Orthop.* **2007**, *27*, 253–259. [CrossRef] [PubMed]
7. Sinha, R.; Weigl, D.; Mercado, E.; Becker, T.; Kedem, P.; Bar-On, E. Eight-Plate Epiphysiodesis: Are We Creating an Intra-Articular Deformity? *Bone Jt. J.* **2018**, *100-B*, 1112–1116. [CrossRef]
8. Raab, P.; Wild, A.; Seller, K.; Krauspe, R. Correction of Length Discrepancies and Angular Deformities of the Leg by Blount's Epiphyseal Stapling. *Eur. J. Pediatr.* **2001**, *160*, 668–674. [CrossRef]
9. Courvoisier, A.; Eid, A.; Merloz, P. Epiphyseal Stapling of the Proximal Tibia for Idiopathic Genu Valgum. *J. Child. Orthop.* **2009**, *3*, 217–221. [CrossRef]
10. Vogt, B.; Tretow, H.; Schuhknecht, B.; Horter, M.; Schiedel, F.; Rödl, R. Coronal and Sagittal Axis Deviation Following Temporary Epiphysiodesis Using Blount-Staple or Eight-Plate for Treatment of Leg Length Discrepancy. *Arch. Orthop. Trauma. Surg.* **2014**, *134*, 421–447.

11. Blount, W.P.; Clarke, G.R. Control of Bone Growth by Epiphyseal Stapling; a Preliminary Report. *J. Bone Joint Surg. Am.* **1949**, *31A*, 464–478. [CrossRef]
12. Gorman, T.M.; Vanderwerff, R.; Pond, M.; MacWilliams, B.; Santora, S.D. Mechanical Axis Following Staple Epiphysiodesis for Limb-Length Inequality. *J. Bone Jt. Surg.-Am. Vol.* **2009**, *91*, 2430–2439. [CrossRef]
13. Schroerlucke, S.; Bertrand, S.; Clapp, J.; Bundy, J.; Gregg, F.O. Failure of Orthofix Eight-Plate for the Treatment of Blount Disease. *J. Pediatr. Orthop.* **2009**, *29*, 57–60. [CrossRef]
14. Wiemann, J.M.; Tryon, C.; Szalay, E.A. Physeal Stapling Versus 8-Plate Hemiepiphysiodesis for Guided Correction of Angular Deformity about the Knee. *J. Pediatr. Orthop.* **2009**, *29*, 481–485. [CrossRef] [PubMed]
15. Métaizeau, J.P.; Wong-Chung, J.; Bertrand, H.; Pasquier, P. Percutaneous Epiphysiodesis Using Transphyseal Screws (PETS). *J. Pediatr. Orthop.* **1998**, *18*, 363–369. [CrossRef] [PubMed]
16. Ballal, M.S.; Bruce, C.E.; Nayagam, S. Correcting Genu Varum and Genu Valgum in Children by Guided Growth: TEMPORARY HEMIEPIPHYSIODESIS USING TENSION BAND PLATES. *J. Bone Jt. Surg. Br.* **2010**, *92-B*, 273–276. [CrossRef] [PubMed]
17. Burghardt, R.D.; Herzenberg, J.E.; Standard, S.C.; Paley, D. Temporary Hemiepiphyseal Arrest Using a Screw and Plate Device to Treat Knee and Ankle Deformities in Children: A Preliminary Report. *J. Child. Orthop.* **2008**, *2*, 187–197. [CrossRef] [PubMed]
18. Gaumétou, E.; Mallet, C.; Souchet, P.; Mazda, K.; Ilharreborde, B. Poor Efficiency of Eight-Plates in the Treatment of Lower Limb Discrepancy. *J. Pediatr. Orthop.* **2016**, *36*, 715–719. [CrossRef]
19. Gottliebsen, M.; Møller-Madsen, B.; Stødkilde-Jørgensen, H.; Rahbek, O. Controlled Longitudinal Bone Growth by Temporary Tension Band Plating: An Experimental Study. *Bone Jt. J.* **2013**, *95-B*, 855–860. [CrossRef] [PubMed]
20. Lauge-Pedersen, H.; Hägglund, G. Eight Plate Should Not Be Used for Treating Leg Length Discrepancy. *J. Child. Orthop.* **2013**, *7*, 285–288. [CrossRef] [PubMed]
21. Borbas, P.; Agten, C.A.; Rosskopf, A.B.; Hingsammer, A.; Eid, K.; Ramseier, L.E. Guided Growth with Tension Band Plate or Definitive Epiphysiodesis for Treatment of Limb Length Discrepancy? *J. Orthop. Surg.* **2019**, *14*, 99. [CrossRef]
22. Karbowski, A.; Camps, L.; Matthia, H.H. Histopathological Features of Unilateral Stapling in Animal Experiments. *Arch. Orthop. Trauma Surg.* **1989**, *108*, 353–358. [CrossRef]
23. Golightly, Y.M.; Allen, K.D.; Helmick, C.G.; Renner, J.B.; Jordan, J.M. Symptoms of the Knee and Hip in Individuals with and without Limb Length Inequality. *Osteoarthr. Cartil.* **2009**, *17*, 596–600. [CrossRef]
24. Golightly, Y.M.; Allen, K.D.; Renner, J.B.; Helmick, C.G.; Salazar, A.; Jordan, J.M. Relationship of Limb Length Inequality with Radiographic Knee and Hip Osteoarthritis. *Osteoarthr. Cartil.* **2007**, *15*, 824–829. [CrossRef] [PubMed]
25. Sanders, J.O.; Howell, J.; Qiu, X. Comparison of the Paley Method Using Chronological Age with Use of Skeletal Maturity for Predicting Mature Limb Length in Children. *J. Bone Jt. Surg.* **2011**, *93*, 1051–1056. [CrossRef]
26. Gottliebsen, M.; Shiguetomi-Medina, J.M.; Rahbek, O.; Møller-Madsen, B. Guided Growth: Mechanism and Reversibility of Modulation. *J. Child. Orthop.* **2016**, *10*, 471–477. [CrossRef] [PubMed]
27. Lee, W.-C.; Kao, H.-K.; Yang, W.-E.; Chang, C.-H. Tension Band Plating Is Less Effective in Achieving Equalization of Leg Length. *J. Child. Orthop.* **2018**, *12*, 629–634. [CrossRef] [PubMed]
28. Bayhan, I.A.; Karatas, A.F.; Rogers, K.J.; Bowen, J.R.; Thacker, M.M. Comparing Percutaneous Physeal Epiphysiodesis and Eight-Plate Epiphysiodesis for the Treatment of Limb Length Discrepancy. *J. Pediatr. Orthop.* **2017**, *37*, 323–327. [CrossRef]

Disclaimer/Publisher's Note: The statements, opinions and data contained in all publications are solely those of the individual author(s) and contributor(s) and not of MDPI and/or the editor(s). MDPI and/or the editor(s) disclaim responsibility for any injury to people or property resulting from any ideas, methods, instructions or products referred to in the content.

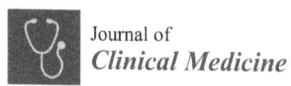

Article

Primary Radial Nerve Lesions in Humerus Shaft Fractures—Revision or Wait and See

Alexander Böhringer *, Raffael Cintean, Konrad Schütze and Florian Gebhard

Department of Trauma Hand and Reconstructive Surgery, Ulm University, Albert-Einstein-Allee 23, 89081 Ulm, Germany
* Correspondence: alexander.boehringer@uniklinik-ulm.de; Tel.: +49-73150054561; Fax: +49-731-500-54502

Abstract: Background: This study investigates the surgical state-of-the-art procedure for humeral shaft fractures with primary radial nerve palsy based on its own case series in relation to the current and established literature. **Methods**: Retrospective review of treated cases between January 2018 and December 2022 describing radial nerve palsy after humerus shaft fractures, radiological fracture classification, intraoperative findings, surgical procedure, patient follow-up and functional outcome. **Results**: A total of 804 patients (463 women and 341 men) with humerus shaft fractures were identified. A total of 33 patients showed symptomatic lesions of the radial nerve (4.1%). The primary lesion was identified in 17 patients (2.1%). A broad and inhomogeneous distribution of fractures according to the AO classification was found. According to the operative reports, the distraction of the radial nerve was found eleven times, bony interposed three times and soft tissue constricted/compressed three times. In every case the radial nerve was surgically explored, there was no case of complete traumatic nerve transection. Four intramedullary nails and thirteen locking plates were used for osteosynthesis. Complete recovery of nerve function was seen in 12 cases within 1 to 36 months. Three patients still showed mild hypesthesia in the thumb area after 18 months. Two patients were lost during follow-up. **Conclusions**: With this study, we support the strategy of early nerve exploration and plate osteosynthesis in humeral fractures with primary radial nerve palsy when there is a clear indication for surgical fracture stabilisation. In addition, early exploration appears sensible in the case of palsies in open fractures and secondary palsy following surgery without nerve exposure as well as in the case of diagnostically recognisable nerve damage. Late nerve exploration is recommended if there are no definite signs of recovery after 6 months. An initial wait-and-see strategy with clinical observation seems reasonable for primary radial nerve palsies without indication for surgical fracture stabilisation.

Keywords: humeral shaft fractures; primary radial nerve palsy; early nerve exploration; peripheral nerve lesions; nerve recovery; wait-and-see strategy

Citation: Böhringer, A.; Cintean, R.; Schütze, K.; Gebhard, F. Primary Radial Nerve Lesions in Humerus Shaft Fractures—Revision or Wait and See. *J. Clin. Med.* **2024**, *13*, 1893. https://doi.org/10.3390/jcm13071893

Academic Editor: Moshe Salai

Received: 12 February 2024
Revised: 13 March 2024
Accepted: 17 March 2024
Published: 25 March 2024

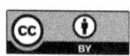

Copyright: © 2024 by the authors. Licensee MDPI, Basel, Switzerland. This article is an open access article distributed under the terms and conditions of the Creative Commons Attribution (CC BY) license (https://creativecommons.org/licenses/by/4.0/).

1. Introduction

With an incidence of $82.1/10^5$ and accounting for 7.4% of all adult fractures, humeral fractures are very common. They are caused by both high-energy and low-energy trauma and are then often associated with osteoporosis due to older age and female gender [1]. Lesions of the radial nerve often occur in fractures of the shaft and distal third [2,3]. Several anatomical peculiarities in these areas have been described as a reason for this. The radial nerve and its accompanying vessels run in the middle of the shaft over a length of 6.2 cm with direct bone contact dorsally on the humerus. It then continues distally through the lateral intermuscular septum. Throughout this course, the nerve is poorly mobile until it crosses the ulnar flexure ventrally of the lateral humeral epicondyle protected by muscle [4–6]. With a reported incidence of 11.8%, these are the most common peripheral nerve lesions associated with bone fractures [2,3,7], whereby the origin of the damage and the appearance of the clinical symptoms can be primary or secondary. Different morphologic stages of the nerve lesion (neuropraxia, axonotmesis and neurotmesis) can cause different degrees of functional impairment in terms of peripheral numbness and paralysis [8,9]. According to the literature, the overall recovery rate is 88.1%, with 70.7% achieved by conservative therapy [3]. Significant differences are found in the fracture morphology between complete (77.6%) and incomplete (98.2%), open (85.7%) and closed (97.1%) fractures [3]. In the case of nerve healing, the brachioradialis muscle is the first to recover, followed by the extensor carpi radialis longus, which extends and radially abducts the wrist. In addition, the Hoffmann–Tinel sign gradually distalises [10,11]. There is general consensus regarding the treatment recommendation for extremely displaced and open humeral shaft fractures with vascular or nerve lesions for early surgical exploration. However, in the grey area of less complex trauma and milder nerve deficits, controversial treatment concepts are recommended and different algorithms are proposed [12,13]. The questions remain: Which combination of fracture morphology (according to the AO = OTA/ASIF (Arbeitsgemeinschaft für Osteosynthesefragen/Orthopaedic Trauma Association/Association of the Study of Internal Fixation) classification) and nerve lesion (is the nerve torn?—interposed, constricted, distracted or compressed?) should be surgically explored at an early stage and, if so, which fixation method (plate, screws, cerclage, external fixator, or nail) should be chosen? With this retrospective case study, we investigate the relationship between fracture morphology and nerve findings in our own collective and show suitable treatment methods to contribute to decision-making in everyday surgical practice.

2. Materials and Methods

This case study has been approved by the institutional ethical committee. It is a retrospective review of patients with humeral shaft fracture and accompanying radial nerve lesions from Ulm University Medical Center from 2018 to 2022. The number of cases was determined by our statistics department for a period of five years. The data collection was based on our hospital information system (SAP IS-H, Germany). The case search was performed with the following ICD-10 codes:

- S42.3—Fracture of humeral shaft incl. humerus o.n.a., multiple shaft fractures, humerus o.n.a.
- S42.40—Part unspecified, incl. distal end o.n.a.
- S42.41—Supracondylar.
- S44.2—Injury of the radial nerve at the level of the upper arm.

Inclusion criteria were all acute traumatic cases of simultaneous humeral shaft fracture and symptomatic nerve lesion according to the above-mentioned ICD 10 codes from a patient age of 18 years. Exclusion criteria were patients under the age of 18, polytraumatised patients, open and pathological fractures, amputation injuries, unassessable central or peripheral neurology and underlying neurological diseases, pre-existing extremity injuries and diseases as well as functional impairment of the arm in question, known lesions of the radial nerve or brachial plexus, local infections and tumour manifestations as well as incompliance.

A descriptive data collection with statistical formation of mean values and percentages as well as tabular and graphical representation with comparative distribution was carried out. Demographic characteristics such as patient age and gender were analysed. The clinical symptoms of the radial nerve lesion, such as hypaesthesia and palsy, were recorded. Humeral shaft fractures were categorised according to the AO classification. In addition, the intraoperative macroscopic nerve findings (severed or injured—interposed, constricted, distracted or compressed) were found. The surgical procedures used with regard to nerve findings (neurolysis, nerve grafting or tendon transfer) and fracture characteristics (fixation by nail, plate, screw, cerclage or external fixator) were recorded. In addition, nerve healing was followed up with the time of restitutio ad integrum or last consultation with remaining deficit.

With regard to the retrospective study design, the follow-up of the cases was based on the available records. The follow-up treatment included physiotherapy, ergotherapy, positioning splints and electrotherapy. Patients were usually followed up at 2, 4, 6 and 12 weeks postoperatively. A clinical examination was performed routinely, with suture traction after 2 weeks and with X-ray control after 6 and 12 weeks. In addition, measurements of nerve conduction velocity and electromyography were repeated within these periods. Further follow-up controls were carried out if complaints persisted or if there was a residual functional deficit.

Fracture classification was based on preoperative radiographs and computed tomography scans according to the AO as shown in Figure 1.

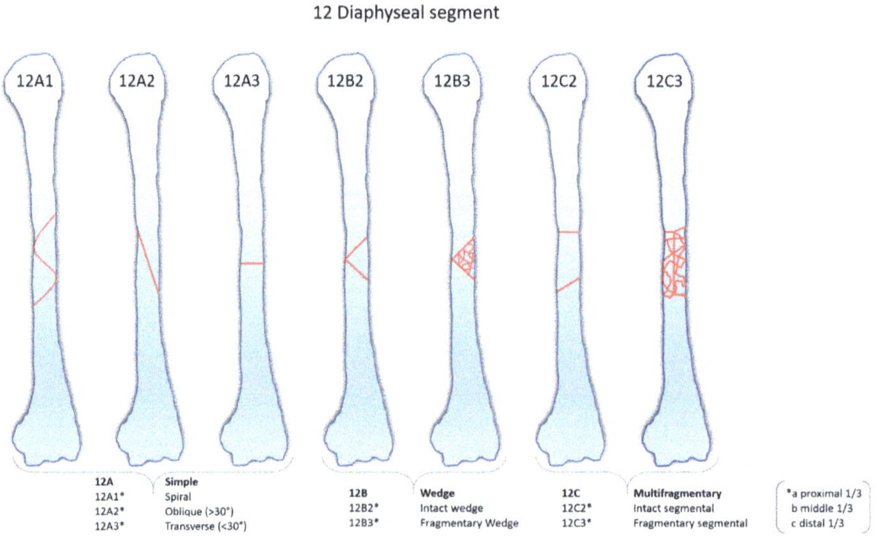

Figure 1. Classification of humeral shaft fractures (12 diaphyseal segments) according to the AO.

To illustrate some cases, the Section 3 shows composite figures of preoperative X-ray, CT examination, intraoperatively photographed nerve findings and fracture osteosynthesis as well as postoperative X-ray control.

3. Results

From January 2018 to December 2022, a total of 804 patients (463 women and 341 men) with humerus shaft fractures were treated at our hospital. A symptomatic lesion of the radial nerve was found in 33 patients (4.1%). In 17 of the 33 patients (2.1% of the 804 patients), the clinical symptoms of the nerve lesion were found to be clearly primary, existing since the accident.

AO classification showed three 12B2c fractures, two 12A1c fractures, two 12A3b fractures and one each of 12A1b, 12A2a, 12A2b, 12A2c, 12A3c, 12B2a, 12B2b, 12B3b, 12B3c and 12C3a fractures. The distribution is shown in Figure 2.

Preoperatively, seventeen patients had hypesthesia and palsy. According to the operative reports, the radial nerve was found to be distracted eleven times, bony interposed three times and soft tissue constricted/compressed three times.

The radial nerve was always surgically explored and a neurolysis was performed. In three cases, the fracture was fixed with closed reduction and intramedullary nailing, and one case of open reduction and intramedullary nailing was found. Open reduction and internal fixation with a locking plate were performed in 13 cases. In addition, cerclage wiring was performed in four cases. In one case, the fracture was initially stabilised with external fixation.

There was no case of traumatic nerve transection. After surgical exploration and neurolysis, all patients underwent physiotherapy and clinical neurological follow-up.

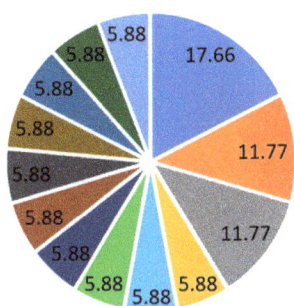

Figure 2. The diagram illustrates the broad and inhomogeneous distribution of AO fracture types in the 17 patients in percentages.

Complete recovery of nerve function was seen in 12 cases within 1 to 36 months. Two patients were lost in follow-up, and three patients still showed mild hypesthesia in the thumb area after 18 months. The patient data are shown in Table 1. Figure 3 shows the recovery of nerve function in the 15 patients over time.

Table 1. The results of the 17 patients with primary radial palsy are shown. Age, sex and clinical symptoms are listed, as well as the exact fracture classification according to AO, the respective intraoperative findings of the affected nerve, surgical treatment, and time to recovery of nerve function. Two patients could not be followed up (LOFU = loss of follow-up). In three patients, mild hypesthesia in the thumb area remained until 18 months after trauma.

Patient Sex and Age (F = Female, M = Male)	Initial Radial Nerve Symptoms	AO Fracture Classification	Radial Nerve Findings Intraoperative	Fracture Treatment Method	Nerve Recovery (Restitutio Ad Integrum) in Months
F, 56	Hypesthesia + palsy	12C3a	Interposed	Neurolysis, cerclage, nail	12
M, 37	Hypesthesia + palsy	12B3b	Constricted	1. Neurolysis + fixator 2. Nail	24
F, 72	Hypesthesia + palsy	12A1b	Distracted	Neurolysis, plate	6
M, 66	Hypesthesia + palsy	12B2a	Distracted	Neurolysis, nail	1
F, 84	Hypesthesia + palsy	12A2c	Distracted	Neurolysis, plate	LOFU
F, 42	Hypesthesia + palsy	12B2c	Distracted	Neurolysis, plate	36
F, 33	Hypesthesia + palsy	12A3c	Distracted	Neurolysis, plate	1
F, 47	Hypesthesia + palsy	12A3b	Distracted	Neurolysis, plate	LOFU
F, 79	Hypesthesia + palsy	12A1c	Interposed	Neurolysis, screw, plate	18 (res. Hyp D1)
F, 22	Hypesthesia + palsy	12B2c	Distracted	Neurolysis, cerclage, screw, plate	18 (res. Hyp D1)

Table 1. Cont.

Patient Sex and Age (F = Female, M = Male)	Initial Radial Nerve Symptoms	AO Fracture Classification	Radial Nerve Findings Intraoperative	Fracture Treatment Method	Nerve Recovery (Restitutio Ad Integrum) in Months
F, 80	Hypesthesia + palsy	12B2b	Distracted	Nail, neurolysis	12
F, 18	Hypesthesia + palsy	12B3c	Compressed	Neurolysis, plate	1
M, 36	Hypesthesia + palsy	12A2b	Constricted	Neurolysis, plate	1
F, 72	Hypesthesia + palsy	12A1c	Interposed	Neurolysis, cerclage, plate	18 (res. Hyp D1)
M, 27	Hypesthesia + palsy	12A3b	Distracted	Nail, neurolysis	3
F, 75	Hypesthesia + palsy	12A2a	Distracted	Neurolysis, cerclage, plate	12
F, 24	Hypesthesia + palsy	12B2c	Distracted	Neurolysis, plate	1

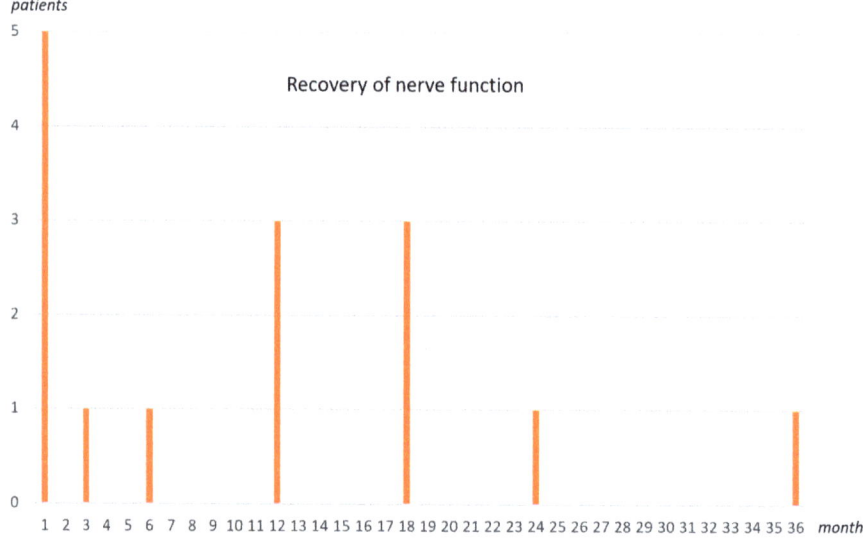

Figure 3. This diagram shows the recovery of nerve function over time. Three of the fifteen patients still had mild hypesthesia in the thumb area after 18 months.

The following images (Figures 4–7) illustrate the intraoperative situation in radial nerve affections with distraction, interposition and constriction/compression due to axial deviation, bone fragments and connective tissue strands/hematomas.

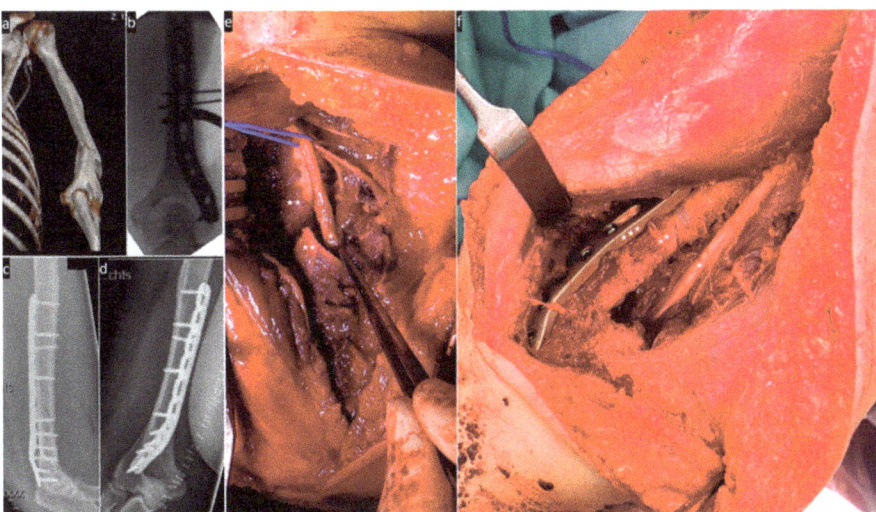

Figure 4. (**a**) Shows the fracture in 3D reconstruction; (**b**) intraoperative X-ray control; (**c**,**d**) postoperative X-ray control; (**e**) the radial nerve (one asterisk) is interposed between the fracture fragments (two asterisks); and (**f**) the fracture (two asterisks) is stabilised with a locking plate (three asterisks) and suture cerclages and the nerve (one asterisk) is neurolysed.

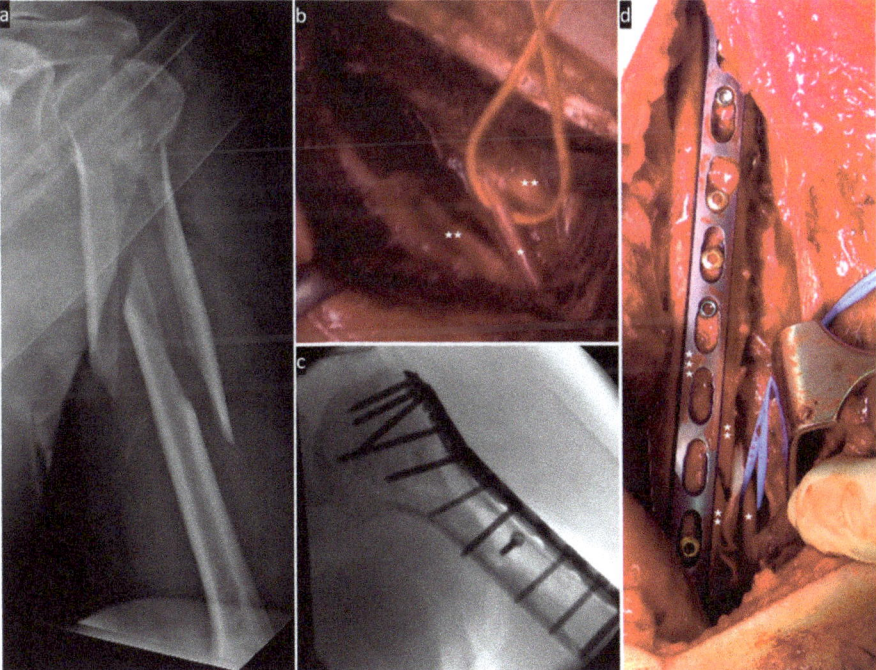

Figure 5. (**a**) Preoperative X-ray of the proximal fracture; (**b**) the nerve (one asterisk) is interposed between the bone fragments (two asterisks); (**c**) intraoperative X-ray control; and (**d**) the nerve (one asterisk) is now neurolysed and separated from the fracture (two asterisks) stabilised with a locking plate (three asterisks) by an absorbable mesh.

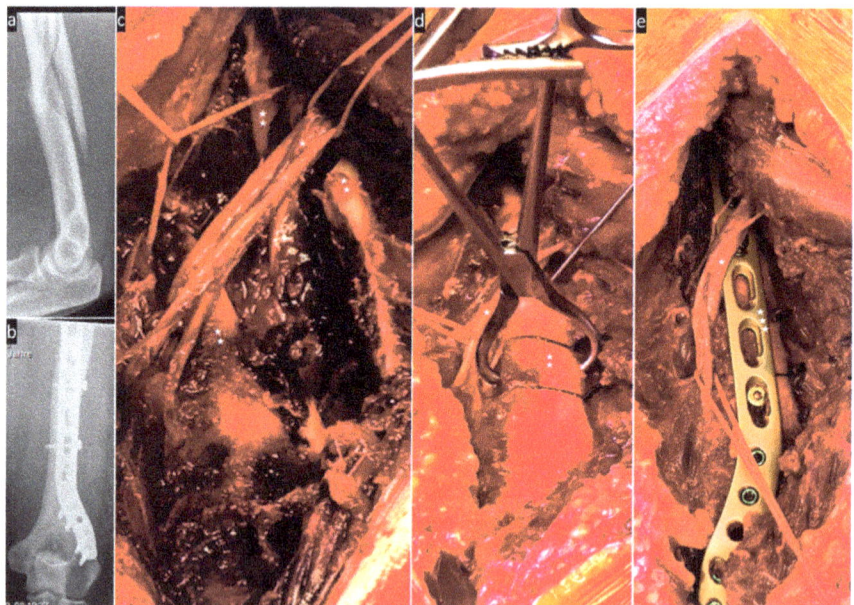

Figure 6. (**a**) Preoperative X-ray of the fracture; (**b**) postoperative X-ray control; (**c**) posterior approach. The interposed nerve (one asterisk) is lifted out of the multi-fragment fracture (two asterisks). (**d**) The nerve (one asterisk) lies relaxed on the repositioned fracture (two asterisks), which is temporarily secured with a clamp, a wire and two resorbable suture cerclages. (**e**) The nerve (one asterisk) crosses the locking plate (three asterisks) without tension.

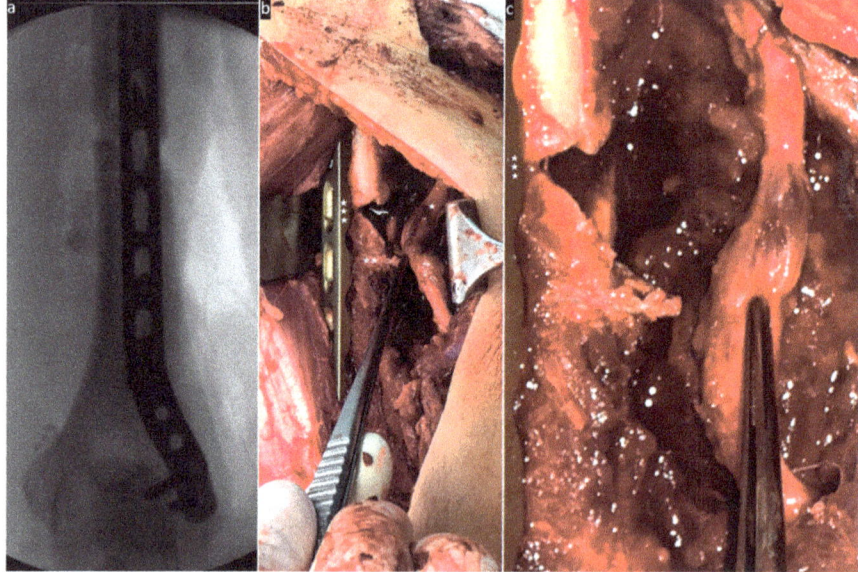

Figure 7. (**a**) Intraoperative X-ray control of the locking plate osteosynthesis. (**b**) The nerve (one asterisk) is clearly constricted by a periosteal cord (two asterisks) in the fracture area with plate osteosynthesis in place (three asterisks). (**c**) The connective tissue cord (two asterisks) in the fracture area next to the plate osteosynthesis (three asterisks) was severed. The neurolysed nerve (one asterisk) is intact in its continuity, but injured by the constriction.

4. Discussion

The incidence of primary radial palsy in humeral shaft fractures is about 11.8% (but varies widely from 2 to 17%) [2,3,7]. The literature recommends various surgical and conservative treatment methods, but one searches in vain for a guideline [12]. From January 2018 to December 2022, a total of 804 patients (463 women and 341 men) with humerus shaft fractures were treated at our hospital. Symptomatic lesions of the radial nerve were found in 33 patients (4.1%). A definite primary lesion with documented radial nerve palsy directly following the accident was found in only 17 patients (2.1%), which is less than reported in the literature. In the remaining 16 patients of our collective, the nerve lesion was secondary, detected/documented in the course of treatment. Hendrickx et al. report a secondary radial nerve palsy of 3% in their study, which is in line with our findings [7].

The distribution of primary to secondary radial palsies is reported in the literature to be 80% to 20% [14]. However, identifying and specifying clinical symptoms can sometimes be challenging. Initial examination may be obscured by pain, shock and fear; on the other hand, severe accompanying injuries may make selective detection of nerve damage difficult. The human factor is another variable for the identification of nerve damage in both the patient and the physician. In addition, nerve damage may be worsened by instability and hematoma in the fracture area. Evidence of this is lacking in the current literature.

According to the literature, radial palsy occurs most frequently in humerus fractures in the middle of the shaft and the transition to the distal third [3]. In addition, the risk is significantly increased for spiral and transverse fractures compared to oblique and comminuted fractures [3]. In our study, fracture classification by AO revealed three 12B2c fractures, two 12A1c fractures, two 12A3b fractures and one each of 12A1b, 12A2a, 12A2b, 12A2c, 12A3c, 12B2a, 12B2b, 12B3b, 12B3c and 12C3a fractures. We hereby see a broad, inhomogeneous distribution. Although the current literature no longer reports a significantly increased incidence of radial palsy in Holstein–Lewis fractures (12A1c), this fracture type is among the second most common in our small collective [3,15].

Primary radial palsies can be caused by distraction, interposition, constriction/compression and transection of the radial nerve [7]. Bony nerve interposition is reported with an incidence of 6–25% and nerve laceration with an incidence of 20–40% [3]. In 2020, Hegemann et al. reviewed 200 cases of nerve palsy in humeral shaft fractures with an intraoperative finding of 35% with no obvious lesions, 30% with neurapraxia and structural damage in 35% [16]. According to the operative reports in our collective, the radial nerve was found to be distracted eleven times, bony interposed three times and soft tissue constricted/compressed three times. This confirmed the indication for early exploration and neurolysis. Open reduction and locking plate osteosynthesis were chosen as the most common surgical procedures because the surgical approach was already given by nerve exploration and neurolysis. In addition, no complete traumatic nerve transection was found in any case.

In the literature, the spontaneous recovery rate is described as high. While a 98% recovery rate is indicated for frequent low-energy traumas, 71% is reported for high-energy trauma and open fractures [3,17]. The recovery rate of the radial nerve after surgical neurolysis and subsequent physiotherapy was also high in our study. Complete recovery of nerve function was seen from 1 to 36 months in 12 cases. Two patients could not be followed up and three patients still showed mild hypesthesia in the thumb area after 18 months. The overall convalescence time was very variable and, in some cases, quite long.

When an indication for osteosynthesis exists with primary nerve palsy, open reduction and plate fixation with nerve exposure are recommended by some authors [7,16]. Indications for humeral shaft fracture fixation include open and pathological fractures, massive soft tissue damage or bone defects, penetrating injuries and gunshot wounds, and significant deformities with shortening at ad latus displacement and axial deviations greater than 20°. In addition, osteosynthesis is recommended for polytrauma, bilateral fractures, vascular injuries and floating elbows [18]. Other indications for early nerve exploration include avoiding further nerve damage (laceration, entrapment) by stabilising the mobile fracture ends and minimising excessive fibrosis [19].

If there is no indication for immediate surgical fracture stabilisation in an acute traumatic humerus fracture with primary radial nerve palsy, such as in closed, nondisplaced fractures without significant axial or rotational deviation, there are both the options of early surgical nerve exploration and expectant observation. In favour of early exploration is the above-mentioned possibility of preventing secondary nerve damage as well as the precise assessment of the existing nerve lesion with direct possible repair, which in such a case leads to a significantly better outcome (90% recovery < 3 weeks vs. 68% recovery > 8 weeks) [19]. The high rate of spontaneous recovery (whether with or without neurolysis with rates from 73 to 92%) and the avoidance of surgical complications including secondary nerve damage such as neurapraxia or injury to the accompanying vessels/neurilemma sheath are arguments for a wait-and-see strategy [7]. In addition, ultrasound can be used to gently examine and evaluate the radial nerve with a sensitivity of up to 89% and a specificity of up to 95% [20,21]. For clinical assessment of nerve recovery, Tinel's sign can be performed every 4 weeks [10] and an EMG examination of the brachioradialis can be performed at 3, 12 and 24 weeks [3,8,22,23]. If signs of nerve recovery remain absent until 6 months after trauma, late exploration with neurolysis, direct neurography, nerve graft, nerve transfer or tendon transfer may be indicated [13,23]. Care should be taken to ensure a tension-free situation in all circumstances.

Furthermore, there is broad consensus on the indication for early nerve exploration in secondary nerve palsies in which the radial nerve was not visualised during the initial surgery.

Due to the retrospective design and the relatively small number of cases in this study, there are of course limitations to the generalisability of the results.

5. Conclusions

With this study, we support the strategy of early nerve exploration and plate osteosynthesis in humeral fractures with primary radial nerve palsy when there is a clear indication for surgical fracture stabilisation. In addition, early exploration appears sensible in the case of palsies in open fractures and secondary palsy following surgery without nerve exposure as well as in the case of diagnostically recognisable nerve damage. Late nerve exploration is recommended if there are no definite signs of recovery after 6 months. An initial wait-and-see strategy with clinical observation seems reasonable for primary radial nerve palsies without indication for surgical fracture stabilisation.

Author Contributions: Conceptualization, F.G.; Writing—original draft, A.B.; Writing—review & editing, R.C. and K.S. All authors have read and agreed to the published version of the manuscript.

Funding: This research received no external funding.

Institutional Review Board Statement: This retrospective study involving human participants was in accordance with the ethical standards of the institutional and national research committee and with the 1964 Helsinki Declaration and its later amendments or comparable ethical standards. The local Human Investigation Committee (IRB) approved this study, approval number 344/23, approval date 20 November 2023.

Informed Consent Statement: In accordance with the local ethics committee, due to the retrospective design, consent to participate and publication were not necessary.

Data Availability Statement: All authors decided that the data and material would not be deposited in a public repository.

Conflicts of Interest: The authors declare that there are no conflicts of interest. No company had influence in the collection of data or contributed to or had influence on the conception, design, analysis and writing of the study. No further funding was received.

References

1. Court-Brown, C.M.; Caesar, B. Epidemiology of adult fractures: A review. *Injury* **2006**, *37*, 691–697. [CrossRef] [PubMed]
2. Holstein, A.; Lewis, G.M. Fractures of the Humerus with Radial-Nerve Paralysis. *J. Bone Jt. Surg. Am.* **1963**, *45*, 1382–1388. [CrossRef]
3. Shao, Y.C.; Harwood, P.; Grotz, M.R.W.; Limb, D.; Giannoudis, P.V. Radial nerve palsy associated with fractures of the shaft of the humerus: A systematic review. *J. Bone Jt. Surg. Br.* **2005**, *87*, 1647–1652. [CrossRef] [PubMed]
4. Bono, C.M.; Grossman, M.G.; Hochwald, N.; Tornetta, P. Radial and axillary nerves. Anatomic considerations for humeral fixation. *Clin. Orthop.* **2000**, 259–264. [CrossRef]
5. Carlan, D.; Pratt, J.; Patterson, J.M.M.; Weiland, A.J.; Boyer, M.I.; Gelberman, R.H. The radial nerve in the brachium: An anatomic study in human cadavers. *J. Hand Surg.* **2007**, *32*, 1177–1182. [CrossRef] [PubMed]
6. Kato, N.; Birch, R. Peripheral nerve palsies associated with closed fractures and dislocations. *Injury* **2006**, *37*, 507–512. [CrossRef]
7. Hendrickx, L.A.M.; Hilgersom, N.F.J.; Alkaduhimi, H.; Doornberg, J.N.; van den Bekerom, M.P.J. Radial nerve palsy associated with closed humeral shaft fractures: A systematic review of 1758 patients. *Arch. Orthop. Trauma Surg.* **2021**, *141*, 561–568. [CrossRef]
8. Seddon, H.J. Three Types of Nerve Injury. *Brain* **1943**, *66*, 237–288. [CrossRef]
9. Sunderland, S. A classification of peripheral nerve injuries producing loss of function. *Brain J. Neurol.* **1951**, *74*, 491–516. [CrossRef]
10. Elton, S.G.; Rizzo, M. Management of radial nerve injury associated with humeral shaft fractures: An evidence-based approach. *J. Reconstr. Microsurg.* **2008**, *24*, 569–573. [CrossRef]
11. Lowe, J.B.; Sen, S.K.; Mackinnon, S.E. Current approach to radial nerve paralysis. *Plast. Reconstr. Surg.* **2002**, *110*, 1099–1113. [CrossRef] [PubMed]
12. Heckler, M.W.; Bamberger, H.B. Humeral shaft fractures and radial nerve palsy: To explore or not to explore…That is the question. *Am. J. Orthop.* **2008**, *37*, 415–419.
13. Rocchi, M.; Tarallo, L.; Mugnai, R.; Adani, R. Humerus shaft fracture complicated by radial nerve palsy: Is surgical exploration necessary? *Musculoskelet. Surg.* **2016**, *100*, 53–60. [CrossRef]
14. Niver, G.E.; Ilyas, A.M. Management of radial nerve palsy following fractures of the humerus. *Orthop. Clin. N. Am.* **2013**, *44*, 419–424. [CrossRef] [PubMed]
15. Ekholm, R.; Ponzer, S.; Törnkvist, H.; Adami, J.; Tidermark, J. Primary radial nerve palsy in patients with acute humeral shaft fractures. *J. Orthop. Trauma* **2008**, *22*, 408–414. [CrossRef] [PubMed]
16. Hegeman, E.M.; Polmear, M.; Scanaliato, J.P.; Nesti, L.; Dunn, J.C. Incidence and Management of Radial Nerve Palsies in Humeral Shaft Fractures: A Systematic Review. *Cureus* **2020**, *12*, e11490. [CrossRef]
17. Laulan, J. High radial nerve palsy. *Hand Surg. Rehabil.* **2019**, *38*, 2–13. [CrossRef]
18. Carroll, E.A.; Schweppe, M.; Langfitt, M.; Miller, A.N.; Halvorson, J.J. Management of humeral shaft fractures. *J. Am. Acad. Orthop. Surg.* **2012**, *20*, 423–433. [CrossRef]
19. Ilyas, A.M.; Mangan, J.J.; Graham, J. Radial Nerve Palsy Recovery with Fractures of the Humerus: An Updated Systematic Review. *J. Am. Acad. Orthop. Surg.* **2020**, *28*, e263–e269. [CrossRef]
20. Cartwright, M.S.; Chloros, G.D.; Walker, F.O.; Wiesler, E.R.; Campbell, W.W. Diagnostic ultrasound for nerve transection. *Muscle Nerve* **2007**, *35*, 796–799. [CrossRef]
21. Esparza, M.; Wild, J.R.; Minnock, C.; Mohty, K.M.; Truchan, L.M.; Taljanovic, M.S. Ultrasound Evaluation of Radial Nerve Palsy Associated with Humeral Shaft Fractures to Guide Operative Versus Non-Operative Treatment. *Acta Medica Acad.* **2019**, *48*, 183–192. [CrossRef] [PubMed]
22. Postacchini, F.; Morace, G.B. Fractures of the humerus associated with paralysis of the radial nerve. *Ital. J. Orthop. Traumatol.* **1988**, *14*, 455–464. [PubMed]
23. Venouziou, A.I.; Dailiana, Z.H.; Varitimidis, S.E.; Hantes, M.E.; Gougoulias, N.E.; Malizos, K.N. Radial nerve palsy associated with humeral shaft fracture. Is the energy of trauma a prognostic factor? *Injury* **2011**, *42*, 1289–1293. [CrossRef] [PubMed]

Disclaimer/Publisher's Note: The statements, opinions and data contained in all publications are solely those of the individual author(s) and contributor(s) and not of MDPI and/or the editor(s). MDPI and/or the editor(s) disclaim responsibility for any injury to people or property resulting from any ideas, methods, instructions or products referred to in the content.

MDPI
St. Alban-Anlage 66
4052 Basel
Switzerland
www.mdpi.com

Journal of Clinical Medicine Editorial Office
E-mail: jcm@mdpi.com
www.mdpi.com/journal/jcm

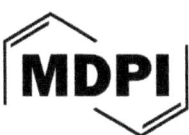

Disclaimer/Publisher's Note: The statements, opinions and data contained in all publications are solely those of the individual author(s) and contributor(s) and not of MDPI and/or the editor(s). MDPI and/or the editor(s) disclaim responsibility for any injury to people or property resulting from any ideas, methods, instructions or products referred to in the content.

www.ingramcontent.com/pod-product-compliance
Lightning Source LLC
LaVergne TN
LVHW070439100526
838202LV00014B/1628